Complications in Acute Care Surgery

Jose J. Diaz · David T. Efron
Editors

Complications in Acute Care Surgery

The Management of Difficult Clinical Scenarios

Springer

Editors
Jose J. Diaz
R Adams Cowley Shock Trauma Center
Acute Care Surgery
University of Maryland School of Medicine
Baltimore, MD
USA

David T. Efron
Acute Care Surgery
John Hopkins Hospital Acute Care Surgery
Baltimore, MD
USA

ISBN 978-3-319-42374-6 ISBN 978-3-319-42376-0 (eBook)
DOI 10.1007/978-3-319-42376-0

Library of Congress Control Number: 2016946623

Printed on acid-free paper

This Springer imprint is published by Springer Nature
The registered company is Springer International Publishing AG Switzerland

To my wife, Dinah, and children, Gabriella, Veronica, and Alejandro, who have been my inspiration to achieve more that I could have ever expected. To my father, J. Jesus Diaz, MD, the community general surgeon, who sparked my life long commitment to the surgical patient.

—Jose J. Diaz

To my father, Gershon Efron, MD, FACS. The consummate master surgeon and clinician.

—David T. Efron

Contents

Contributors

Charles A. Adams, Jr. Division of Trauma and Surgical Critical Care, Rhode Island Hospital, Warren Alpert Medical School of Brown University, Providence, RI, USA

Danielle L. Barnard Department of Surgery, The University of Tennessee Health Science Center, Memphis, TN, USA

James H. Black, III Division of Vascular and Endovascular Surgery, Johns Hopkins University School of Medicine, Baltimore, MD, USA

L.D. Britt Department of Surgery, Eastern Virginia Medical School, Norfolk, VA, USA

Brandon R. Bruns R Adams Cowley Shock Trauma Center, University of Maryland, Baltimore, MD, USA

Michael L. Cheatham Orlando Health Surgical Group, Orlando Regional Medical Center, Orlando, FL, USA

William G. Cioffi Department of Surgery, Rhode Island Hospital, Warren Alpert Medical School of Brown University, Providence, RI, USA

Raul Coimbra Division of Trauma, Surgical Critical Care, Burns and Acute Care Surgery, University of California, San Diego Health Sciences, San Diego, CA, USA

Bryan R. Collier Acute Care Surgery: Trauma, Surgical Critical Care, Emergency General Surgery, Virginia Tech Carilion School of Medicine, Roanoke, VA, USA

Zara Cooper Harvard Medical School, Boston, MA, USA

Edward E. Cornwell, III Department of Surgery, Howard University Hospital, Washington, DC, USA; The LaSalle D. Leffall, Jr., Professor & Chairman of Surgery, Howard University College of Medicine, Department of Surgery, Howard University Hospital, Washington, DC, USA

Martin A. Croce Department of Surgery, Elvis Presley Memorial Trauma Center, University of Tennessee Health Science Center, Memphis, TN, USA

Jose J. Diaz Division of Acute Care Surgery, R Adams Cowley Shock Trauma Center, University of Maryland Medical Center, Baltimore, MD, USA

David T. Efron Division of Acute Care Surgery, Johns Hopkins University School of Medicine, Baltimore, MD, USA

Gregory R. English UPMC Hamot, Erie, PA, USA

Eric W. Etchill Department of Surgery, University of Pittsburgh, Pittsburgh, PA, USA

Timothy C. Fabian Department of Surgery, The University of Tennessee Health Science Center, Memphis, TN, USA

David V. Feliciano IU Division of General Surgery, Indiana University Hospital, Indiana University Medical Center, Indianapolis, IN, USA

Glen A. Franklin Department of Surgery, University of Louisville, Louisville, KY, USA

Nicole M. Garcia Department of Surgery, University of Louisville, Louisville, KY, USA

Andrew Gaugler Jackson Memorial Hospital, Ryder Trauma Center, Miami, FL, USA

Stephen P. Gondek Division of Trauma and Surgical Critical Care, Vanderbilt University Medical Center, Nashville, TN, USA

Sharon M. Henry Program in Trauma, University of Maryland School of Medicine, University of Maryland Medical Center R A Cowley Shock Trauma Center, Baltimore, MD, USA

Sergio E. Hernandez Department of Surgery, University of Pittsburgh, Pittsburgh, PA, USA

Beth R. Hochman Columbia University Medical Center, New York, NY, USA

Joy Hughes Department of Surgery, Mayo Clinic College of Medicine, Rochester, MN, USA

Rao R. Ivatury Department of Surgery, Virginia Commonwealth University, Richmond, VA, USA

Gregory J. Jurkovich Department of Surgery, University of Colorado, Aurora, CO, USA

Steven A. Kahn Department of Surgery, University of South Alabama Medical Center, Mobile, AL, USA

Todd Kellogg Department of Surgery, Mayo Clinic College of Medicine, Rochester, MN, USA

Leslie Kobayashi Division of Trauma, Surgical Critical Care, Burns and Acute Care Surgery, University of California, San Diego Health Sciences, San Diego, CA, USA

Lisa M. Kodadek Department of Surgery, Johns Hopkins University School of Medicine, Baltimore, MD, USA

Narong Kulvatunyou Division of Acute Care Surgery, Department of Surgery, University of Arizona, Tucson, AZ, USA

Alaina M. Lasinski Department of Surgery, Loyola University Medical Center, Maywood, IL, USA

Elizabeth Lilley The Center for Surgery and Public Health at Brigham and Women's Hospital, Boston, MA, USA

Pamela A. Lipsett Department of Surgery, Department of Anesthesiology and Critical Care Medicine, Johns Hopkins University School of Medicine, Baltimore, MD, USA

Katie M. Love Acute Care Surgery: Trauma, Surgical Critical Care, Emergency General Surgery, Virginia Tech Carilion School of Medicine, Roanoke, VA, USA

Fred A. Luchette Department of Surgery, Loyola University Medical Center, Maywood, IL, USA

Addison K. May Division of Trauma and Surgical Critical Care, Vanderbilt University Medical Center, Nashville, TN, USA

Ernest E. Moore Department of Surgery, University of Colorado Denver, Denver, CO, USA

Hunter B. Moore Department of Surgery, University of Colorado, Aurora, CO, USA

Nicholas Namias Daughtry Family Department of Surgery, Jackson Memorial Hospital, Ryder Trauma Center, University of Miami Miller School of Medicine, Miami, FL, USA

Mayur Narayan Division of Acute Care Surgery, Clements University Hospital, UT-Southwestern Medical Center, Dallas, TX, USA

Andrew B. Peitzman Department of Surgery, University of Pittsburgh Medical Center, UPMC Presbyterian, Pittsburgh, PA, USA

Joseph Posluszny Department of Surgery, Loyola University Medical Center, Maywood, IL, USA

Patrick M. Reilly Perelman School of Medicine, University of Pennsylvania, Philadelphia, PA, USA

Peter Rhee Division of Acute Care Surgery, Department of Surgery, University of Arizona, Tucson, AZ, USA

Michael Rotondo Department of Surgery, University of Rochester Medical Center, Rochester, NY, USA

Alaa Sada Department of Surgery, Mayo Clinic College of Medicine, Rochester, MN, USA

Karen Safcsak Orlando Health Surgical Group, Orlando Regional Medical Center, Orlando, FL, USA

Michael Sarr Department of Surgery, Mayo Clinic College of Medicine, Rochester, MN, USA

Thomas M. Scalea R Adams Cowley Shock Trauma Center, University of Maryland, Baltimore, MD, USA

Jason W. Smith Department of Surgery, University of Louisville, Louisville, KY, USA

Jason A. Snyder Department of Surgery, Elvis Presley Memorial Trauma Center, University of Tennessee Health Science Center, Memphis, TN, USA

Nicole Stassen Department of Surgery, University of Rochester Medical Center, Rochester, NY, USA

Carrie Valdez R Adams Cowley Shock Trauma Center, University of Maryland Medical School, Baltimore, MD, USA

Jason B. Young Division of Trauma and Surgical Critical Care, Vanderbilt University Medical Center, Nashville, TN, USA

Syed Nabeel Zafar Department of Surgery, Howard University Hospital, Washington, DC, USA

Brian S. Zuckerbraun Department of Surgery, University of Pittsburgh, Pittsburgh, PA, USA; VA Pittsburgh Healthcare System, Pittsburgh, PA, USA

Chapter 1
Challenging IV Access in the Patient with Septic Shock

Jason B. Young, Stephen P. Gondek, Steven A. Kahn and Addison K. May

Types of Intravenous Access

Decisions regarding the type and location of access must take into account several factors including whether there is a need for hemodynamic monitoring, the rate of fluid administration required, the type of infusion required, availability of accessible site, and the risk/benefit ratio for insertion and maintenance. The need for hemodynamic monitoring and the instillation of fluids that are injurious or caustic if given peripherally may require the placement of central venous access.

The flow of fluids through any IV catheter can be described by Poiseuille's law which states that the flow (Q) of fluid is related to the viscosity (n) of the fluid, the pressure gradient across the tubing (P), the length (L) of the tubing, and the radius (r) of the tubing [12]. Increasing the viscosity of the fluid (blood products being more viscous than crystalloid solutions) or the length of the IV catheter tubing will decrease the flow rate. Increasing the pressure gradient across the tubing will increase the flow rate. Most importantly, increasing the radius of the tubing will increase the flow rate to the fourth power. The size of an IV catheter is measured as a gauge; the smaller the gauge, the larger the diameter of the catheter. Due to the short length of catheter

J.B. Young (✉) · S.P. Gondek · A.K. May
Division of Trauma and Surgical Critical Care, Vanderbilt University Medical Center,
1211 21st Ave S, 404 Medical Arts Building, Nashville, TN 37212, USA
e-mail: jason.b.young@vanderbilt.edu

S.P. Gondek
e-mail: stephen.p.gondek@vanderbilt.edu

A.K. May
e-mail: addison.may@vanderbilt.edu

S.A. Kahn
Department of Surgery, University of South Alabama Medical Center,
2451 Fillingim Street, Suite 10-I, Mobile, AL 36617, USA
e-mail: skahn@health.southalabama.edu

J.J. Diaz and D.T. Efron (eds.), *Complications in Acute Care Surgery*,
DOI 10.1007/978-3-319-42376-0_1

Table 1.1 Peripheral IV[a] flow rates

Gauge	Length (mm)	Flow rate (ml/min)[b]
14	32	325
16	30	215
18	30	110
20	30	63

[a]Jelco Protectiv Plus-W Safety IV Catheter, Smiths Medical ASD, Inc., Southington, CT
[b]Flow rates are by gravity at 1 m height

required to achieve peripheral access, flow rates are more rapid than through longer, centrally placed catheters. Fluids can be run at a remarkably rapid rate through various peripheral IV gauges (Table 1.1). Additionally, for red blood cell infusion, cells may lyse if transfused through a smaller gauge IV catheter (less than 24 gauge).

Peripheral Intravenous Access

Obtaining vascular access in critically ill patients is one of the most important elements of clinical care, second only to managing the airway. The peripheral IV is often the first, inexpensive, and least invasive device utilized to obtain intravenous access. Two "large bore," peripheral IVs remain the gold standard for resuscitation of the exsanguinating trauma patient.

Unfortunately, critically ill patients often have factors that complicate obtaining peripheral access, such as hypovolemia, edema, obesity, a history of IV drug abuse, chronic kidney disease, vasculopathy, diabetes, and/or other chronic disease [5]. The placement of the peripheral IV in normal adults is relatively simple and may be performed by nurses, technicians, and physicians. However, in emergency and critical settings, the clinical setting and the need for larger bore catheters frequently requires more experienced care providers and may be aided by adjunctive technologies, such as ultrasound and hand-held venous illumination/visualization devices. The use of ultrasound has been shown to improve success in obtaining access expeditiously compared to standard approaches [12]. Initially shown to be beneficial for central venous catheter placement, ultrasound has now been widely studied for peripheral venous access as well. One downside is that it does require additional training. Both single- and double-operator techniques have been described. The double-operator technique where one provider holds the probe, and the other provider cannulates the vein is associated with higher success rates. Fewer skin punctures and increased patient satisfaction has also been described with this method of IV placement.

Other light-based hand-held devices have been developed to illuminate veins to ease cannulation [2]. These commonly utilize near-infrared light to highlight hemoglobin and visualize the vein. Veins containing hemoglobin appear dark on a red background. Although multiple devices have been developed, currently there is limited literature that demonstrates a clear benefit for their use.

Sincc pcriphcrally placcd short IV catheters infuse into smaller peripheral veins, the complications of infiltration and phlebitis increase dramatically with catheter dwell time. In order to limit the incidence of phlebitis, the Centers for Disease Control and Prevention recommends replacing peripheral venous catheters and rotating the site at least every 72–96 h [7]. In critically ill patients, the ability to maintain adequate access with this schedule may be very limited.

Peripherally Inserted Central Catheter (PICC)

The management of certain patients may require access to the central venous system or may require prolonged dwell time. One alternative to a conventional central line in this setting is a peripherally inserted central venous catheter (PICC). The catheter enters a peripheral vein, then traverses the deep venous system, and is therefore able to remain longer compared to conventional, short peripheral venous catheters. PICC lines are often used for long-term access for antibiotics, chemotherapy, and total parenteral nutrition (TPN) [1]. For placement, a peripheral vein in the arm is accessed and cannulated via a percutaneous approach and the line is advanced under ultrasonic, fluoroscopic, or radiographic guidance until the line reaches the superior vena cava. When compared to conventional central venous catheters, PICCs are longer and have smaller lumens therefore slower flow rates (Table 1.2), and may not be ideal for administration of blood. Placement of PICC lines is associated with a lower rate of major complications such as pneumothorax, air

Table 1.2 Central venous catheter[a] flow rates

Type	Size	Lumens	Lumen size	Flow rate (ml/h)[b]
MAC introducer	9 Fr × 11.5 cm	Distal	9 Fr	30,450
		Proximal	12 gauge	11,950
PSI (cordis)	8.5 Fr × 10 cm	Single	8.5 Fr	7560
Triple lumen	7 Fr × 30 cm	Distal	16 gauge	2300
		Medial	18 gauge	1000
		Proximal	18 gauge	1100
PICC	5 Fr × 70 cm	Single	16 gauge	1300
PICC	5 Fr × 70 cm	Distal	18 gauge	440
		Proximal	20 gauge	120

[a]Arrow International, Inc, Asheboro, NC
[b]Flow rates are by gravity at 1 m height
MAC Multi-lumen access catheter; *PICC* Peripherally inserted central catheter; *PSI* Percutaneous sheath introducer

embolization, and cardiac dysrhythmias than conventional central venous catheters, but may be associated with higher rates of phlebitis, thrombosis with subsequent loss of venous access for hemodialysis, and infection rates [12]. Complications dramatically increase with extended periods of use, and increase in frequency after 30 days of dwell time. Additional complications include infection, breakage, and leakage. Some PICC lines with small tubing diameters may pose problems with administration of red blood cells secondary to lysis. Additionally, when giving blood through a single-lumen PICC line, this may be incompatible with other administered medications; therefore, a double-lumen PICC line may be preferable if red blood cell transfusions will be performed. When using PICC lines in patients that might need long-term dialysis, one should keep in mind that they have the potential to exhaust potential fistula options down the road. As PICC lines are usually inserted by specially trained nurses or radiologists in the USA, the exact steps and techniques of insertion are outside the scope of this chapter.

Central Intravenous Access

Peripheral IV access may be unobtainable or insufficient in a multitude of clinical scenarios, notably including patients who require immediate IV access where a peripheral IV has failed, patients requiring infusion with high osmolarity solutions (i.e., TPN), caustic solutions (i.e., chemotherapeutic agents, antibiotics), patients requiring many vasoactive solutions, and patients requiring hemodynamic monitoring. Central venous access offers the benefit of durable IV access with a lower frequency of accidental catheter removal, infiltration, and loss of access, but is not without its own added risks of placement-related complications, thrombus formation, stenosis, and increased risk of infection [14]. Of note, multi-lumen catheters may be associated with a slightly higher risk of infection in comparison with single-lumen catheters [3].

There are a number of additional benefits of central venous catheters (CVCs) over a peripheral IV (PIV). Traditional teaching dictates that in situations requiring rapid infusions, bilateral large bore IVs will offer a greater flow rate than a single CVC because the length of the CVC will reduce flow rates and require prohibitively high infusion pressures. In the case of triple-lumen catheters, this is true; however, shorter and larger CVCs have become available that can overcome flow rate limitations (Table 1.2). Although beyond the scope of discussion in this chapter, CVCs also offer the added benefit of additional hemodynamic monitoring in the form of central venous pressure or even pulmonary artery catheter access as well as biochemical data such as central venous O_2.

Three access points are commonly used for central venous catheterization: femoral vein, subclavian (SC) vein, and internal jugular (IJ) vein. Site selection is unique to each patient, and no single site is inherently better for all comers. Site selection should weigh these risks and benefits for each patient. Additionally, while there are no absolute contraindications to a given site, relative contraindications include burn, preexisting infection, coagulopathy, and anatomic abnormalities. One meta-analysis reported the average catheter-related bloodstream infection density of 2.5 per 1000 catheter days with all three sites combined [11].

Femoral

Femoral vein access has the distinct advantage of eliminating any of the risk of pneumothorax, hemothorax, and arrhythmias associated with IJ and SC CVCs. Additionally, both the femoral artery and vein are easily accessible and easily compressed with manual pressure, giving this access a distinct advantage in the case of coagulopathic patients or in inadvertent arterial sticks. Unfortunately, the Clinical Infectious Disease Society discourages the use of femoral catheters due to increased infectious risk [14]. Complications associated with femoral central venous catheters include infection, thrombosis, and arterial puncture.

Internal Jugular

Internal jugular vein access is commonplace and easily obtained with the aid of bedside ultrasound. Blind technique should be discouraged due to the risk of carotid injury. The use of ultrasound can drastically reduce this risk, but does require proper training in its technique. While the infectious risk in IJ catheterization is reduced when compared to femoral access, SC access has the lowest of the three sites. IJ access is preferred in patients who are undergoing or expected to require long-term hemodialysis to avoid the risk of SC vein stenosis and potential loss of hemodialysis access; however, the infectious risk may be higher secondary to difficulty maintaining a dressing. Complications associated with IJ central venous catheters include infection, thrombosis, non-compressible arterial puncture, pneumothorax, hemothorax, nerve injury, and lymphatic injury.

Subclavian

Subclavian vein access has the lowest infectious risk of any of the access sites because of significantly less skin organism counts at the insertion site and is the recommended site by the Clinical Infectious Disease Society in the absence of other factors [14]. While ultrasound can be used in the placement of subclavian catheters, these authors prefer a landmark-based technique. Compression of the subclavian artery is extremely difficult, and care must be taken to avoid injury. Prior to dilation of the vein, the return of dark blood should be observed, and the needle should be transduced with a venous pressure observed. Complications associated with SC central venous catheters include infection, thrombosis, stenosis, arterial puncture, pneumothorax, and hemothorax.

Intraosseous Access

Establishing timely IV access is a challenging task with patients in extremis or profoundly hypovolemic yet is crucial for adequate resuscitation. In patients with circulatory collapse, intraosseous (IO) needle placement provides a rapid alternative and effective route for administering crystalloid solutions, medications, and blood products [6].

Any medication that can be administered safely via a central venous catheter can be administered via an IO line at the equivalent dose. Contraindications to placement of an IO line are local infection at insertion site, fracture of the targeted bone, prosthesis of the targeted bone, recent IO in the same extremity, and absence of anatomic landmarks or excessive tissue.

Several complications of IO needle placement can occur. Fluid extravasation occurs from a misplaced needle or from excessive movement of the needle after placement leading to enlargement of the entry site. Compartment syndrome may occur when the IO needle passes through the opposite cortex, thereby infusing fluids into the calf rather than the venous system. For this reason, it is essential to perform frequent compartment checks when an IO is in use. Additional complications of IO catheters include myonecrosis from extravasation of caustic medications, infection such as cellulitis and osteomyelitis, hematoma, fracture, fat microemboli, and pain. It is imperative that IV access be established and the IO catheter be removed as soon as possible (no later than 72–96 h) to avoid the aforementioned complications.

Common sites for placement of IO needles include the proximal tibia, distal tibia, humeral head, distal femur, and sternum. The humeral head may be the preferred site when obtaining emergent vascular access in the trauma patient as there may be an undiagnosed lower extremity venous injury or IVC injury that would preclude administering medications, IV fluids, or blood products from an access site below the level of venous injury.

Proximal Tibia Insertion

After extending the leg, the tibial tuberosity is palpated and identified. The insertion site is 2 cm medial to the tibial tuberosity, or two finger widths below the patella and 2 cm medial, along the flat aspect of the tibia. The IO needle is inserted through the skin and subcutaneous tissue until the bone is reached. Advance the needle through the cortex until reaching the marrow space, at which point a “pop” or “give” sensation (lack of resistance) is felt. The inner trocar is removed, then a syringe is attached to the needle, and bone marrow is aspirated to confirm correct placement. The flow with a 10 ml push of normal saline is confirmed without resistance or extravasation. In fresh human cadavers, tibial flow rates can reach 30.7 mL/min when using a pressure bag (EZ-IO device) [15].

Humeral Head Insertion

The patient is positioned, so the shoulder is adducted and the greater tuberosity is prominent by lying the patient supine with the palm overlying the abdomen. The proximal humerus and the greater tuberosity is palpated. The needle at a 90° angle directly into the greater tuberosity is inserted. The directions as described above are followed. In fresh human cadavers, humeral flow rates may reach 57.1 mL/min when using a pressure bag (EZ-IO catheter) [15]. This location is the most common site of IO insertion at our institution.

Venous Cutdown

When peripheral IV access is unable to be obtained during resuscitation of critically ill or injured patients, alternative routes of access must be secured rapidly in order to administer crystalloid fluids, blood products, and medications. Alternatives include central venous and IO access; however, these routes are not always feasible. An additional alternative for venous access is that of venous cutdown [16]. The greater saphenous vein in the distal leg at the ankle is most commonly used for venous cutdown as its location is superficial and predictable making it ideal for cutdown. At the ankle, it crosses 2 cm anterior to the medial malleolus and continues up the anteromedial aspect of the leg.

To perform a greater saphenous vein cutdown at the ankle, the patient is placed supine and the foot is externally rotated. A 2–3 cm transverse skin incision is made 2 cm cephalad and anterior to the medial malleolus. Care should be taken to incise the skin only as the vein is superficial and can be easily transected by a deep incision. The subcutaneous tissue is dissected parallel to the course of the vein and can be achieved with either a hemostat or gauze. The vein is mobilized and free ties are passed posterior to the vein both proximally and distally. The proximal vein is ligated and a transverse venotomy is made encompassing no more than 50 % of the total diameter of the vein. A catheter is introduced into the vein and secured with the distal tie. IV fluids, blood products, and medications may then be administered. IV tubing may be inserted directly into the vein for more rapid flow rates. The incision site is then closed and dressed around the IV tubing.

Contraindications to venous cutdown include venous thrombosis, overlying cellulitis, and major trauma to the targeted extremity. Complications of venous cutdown include failed cannulation, hemorrhage, thrombosis, embolus, infection, nerve injury, and arterial injury.

Special Considerations in Difficult Clinical Settings

Coagulopathy

In the emergent setting, coagulopathy should have little bearing on the algorithm for obtaining IV access. No limitation exists for the use of peripheral IVs in the coagulopathic patient. While many clinicians mandate reversal of coagulation disorders prior to placement of CVCs, several series demonstrate that doing so is not necessary. In one such series of 100 catheter placements in patients with coagulation disorders, only a single patient with a platelet count of 6000 was not controlled with local measures and received one unit of packed RBCs [4]. Our practice favors IJ or femoral catheters in patients with gross disorders of coagulation due to ease of compression at these sites. Difficult access requiring IO or cutdown venous access should be considered on an individual basis, with the benefits of access dramatically outweighing the risks in the majority of cases.

Deep Venous Thrombosis/Venous Occlusion

In patients with known deep venous thrombosis (DVT), peripheral and central access should be avoided in the affected limb secondary to potential subsequent non-function and venous embolism. Additionally, when a DVT is identified in association with a central line, the American College of Chest Physicians does not recommend routine removal of the catheter and instead suggests therapeutic anticoagulation for the duration of the catheter's placement and three months thereafter; however, some clinicians may opt to reposition an easily movable line with associated significant thrombosis as well as eliminating a possible higher infection risk [10].

Chronic Kidney Disease/Hemodialysis Patients

Establishing IV access in chronic kidney disease (CKD)/hemodialysis (HD) patients can be challenging from both an insertion and location strategy standpoint. It is imperative to preserve the integrity of peripheral and central veins for future HD access in patients with CKD. Creating a high-quality arteriovenous fistula in the presence of prior venous injury may be unattainable. Venous injury from prior peripheral and central access sites can present as phlebitis, sclerosis, stenosis, and thrombosis.

Identifying patients at risk for future HD is crucial when contemplating preservation and protection of venous anatomy. Venous access sites for patients with CKD, as recommended by the American Society of Diagnostic and Interventional Nephrology, include dorsal veins of the hand for phlebotomy and peripheral IV access, internal jugular veins for central IV access, external jugular veins as acceptable alternatives, and to avoid placement of PICC lines or using the subclavian veins for central IV access [9].

Once vascular access for HD has been established, vein preservation must be ongoing as each vascular access site is at risk for subsequent failure.

Morbidly Obese Patients

Obesity may be associated with difficult IV access even for experienced providers. Difficult IV access is defined as multiple attempts and/or the anticipation of more complex interventions required to establish and maintain peripheral IV access. Obtaining vascular access in the critically ill obese patient may be quite challenging, can delay therapy, and can potentially distract the provider from patient monitoring [13]. In obese patients, normal landmarks may be distorted, and visualization of veins may be impossible.

Ultrasonography is an invaluable tool in aiding the practitioner in establishing IV access, particularly in the obese population. Success rates are significantly improved, and patients undergoing ultrasound-guided IV access require less overall time to establish IV access as well as less time to successful cannulation from the first percutaneous puncture.

Central venous, IO, or intramuscular routes for medication and IV fluid administration may be required in the obese patient. Additionally, dose adjustment of medications in the obese patient may need to be considered.

Burn Patients

Vascular access in burn patients is particularly challenging for several reasons: (1) Large burns often require central access for long periods of time. (2) Burn patients are predisposed to infection because of their compromised skin and their overall immunosuppression. (3) Normal landmarks may be obliterated by injury [17]. Thick eschar and scar can also degrade the quality of ultrasound images. Keeping in mind the previously mentioned exceptions, most of the general principles of vascular access for standard ICU patients outlined in this chapter apply to burn patients.

In an emergent setting, vascular access should be obtained in the most expedient fashion that the provider is comfortable with. The IO needle can be useful in this setting, especially if thick burns are complicating access. In general, one should attempt to avoid placing access through burned tissue if possible. However, if not possible, the provider should not hesitate to place a catheter through a burned area. This should be monitored closely as proximity to burned tissue is associated with increased risk of infection, particularly with central lines. Central venous catheters are particularly useful for burn patients with a large total body surface area burn (>30 %) who will require a large volume of resuscitation and continuous infusions of multiple drugs.

Catheter-related infection is one of the most common sources of sepsis in the burn patient. Infection rates up to 23 % have been reported in the literature and are associated with high mortality (approximately 15 %) when they occur. Thus, careful attention should be paid to sterile technique, as outlined by the CDC. Some of these measures include chlorhexidine prep, cap, mask, sterile gown, sterile gloves, large sterile drape with a small opening, close monitoring of the site, and routine maintenance and dressing changes. Given the complexities outlined above, there is some controversy regarding the duration that central lines should be left in place in this patient population. In general, the literature has evolved to support leaving catheters in place for longer periods of time and does not show a benefit to routine changes over a wire. Multiple large randomized trials have shown no difference in the incidence of catheter-related infections in patients who had lines placed at a new site every 7 days and those who had their lines changed over a wire every 7 days. Lower rates of infection have been reported with antibiotic impregnated catheters, a subclavian approach, a percutaneous approach (as opposed to an open cutdown), and single-lumen catheters. It is often necessary to suture IV lines in place (peripheral and central) as burn wound exudate often makes it difficult to keep standard adhesive dressings in place.

Unobtainable Intravenous Access

In the setting of difficult access, the provider should consider the use of the techniques and devices listed previously in this chapter. During an emergency, however, if one cannot achieve IV or IO access, several common resuscitation medications can be instilled through an endotracheal tube [8]. Keep in mind that this method of medication administration results in significantly lower blood concentrations than when given via an IV or IO route. Most of the experts and texts recommend administering at least 2–2½ times the IV dosages. Giving standard IV doses through an endotracheal tube may not be effective. Medications that can be instilled via an endotracheal tube for adult patients include naloxone, atropine, vasopressin, epinephrine, and lidocaine (mnemonic: NAVEL).

Clinical Scenario

A 60-year-old man is admitted to the SICU status post-head and neck operative intervention for cervical esophageal squamous cell carcinoma with tracheostomy and left-sided pectoralis flap 1 week ago. He now is septic from an unknown source. He is requiring norepinephrine infusion for blood pressure support. His creatinine is 3.4 mg/dL with marginal urine output.

Blood cultures are positive for gram-negative rods. The patient has a left lower extremity DVT, a history of PE, and an IVC filter in place.

Author Response:

Obtaining adequate and appropriate vascular access in this critically ill patient is of utmost importance for a multitude of reasons including the administration of intravenous fluids and medications, hemodynamic monitoring (trending CVP, especially in a patient with acute kidney injury and marginal urine output, and central venous O_2 saturation), and drawing blood. Additional factors that go into the decision-making process for the type and location of access include the rate of fluid administration required, the type of infusion required, availability of access site, and the risk/benefit ratio for insertion and maintenance. This patient is requiring vasopressor administration, specifically norepinephrine, which is injurious/caustic if given peripherally; therefore, he will require placement of central venous access. He is in septic shock, will likely require simultaneous administration of multiple intravenous fluids and medications, and will likely not require a significantly high flow rate of volume administration such as a patient in hemorrhagic shock requiring massive blood product transfusion; therefore placement of a central venous triple-lumen catheter would be appropriate. Several factors may preclude placement of a triple-lumen catheter in particular locations such as the left femoral vein and left internal jugular vein given the left lower extremity DVT and recent head and neck operative intervention with left-sided pectoralis flap, respectively. Additionally, the right internal jugular vein may not be an option given bulky dressings at the operative site. The subclavian veins have adequate options given the lowest infectious risk of the three access sites and distance from incision site and deep vein thrombosis in this patient. One consideration with subclavian vein access in this patient, however, is his acute kidney injury in the face of sepsis which increases his risk of chronic kidney disease requiring permanent dialysis. It is imperative to preserve the integrity of central veins for future hemodialysis access in patients with chronic kidney disease. Venous injury from central access sites, particularly with the subclavian vein, can present as venous stenosis which may preclude permanent hemodialysis access in the affected extremity. Identifying patients at risk for future hemodialysis is crucial when contemplating preservation and protection of venous anatomy. Lastly, the patient is bacteremic and therefore will likely require frequent central venous catheter changes secondary to bacterial seeding regardless of access site. The indication and access site for placement of a central venous catheter should be guided by the risk/benefit ratio and by the most current evidence or guidelines.

Key Questions

1. *In patients with an inferior vena cava filter, does one change or alter the approach to central intravenous access?*
2. *In the era of ultrasound guidance for central line placement, what is the relative risk/benefit of subclavian line placement?*

References

1. Bhullar IS, Block E. Vascular cannulation. In: Gabrielli A, layon AJ, Yu M, editors. Civetta, Taylor, & Kirby's critical care. 4th ed. Philadelphia: Lippincott Williams & Wilkins; 2009. p. 409–28.
2. De Graaff JC, Cuper NJ, Mungra RA, et al. Near-infrared light to aid peripheral intravenous cannulation in children: a cluster randomized clinical trial of three devices. Anaesthesia. 2013;68(8):835–45. doi:10.1111/anae. 12294. Epub 14 June 2013.
3. Dezfulian C, Lavelle J, Nallamothu BK, et al. Rates of infection for single-lumen versus multi-lumen central venous catheters: a meta-analysis. Crit Care Med. 2003;31(9):2385–90.
4. Doerfler MD, Kaufman B, Goldenberg AS. Central venous catheter placement in patients with disorders of hemostasis. Chest. 1996;110(1):185–8.
5. Emergency Nurses Association Clinical Practice Guideline: Difficult Intravenous Access. https://www.ena.org/practice-research/research/CPG/Documents/DifficultIVAccessCPG.pdf. Accessed 7 July 2015.
6. EZ-IO Intraosseous Vascular Access System. Clinical education resources. http://www.teleflex.com/en/usa/ezioeducation/index.html. Accessed 7 July 2015.
7. Guidelines for the Prevention of Intravascular Catheter-Related Infections. http://www.cdc.gov/mmwr/preview/mmwrhtml/rr5110a1.htm. Accessed 10 July 2015.
8. Haque IU, Gabrielli A, Zaritsky AL. Fundamentals of cardiopulmonary resuscitation. In: Gabrielli A, layon AJ, Yu M, editors. Civetta Taylor, & Kirby's critical care. 4th ed. Philadelphia: Lippincott Williams & Wilkins; 2009. p. 697–720.
9. Hoggard J, Saad T, Schon D, et al. Guidelines for venous access in patients with chronic kidney disease. A position statement for the American Society of Diagnostic and interventional nephrology, Clinical Practice Committee and the Association for Vascular Access. Semin Dial. 2008;21(2):186–91.
10. Kearon C, Akl EA, Comerota AJ, et al. Antithrombotic therapy for VTE disease: antithrombotic therapy and prevention of thrombosis, 9th ed: American College of chest physicians evidence-based clinical practice guidelines. Chest. 2012;141 suppl 2:e419S–94S.
11. Marik PE, Flemmer M, Harrison W. The risk of catheter-related bloodstream infection with femoral venous catheters as compared to subclavian and internal jugular venous catheters: a systematic review of the literature and meta-analysis. Crit Care Med. 2012;40(8):2479–85.
12. Marino PL. Establishing venous access. In: Marino PL, editor. The ICU book. 3rd ed. Philadelphia: Lippincott Williams & Wilkins; 2006. p. 107–28.
13. Nafiu OO, Burke C, Cowan A, et al. Comparing peripheral venous access between obese and normal weight children. Pediatr Anesth. 2010;20:172–6.
14. O'Grady NP, Alexander M, Burns LA, et al. Summary of recommendations: guidelines for the prevention of intravascular catheter-related infections. Clin Infect Dis. 2011;52(9):1087–99.
15. Pasley J, Miller CH, DuBose JJ, et al. Intraosseous infusion rates under high pressure: a cadaveric comparison of anatomic sites. J Trauma Acute Care Surg. 2015;78(2):295–9.

16. Westfall MD, Price KR, Lambert M, et al. Intravenous access in the critically ill trauma patient: a ulticentered, prospective, randomized trial of saphenous cutdown and percutaneous femoral access. Ann Emerg Med. 1994;23(3):541–5.
17. Woodson L, Sherwood E, Aarsland A, et al. In: Herndon DN, editors. Total burn care. 4th ed. Elsevier Inc., China; 2012. p. 173–98.

Chapter 2
Fluids in Septic Shock: Crystalloid, Colloids, or Blood?

Nicholas Namias and Andrew Gaugler

Crystalloids

Crystalloid fluids are true solutions, those whose particles are dissolved into their ionic forms and able to pass through a semipermeable membrane. For the purpose of this chapter, they are isotonic solutions, namely 0.9 % saline and lactated Ringers. Crystalloids have long been the "work horse" intravenous fluids of medicine. They are relatively inexpensive, readily available, have a long shelf life, and require no special preparation other than warming.

The origin of intravenous crystalloid therapy can be traced to the landmark observations of William O'Shaughnessy in the early nineteenth century. While combating the Indian cholera pandemic that devastated the former British Empire in the 1830s, O'Shaughnessy observed that blood samples of cholera patients had lost large amounts of water, salt, and alkaline content. Additionally, he wrote "Urea exists in those cases where suppression of urine has been a marked symptom." Despite his accurate description of the fluid depleted state of his patients, O'Shaughnessy never applied this knowledge to treatment in humans.

Drawing upon these observations, Thomas Latta, a contemporary of O'Shaughnessy, pioneered the development of fluid resuscitation. Frustrated by his initial failures with rectal and oral hydration, Latta published the first known report of intravenous resuscitation when he infused six pints of a salt-containing solution

N. Namias (✉)
Daughtry Family Department of Surgery, Jackson Memorial Hospital,
Ryder Trauma Center, University of Miami Miller School of Medicine,
PO Box 016960 D-40, Miami, FL 33101, USA
e-mail: nnamias@miami.edu

A. Gaugler
Jackson Memorial Hospital, Ryder Trauma Center, 1800 NW 10th Avenue,
Suite 227, Miami, FL 33136, USA
e-mail: andrew.gaugler@gmail.com

J.J. Diaz and D.T. Efron (eds.), *Complications in Acute Care Surgery*,
DOI 10.1007/978-3-319-42376-0_2

into an elderly woman dying of cholera in May of 1832. Though he described an appropriate clinical response, the patient expired due to continued fluid losses. Latta continued his efforts with three additional cholera patients, one of whom survived the disease and recovered.

Though their work laid the foundation for modern intravenous fluid therapy, as the cholera pandemic subsided, so did the early interest in fluid therapy, and their contribution was largely forgotten by history. Though early efforts in fluid resuscitation held promise, it would take another 50 years for a resurgence of interest. With Jennings report of intravenous resuscitation in shock due to obstetrical hemorrhage in the 1880s, interest re-emerged. By the turn of the century, saline solutions appear to have become standard practice in hospital-based medicine [1].

Albumin

In the human body, albumin exists as the most common plasma protein, making up about 50 % of all plasma protein content and accounting for 80 % of intravascular oncotic pressure. The liver synthesizes 10–12 g of albumin daily, which is not stored, and is degraded continuously. Intravascular oncotic pressure, based on albumin content, is one of the many mechanisms by which the body maintains a state of homeostatic organ perfusion, but likely the simplest.

Clinical use of albumin as a volume expander was first reported during the Second World War, where it was widely used in its freeze-dried form. Since that time, albumin has been widely used to expand intravascular volume and increase plasma oncotic pressure. Albumin usage has also been championed as a resuscitative fluid due to its ability to serve as a carrier of pharmacologic compounds, scavenge reactive oxygen species, and serve as an acid-base buffer. The clinical efficacy and safety, especially compared to crystalloid fluids, have been the subject of much interest in the medical literature in recent years.

Albumin Versus Crystalloids in Sepsis

The ideal choice of fluid for resuscitation in sepsis and septic shock has been the subject of much debate over the last decade. While there is little doubt that effective fluid resuscitation is paramount to the care of the septic patient, the studies published in recent years have attempted to determine whether the choice of fluid influences patient outcomes. The first large study published regarding this was the SAFE study in 2004. Nearly 7000 ICU patients requiring intravenous fluid resuscitation were randomized to receive either 0.9 % saline or 4 % albumin. The authors reported no difference in a 28-day mortality in the study population as a whole (20.9 % vs. 21.1 %, $p = 0.87$). Additionally, there were no differences in mechanical ventilation days, renal replacement therapy, and ICU length of stay. In their subgroup analysis, patients with severe sepsis showed a trend toward decreased mortality in the albumin group (30.7 %) when compared to those receiving saline only (35.3 %), but the study was underpowered to determine any true benefit to albumin [2].

In the 2013 CRISTAL study, Annane et al. looked at 28-day mortality in ICU patients requiring fluid resuscitation for hypovolemia. Unlike the SAFE trial, the CRISTAL trial focused on patients who presented to the ICU with hypotension and lactic acidosis. Nearly 3000 patients were randomized to either colloids (4 or 20 % albumin or HES) versus crystalloids. The primary endpoint of 28-day mortality (25.4 % vs. 27 %, $p = 0.26$) did not reveal a difference between colloids and crystalloids. When analyzed for 90-day mortality, the colloid group exhibited increased survival (30.7 % vs. 34.2 %, $p = 0.03$). The authors felt this result was "exploratory" and should spur further study, and did not conclude that there is a definitively lower mortality at 90 days. The study shows that colloid and crystalloid resuscitation are likely equivalent in terms of overall mortality. However, when interpreting the results of the CRISTAL trial in the context sepsis, it should be noted that the majority of colloid solutions administered were hydroxyethyl starches (70 %), which have been shown to have deleterious effects [3].

The previous studies clearly demonstrated the need for a study to evaluate the potential difference in albumin and crystalloid in patients with severe sepsis and septic shock. To address this population, the ALBIOS trial was conducted as a large open-label study of more than 1800 patients at 100 different ICU's across Italy. Patients were randomized to receive both crystalloids and albumin boluses to maintain a serum albumin level >30 g/L versus crystalloid alone. As in the previous studies, 28-day mortality was chosen as the primary outcome and the two arms failed to show a significant difference in survival (31.8 % vs. 32 %, $p = 0.94$). Secondary outcomes of 90-day mortality, organ dysfunction, and length of stay were also equivalent [4].

Albumin and crystalloid have also been evaluated with respect to lung injury, pulmonary edema, and organ injury. Differences have not been shown definitively. Interestingly, albumin was shown to increase cardiac index in a more linear fashion than crystalloid, but the clinical significance of this remains unclear.

What can be inferred from these studies? In the authors' opinions, while albumin is a safe and effective resuscitative fluid in severe sepsis and septic shock, it has not shown any clear superiority over crystalloid. However, the endpoint of mortality may be the wrong endpoint to research. Few interventions have an effect of such magnitude that it carries through to mortality. It may be enough that clinical endpoints can be achieved with lower volumes. It is unlikely that there will ever be a study powered to detect a difference in PF ratio, compartment syndromes, or ventilator days as a primary outcome. Therefore, given the increased cost associated with albumin usage, crystalloid should be the primary resuscitative fluid in sepsis. When additional or adjunctive fluids are needed, albumin still appears to be safe.

Starches

Hydroxyethyl starch is a commonly used fluid for volume expansion in the ICU worldwide. Several recent randomized controlled trials have been published evaluating 6 % hydroxyethyl starch (HES) solutions in septic patients. In 2012, the CRYSTMAS study was published, evaluating the safety and efficacy of HES versus 0.9 % saline. The study reported no difference in mortality (31 % vs. 25.3 %, $p = 0.37$) or acute renal failure (24.5 % vs. 20 %, $p = 0.454$). The primary outcome of this trial was resuscitative volume infused, not mortality or renal failure, and was underpowered to detect the 6 % observed nominal difference in mortality. The CHEST trial in 2012 evaluated the 90-day mortality in a mixed population of 7000 ICU patients randomized to either HES or 0.9 % saline. Although no difference in 90-day mortality was detected (18 % vs. 17 %, $p = 0.26$), a significant risk of kidney injury requiring renal replacement therapy was detected (7 % vs. 5.8 %, $p = 0.04$). The 6S group from Scandinavia also provides additional evidence for caution in their study of HES versus Ringer's acetate in severe sepsis. The study of 798 patients revealed an increased risk of 90-day mortality, renal failure, and bleeding complications associated with HES. Interestingly, while their long-term follow-up data at 6 months and one year did not show a significant increase in mortality risk, post hoc analysis did suggest that the increased risk of death was closely linked to bleeding complications. Due to concerns of increased mortality, bleeding, and renal dysfunction, the use of HES as a resuscitative fluid in sepsis is not recommended [5, 6].

Blood

The transfusion of blood products is a common adjunctive therapy in patients with septic shock. Clearly, patients with ongoing hemorrhage in the setting of septic shock usually require transfusion, but other patients are transfused for anemia without the presence of hemorrhage as well. In the past, patients were routinely transfused to a hematocrit of 30 %, with the belief that increased red cell mass would improve tissue oxygenation and decrease myocardial ischemia. In Rivers Early Goal Directed Therapy (EGDT) study, transfusions were used to target goal-mixed superior vena cava oxygen saturation ($ScVO_2$), regardless of hematocrit. As early as 1999, the Transfusion Requirements in Critical Care (TRICC) study showed no risk in allowing hemoglobin to fall below 7 g/dL before transfusion. These findings were corroborated by the Transfusion Requirements in Septic Shock (TRISS) study, which found that in patients admitted to the ICU with septic shock, there was no benefit in transfusing above hemoglobin of 7 g/dL. The authors do not transfuse unless the hemoglobin falls below 7 g/dL. Given her recent emergent operation and ongoing fluid resuscitation, it would be prudent to follow serial hemoglobin levels to assess for hemodilution or hemorrhage. With the increased recognition of adverse events related to blood transfusion, such as ABO mismatch, increased risk for infection, transfusion-related lung injury (TRALI), and transfusion-associated circulatory overload (TACO), the risk/benefit ratio must be thoroughly assessed by the treating physician prior to initiating transfusion [7].

Fluids and Protocol-Based Care

EGDT is a concept of targeting therapy in the early hours of septic shock to reach certain physiologic endpoints for resuscitation. In his single center trial reported in 2001, Rivers randomized patients to a protocol aimed at using fluids, vasopressors, invasive hemodynamic monitoring, and transfusion to resuscitate to CVP of 8–12, MAP >65, $ScVO_2$ >70 %, and a urine output of greater than 0.5 ml/kg/h, and demonstrated a 16 % reduction in mortality when compared to usual care. The findings of this study caused a dramatic shift in the critical care management of septic shock and heavily lent to the Surviving Sepsis Campaign Guidelines. However, Rivers study was not without criticism. His method of EGDT mandates invasive hemodynamic monitoring with central venous catheters and advocates for resuscitation to supraphysiologic endpoints. What is also unclear is which elements of EGDT were responsible for the dramatic improvement in outcomes [8].

Two recent studies have aimed at comparing EGDT and/or protocol-based resuscitation with usual care at the discretion of the attending critical care physician in patients with severe sepsis and septic shock. The ProCESS study was a multicenter randomized controlled trial with 1341 patients with septic shock, randomized to protocol-based care (that did not require invasive hemodynamic monitoring, inotropes, or transfusions), EGDT, or usual care. The study showed essentially no difference in mortality across all groups at 60 days, 90 days, and 1 year [9].

ARISE 2014 was a similar multicenter international randomized control trial that compared EGDT to usual care in over 1600 patients with severe sepsis or septic shock. Like the Process trial, the ARISE investigators were unable to show any difference in early or late mortality between the two groups. In addition, the subjects randomized to EGDT received a higher volume of IV fluids, more inotropic and vasopressor support, and were more likely to receive transfusions [10].

These two studies have shed new light on numerous aspects of the care of patient with severe sepsis and septic shock. First, invasive hemodynamic monitoring for resuscitation in the septic patient does not appear to improve outcomes. Second, transfusion of packed red blood cells should be used judiciously and only in the setting of symptomatic anemia. Most importantly, the individual judgment of the seasoned critical care physician cannot be replaced by a standardized protocol. In a recent retrospective cohort study of patients undergoing EGDT, 67 % of patients exhibited signs of fluid overload on the first clinical day and 48 % had persistent overload on day three. This fluid overload was linked to an increased number of interventions (thoracentesis, diuresis, mechanical ventilation, etc.) and was associated with an increased risk of in-hospital mortality.

Individualized Approach to Resuscitation in Septic Shock

Septic patients present to the ICU with a unique physiology based on their underlying medical condition and degree and response to critical illness. We recommend an initial fluid challenge and continued resuscitation with crystalloid in most patients. Albumin can safely be used as a resuscitative adjunct at the discretion of the bedside physician, with the understanding that the cost is greater than crystalloid. Hydroxyethyl starches should be abandoned in the treatment of sepsis. Lack of physiologic improvement demands further investigation for the cardiovascular status with echocardiography and/or pulmonary artery catheterization. Other commercially available systems for monitoring hemodynamic parameters from arterial line waveforms may be useful, but like the traditional methods, are limited by a set of suppositions which are difficult to achieve in the real world. In practice, life-threatening hypotension is temporized with norepinephrine while proceeding with hemodynamic investigations. For patients presenting with anemia, red cell transfusion should be reserved for patients with a hemoglobin level less than 7 g/dL. Ultimately the resuscitation of the septic patient in the intensive care unit should be guided not by absolute number and guidelines, but based of the clinician's judgment and titrated to the appropriate clinical response.

Clinical Scenario

A 64 year-old woman is status post emergent subtotal colectomy for *Clostridium difficile* colitis and toxic megacolon that developed one week after coronary artery bypass graft and mitral valve replacement. Her ejection fraction is 45 % at baseline. Upon return from the operating room to the surgical intensive care unit, she is oliguric, febrile to 39 °C, and has a hemoglobin of 7.5 gms/dL.

Beyond a shadow of a doubt, the above patient provides a picture of surgical sepsis, the management of which is complicated by her underlying comorbidities. Though this presentation paints a picture of the organ system dysfunction associated with severe sepsis, the astute clinician must also quickly evaluate for other potential underlying causes, such as cardiac failure, injury to the ureters during colectomy, or ongoing hemorrhage. The keys to managing the septic patient are immediate recognition, fluid and vasopressor resuscitation, early broad-spectrum antibiotic therapy, source control of surgical sepsis, and support of dysfunctional or failed organ systems. For the scope of this chapter, we will focus our efforts on how and why septic patients should be fluid resuscitated.

Supporting end-organ perfusion is critical in combating the deleterious host response to infection. Hypoperfusion from sepsis is multifactorial. Septic shock results in a marked state of vasoplegia, and arterial and venous dilation due to the lack of vascular smooth muscle contractility. This response negatively impacts organ perfusion by two mechanisms: Arterial dilation causes systemic hypotension, while venodilation in splanchnic and cutaneous beds decreases venous return to the right heart, lowering the effective circulating volume and thus cardiac output. In addition, the inflammatory response in sepsis also leads to diffuse endothelial injury, resulting in abnormalities in microvascular blood flow as well as increased capillary permeability and fluid shifts into the interstitial space. Further, intravascular volume can be further depleted by fluid losses from the gastrointestinal tract (i.e., vomiting associated with bowel obstruction or the diarrhea caused by the above patients C. diff infection), evaporative and blood loss during surgery, general anesthesia, and the patients underlying medical comorbidities.

Intravenous fluid resuscitation is the first-line therapy for improving hypotension and end-organ dysfunction in severe sepsis and septic shock. During the resuscitative phase, ensuring adequate intravascular volume and end-organ perfusion is a top priority. In the absence of known or preceding cardiac dysfunction, the Surviving Sepsis Campaign Guidelines suggest a minimum volume of 30 mL/kg challenge of intravenous crystalloid bolus should be used for initial resuscitation and intravenous fluid administration should continue as long as there is evidence of physiologic improvement in hemodynamic parameters [11].

The aforementioned patient certainly requires intravenous fluid resuscitation. Having undergone an emergent operation for toxic megacolon, she not only exhibits signs of end-organ dysfunction related to sepsis, but also may be under resuscitated due to blood and fluid losses in the operating room. The patient's response to this initial fluid challenge should be closely monitored and additional consideration should be given to her known previous cardiac dysfunction. She has recently undergone coronary bypass grafting and a mitral valve replacement and her baseline echocardiogram showed a slightly decreased ejection fraction of 45 %. Although her initial operation was intended to ensure adequate myocardial blood flow and cardiac chamber function, evaluating her cardiac function early in her ICU course is essential for optimizing her resuscitation.

Cardiac dysfunction complicates fluid resuscitation in septic patients. Based on a recent meta-analysis of echocardiographic data, diastolic dysfunction is present in nearly half of patients with sepsis and is associated with significantly increased risk for mortality. The ability of the ventricle to relax and fill with blood during diastole is an important consideration when giving a fluid challenge to a septic patient. Increasing the intravascular volume in the presence of marked diastolic dysfunction will increase cardiac filling pressures as well as venous and pulmonary hydrostatic pressures, without a concurrent beneficial increase in stroke volume or cardiac output.

There are multiple tools at the disposal of the critical care physician to assess cardiac function. A focused clinical exam will reveal overt signs of cardiac dysfunction such as jugular venous distension, third and fourth heart sounds, and peripheral edema. Chest radiographs should be obtained to evaluate for cardiomegaly and vascular congestion. However, given the above patient's past medical history, further objective evidence is warranted. A focused bedside echocardiogram looking for both systolic and diastolic dysfunction (as well as prosthetic valve function) should be performed and followed up with a formal bedside transthoracic echocardiogram. In the presence of major cardiac dysfunction, aggressive fluid resuscitation could further exacerbate end-organ dysfunction and early use of vasopressors and inotropes should be considered.

Without evidence of systolic or diastolic function requiring pharmacotherapy to improve cardiac output, fluid resuscitation should begin upon arrival to the intensive care unit. The initial resuscitative fluid in this patient should be intravenous crystalloid. Though it will be discussed in detail below, based on multiple recent clinical trials, resuscitating septic patients with albumin provides no tangible benefit over crystalloids. The use of hydroxyethyl starches in sepsis has been shown to cause harm and should be avoided. Although the patient in the clinical scenario is anemic, in the absence of ongoing hemorrhage, transfusion should be held unless the hemoglobin falls below 7 g/dL.

In addition to intravenous fluid resuscitation, other causes of this patient's oliguria should be investigated. A renal ultrasound would show dilation of the renal pelvis and collecting system if a ureter was inadvertently ligated. Ascites could represent a urinary leak from an injured, but not ligated ureter. Serum and urine chemistries should be obtained to evaluate electrolyte and creatinine clearance and fractional excretion of sodium. Urine output should be monitored via a Foley catheter, which hopefully would have been placed at or before the operation. Adequate monitoring of cardiopulmonary status and sufficient intravenous access are necessary elements of care in this patient.

The patient's response to resuscitation and the results of clinical investigations should further guide the management of this patient. Early goal-directed therapy and standardized, protocol-based care have not been shown to improve outcomes in severe sepsis and septic shock. Invasive hemodynamic monitoring has not been shown to be efficacious when applied to a broad population of septic patients. However, if the patient in the scenario above failed to respond adequately to fluid resuscitation, the authors would consider using a pulmonary artery catheter to guide the use of vasopressors or inotropes. Further therapy and interventions for this patient should be guided by her clinical response and the seasoned judgment of the bedside physician.

Key Questions

1. *Is it any wonder that sepsis is such a difficult disease to treat with fluids? How is one supposed to perfectly fill a leaking system with only inferential endpoints of fullness?*
2. *Are colloids and crystalloids truly no different or are we lacking adequately powered studies in very selected subgroups like the elderly with congestive heart failure?*

References

1. Baskett TF. William O'Shaughnessy, Thomas Latta and the origins of intravenous saline. Resuscitation. 2002;55(3):231–4.
2. Investigators SS, et al. Impact of albumin compared to saline on organ function and mortality of patients with severe sepsis. Intensive Care Med. 2011;37(1):86–96.
3. Annane D, et al. Effects of fluid resuscitation with colloids vs crystalloids on mortality in critically ill patients presenting with hypovolemic shock: the CRISTAL randomized trial. JAMA. 2013;310(17):1809–17.
4. Caironi P, et al. Albumin replacement in patients with severe sepsis or septic shock. N Engl J Med. 2014;370(15):1412–21.
5. Myburgh JA, et al. Hydroxyethyl starch or saline for fluid resuscitation in intensive care. N Engl J Med. 2012;367(20):1901–11.
6. Perner A, et al. Hydroxyethyl starch 130/0.42 versus Ringer's acetate in severe sepsis. N Engl J Med. 2012;367(2):124–34.
7. Holst LB, et al. Lower versus higher hemoglobin threshold for transfusion in septic shock. N Engl J Med. 2014;371(15):1381–91.
8. Rivers E, et al. Early goal-directed therapy in the treatment of severe sepsis and septic shock. N Engl J Med. 2001;345(19):1368–77.
9. Pro CI, et al. A randomized trial of protocol-based care for early septic shock. N Engl J Med. 2014;370(18):1683–93.
10. Peake SL, et al. Goal-directed resuscitation for patients with early septic shock. N Engl J Med. 2014;371(16):1496–506.
11. Dellinger RP, et al. Surviving sepsis campaign: international guidelines for management of severe sepsis and septic shock: 2012. Crit Care Med. 2013;41(2):580–637.

Chapter 3
Resuscitation of the Patient in Septic Shock

Lisa M. Kodadek and Pamela A. Lipsett

Abbreviations and Acronyms

6S	Scandinavian starch for severe sepsis/septic shock
ALBIOS	Albumin Italian outcome sepsis study
ARISE	Australasian resuscitation in sepsis evaluation
CHEST	Crystalloid versus hydroxyethyl starch trial
CRISTAL	Colloids versus crystalloids for the resuscitation of the critically ill
cu mm	Cubic millimeter
CVP	Central venous pressure
EGDT	Early goal-directed therapy
HES	Hydroxyethyl starch
ICU	Intensive care unit
IL	Interleukin
LPS	Lipopolysaccharide
MAP	Mean arterial pressure
mm Hg	Millimeters mercury
$PaCO_2$	Partial arterial pressure of carbon dioxide
PaO_2/FIO_2	Ratio of arterial oxygen partial pressure to fractional inspired oxygen
PAMPs	Pathogen-associated molecular patterns
ProCESS	Protocolized care for early septic shock
ProMISe	Protocolized management in sepsis
QSOFA	Quick Sequential [Sepsis-Related] Organ Failure Assessment Score
SAFE	Saline versus albumin fluid evaluation
SBP	Systolic blood pressure

L.M. Kodadek (✉)
Department of Surgery, Johns Hopkins University School of Medicine,
600 N Wolfe Street, Tower 110, Baltimore, MD 21287, USA
e-mail: lkodade1@jhmi.edu

P.A. Lipsett
Department of Surgery, Department of Anesthesiology and Critical Care Medicine,
Johns Hopkins University School of Medicine, 600 N Wolfe Street, Osler 603,
Baltimore, MD 21287, USA
e-mail: plipsett@jhmi.edu

J.J. Diaz and D.T. Efron (eds.), *Complications in Acute Care Surgery*,
DOI 10.1007/978-3-319-42376-0_3

$ScvO_2$	Central venous oxygen saturation
SIRS	Systemic inflammatory response syndrome
SOFA	Sequential [Sepsis-Related] Organ Failure Assessment Score
SSC	Surviving sepsis campaign
SvO_2	Mixed venous oxygen saturation
TLR	Toll-like receptor
US	United States
VISEP	Efficacy of volume substitution and insulin therapy in severe sepsis

Introduction

Sepsis is defined as life-threatening organ dysfunction caused by a dysregulated host response to infection. Septic shock is a subset of sepsis in which underlying circulatory and cellular/metabolic abnormalities are profound enough to substantially increase mortality [1–4]. Sepsis has long intrigued the medical community and remains a robust area for both basic science and clinical research. Derived from the Greek word "sepo," meaning "I rot," Hippocrates and other early scientists associated sepsis with decomposition in the presence of bacteria [5, 6]. Germ theory of disease, confirmed by Pasteur, continued to implicate bacteria as the direct cause of sepsis. Contemporary scientists began to reconsider this theory when patients succumbed to sepsis despite appropriate eradication of the causal bacteria with antibiotics. Furthermore, additional etiologies including injured tissue, ischemic tissue, perfusion derangements and antigen–antibody reactions were recognized as causes of similar or identical metabolic and physiologic derangement. It became apparent that the systemic inflammatory response is independent of the insult; the response was, in fact, host-dependent [7].

Treatment of sepsis requires early diagnosis, source control, timely antibiotic administration, and effective resuscitation [8]. Guidelines for management are provided by the Surviving Sepsis Campaign (SSC), which was first published in 2004 and continues to provide updated best practice guidelines every four years [9]. Resuscitation for sepsis and septic shock, with particular respect to quantitative hemodynamic targets of resuscitation, has been an area for ongoing debate and a prodigious body of research. Early goal-directed therapy (EGDT), first introduced in 2001, [10] was a single-center proof-of-concept study that randomized emergency department patients with severe sepsis or septic shock to 6 h of protocolized, quantitative resuscitation versus usual care. The EGDT protocol utilized intravenous fluids, vasopressors, inotropes, and blood transfusions to achieve a balance of oxygen delivery and oxygen demand through real-time adjustments to cardiac preload, afterload, and contractility. This study demonstrated statistically significant decreased in-hospital mortality among those patients treated with EGDT versus usual care (relative risk reduction 42 %).

While EGDT was adopted in international guidelines, [11] concerns remain about the validity of this approach, the complexity of implementation, and resource utilization. A number of recent studies have failed to demonstrate a mortality benefit of EGDT in multisite randomized controlled trials. The ProCESS (Protocolized Care for Early Septic Shock) trial sought to determine whether all aspects of EGDT were necessary and whether the findings were generalizable [12]. The results of this study, conducted in 31 United States (US) emergency departments, failed to show any difference in 90-day and 1-year mortality between patients treated with EGDT and standard therapy. The ARISE (Australasian Resuscitation in Sepsis Evaluation) study evaluated EGDT versus usual care in 51 centers in Australia and New Zealand [13]. The ProMISe (Protocolized Management in Sepsis) study examined EGDT versus usual care in 56 centers in England [14]. Neither of these contemporary multicenter studies showed a mortality benefit for EGDT.

Resuscitation of patients with sepsis and septic shock remains an important area for research with significant implications for clinical care. Best practice guidelines will continue to reflect the most current evidence-based literature, and all clinicians must monitor and adapt their practice to ensure best outcomes for patients.

Definitions

A 1991 consensus conference, under the chairmanship of Roger C. Bone, MD, first published standard definitions for sepsis, severe sepsis and septic shock (Sepsis-1 guidelines) [15]. This committee also coined the systemic inflammatory response syndrome (SIRS) as the clinical manifestation of the hypermetabolic response to infection or a noninfectious insult. SIRS criteria include (1) temperature >38 or <36 °C, (2) heart rate > 90 beats per minute, (3) tachypnea with respiratory rate >20 breaths per minute or hyperventilation with partial arterial pressure of carbon dioxide ($PaCO_2$) <32 mm mercury (mm Hg), and (4) white blood cell count >12,000/cubic milliliter (cu mm) or <4000/cu mm or >10 % immature neutrophils ("bands").

Sepsis-1 guidelines originally defined sepsis as two or more SIRS criteria in the presence of confirmed or suspected infection; severe sepsis was defined as sepsis associated with organ dysfunction, hypoperfusion or sepsis-induced hypotension. Signs of hypoperfusion included lactic acidosis, oliguria, and acute alterations in mental status. Sepsis-induced hypotension was defined as systolic blood pressure (SBP) <90 mm Hg or mean arterial pressure (MAP) <70 mm Hg or a reduction >40 mm Hg from baseline or less than two standard deviations below normal for age in the absence of other causes for hypotension [9]. Septic shock was defined by Sepsis-1 guidelines as sepsis-induced hypotension despite adequate fluid resuscitation with perfusion abnormalities. Of note, patients receiving inotropic or vasopressor therapies who were not hypotensive were, still considered to have septic shock should if perfusion abnormalities persisted. In 2001, a second conference (Sepsis-2 guidelines) met to review the definitions established in 1991 [16]. The signs and symptoms of sepsis were expanded to reflect clinical experience, but no other major changes to the definitions were made.

Risk factors for sepsis and septic shock include chronic disease (including human immunodeficiency virus/acquired immunodeficiency syndrome, chronic obstructive pulmonary disease malignancies), immunosuppressive medication use, and genetic characteristics and predisposition [22]. Recent work highlights a relationship between microbiome disruption, or dysbiosis, and subsequent risk for severe sepsis [27]. Other risk factors include age, sex, and race. Sepsis is more common among infants and older patients, as well as men (compared to women), and black patients (compared to white patients) [22, 23, 28, 29].

Pathogenesis

Sepsis and septic shock result from a complex response to infection involving both pro-inflammatory and anti-inflammatory pathways. The host response ultimately causes clearance of the infection as well as tissue injury leading to organ dysfunction and secondary infections [22]. Pro-inflammatory pathways are thought to cause tissue injury, and anti-inflammatory pathways are responsible for immune suppression and secondary infection. The failure of anti-inflammatory therapies to change outcome in numerous clinical sepsis trials highlights the importance of both pathways in the pathogenesis of sepsis. The outcome in a given case depends on pathogen factors, such as load and virulence, as well as host factors, including genetic characteristics and coexisting illness [30].

Community-acquired and hospital-acquired infections may lead to sepsis. Common sources include pneumonia, urinary tract infections, and intra-abdominal infections [31]. Prior to 1987, gram-negative bacteria were most commonly involved in sepsis [29]. Gram-positive bacteria have now become the most common pathogen; fungal organisms have also increased in incidence. A cross-sectional estimation from the year 2000 reported the causative organism in sepsis to be 52.1 % gram-positive bacteria, 37.6 % gram-negative bacteria, 4.7 % polymicrobial, 4.6 % fungi, and 1 % anaerobes [29]. *Staphylococcus aureus* and *Streptococcus pneumoniae* are the most commonly implicated gram-positive bacteria, and *Escherichia coli*, *Klebsiella* species and *Pseudomonas aeruginosa* are the most commonly implicated gram-negative bacteria [30].

The host response to infectious products, such as lipopolysaccharide (LPS), is a result of signaling through pattern recognition receptors. As part of the innate immune system, pattern recognition receptors recognize preserved pathogen-associated molecular patterns (PAMPs), which are absent in higher eukaryotes. For example, the toll-like receptor (TLR) recognizes PAMPs and causes a cascade of pro-inflammatory cytokines such as interleukin (IL)-1 and IL-6, which subsequently lead to the clinical signs of sepsis [30]. Endogenous products such as mitochondrial DNA and uric acid ("alarmins"), released with necrosis, ischemia, or trauma, also signal through a TLR to cause a similar cytokine release in sterile inflammatory responses [17]. These overlapping signaling pathways explain why the host response to both infection and sterile inflammatory processes may be nearly identical. Accordingly, transcriptome analysis has shown a similar genomic response to endotoxemia and trauma [33].

The specific causes of tissue injury and organ dysfunction in severe sepsis are multifactorial. Disruption of coagulation and fibrinolysis homeostasis and endothelial dysfunction contribute to microvascular thrombi, impaired oxygenation, and in many cases, disseminated intravascular coagulation. Organ failure is thought to be related primarily to tissue hypoxia, which is mediated through both local and systemic physiologic factors [22].

Diagnosis

Sepsis and septic shock are managed emergently; outcomes depend on early diagnosis and appropriate, timely management. The 2016 Sepsis-3 guidelines provide a clear diagnostic approach for identifying patients with sepsis and septic shock [1]. Patients with suspected infection should be assessed using a quick SOFA (qSOFA) score. The qSOFA consists of three clinical criteria easily and quickly assessed at the bedside: altered mentation, systolic blood pressure of 100 mm Hg or less, and respiratory rate of 22/minute or greater. If a patient has 2 or more of these findings, the SOFA score should then be applied to assess for organ dysfunction. If a patient does not meet qSOFA clinical criteria, frequent reassessment for sepsis is warranted when clinically indicated. Organ dysfunction is determined using the SOFA score (Table 3.1). SOFA variables include PaO2/FIO2, Glasgow Coma Scale score, mean arterial pressure, administration of vasopressors, serum creatinine or urine output, bilirubin, and platelet count. An acute change in total SOFA score ≥ 2 points consequent to the infection is diagnostic for sepsis. The baseline SOFA

Table 3.1 Sequential [sepsis-related] organ failure assessment (SOFA) score

System	Score				
	0	1	2	3	4
RespirationPaO2/FIO2, mm Hg (kPa)	≥400 (53.3)	<400 (53.3)	<300 (40)	<200 (26.7) with respiratory support	<100 (13.3) with respiratory support
CoagulationPlatelets, x103/μL	≥150	<150	<100	<50	<20
LiverBilirubin, mg/dL (μmol/L)	<1.2 (20)	1.2-1.9 (20-32)	2.0-5.9 (33-101)	6.0-11.9(102-204)	>12.0 (204)
Cardiovascular	MAP≥ 70 mm Hg	MAP < 70 mm Hg	Dopamine <5 or dobutamine (any dose)a	Dopamine 5.1-15 or epinephrine ≤0.1 or norepinephrine ≤0.1a	Dopamine >15 or epinephrine >0.1 or norepinephrine >0.1a
Central Nervous SystemGlasgow Coma Scale scoreb	15	13–14	10–12	6–9	< 6

(continued)

Table 3.1 (continued)

System	Score				
	0	1	2	3	4
RenalCreatinine, mg/dL (μmol/L)	<1.2 (110)	1.2-1.9 (110-170)	2.0-3.4 (171-299)	3.5-4.9 (300-440)	>5.0(440)
Urine output, mL/d				<500	<200

[*]Organ dysfunction can be identified as an acute change in total SOFA score ≥ 2 points consequent to infection. The baseline SOFA score can be assumed to be zero in patients not known to have preexisting organ dysfunction. Adapted from: Singer M, Deutschman CS, Seymour CW, et al. The Third International Consensus Definitions for Sepsis and Septic Shock (Sepsis-3). JAMA 2016;315(8):801–810

Abbrevations: *PaO2/FIO2* ratio of arterial oxygen partial pressure to fractional inspired oxygen; *mm Hg* millimeters mercury; *kPa, kiloPascal; MAP* mean arterial blood pressure

[a]Catecholamine doses are given as μg/kg/min for at least 1 hour

[b]Glasgow Coma Scale scores range from 3-15; higher score indicates better neurologic function.

score can be assumed to be zero in patients not known to have preexisting organ dysfunction. Septic shock is diagnosed when clinical criteria for sepsis are met and the patient exhibits persistent hypotension requiring vasopressors to maintain MAP≥ 65 mm Hg and a serum lactate level > 2 mmol/L despite adequate volume resuscitation.

Severe sepsis is diagnosed when sepsis-induced tissue hypoperfusion or organ dysfunction is present. Signs of hypoperfusion may include lactate above upper limit of normal and urine output <0.5 mL/kg/h for 2 h despite adequate fluid resuscitation. Signs of organ dysfunction include acute lung injury with a ratio of arterial oxygen partial pressure to fractional inspired oxygen (PaO_2/FIO_2) <250 in the absence of pneumonia, PaO_2/FIO_2 <200 in the presence of pneumonia, creatinine >2.0 mg/dL, bilirubin >2 mg/dL, platelet count <100,000 μL, or coagulopathy with INR >1.5 [6].

Management

Early recognition and diagnosis of sepsis, source control, antibiotic treatment, and effective fluid resuscitation are critical for appropriate management of the septic patient. While many patients may be initially diagnosed and treated in the ED or on the general wards, definitive management in an ICU setting is appropriate for most patients with severe sepsis and septic shock. The SSC provides core sets of recommendations, or "bundles," to guide the care of patients with sepsis and septic shock throughout their courses. The purpose of fluid resuscitation is to correct tissue hypoxia, which may otherwise lead to more severe stages of sepsis, multiorgan dysfunction and death.

Fluid Selection

Resuscitation fluids are generally classified as colloids or crystalloids. Colloids, such as 4–5 % human albumin or hydroxyethyl starches (e.g., Hetastarch), are suspensions of high molecular weight molecules within a carrier solution and are generally unable to cross the semipermeable capillary membrane. Crystalloids, including normal (0.9 %) saline, lactated Ringer's solution, and balanced salt solutions (e.g., PlasmaLyte), are ion solutions that are freely permeable and contain specific sodium and chloride concentrations for precise tonicity.

Historically, physiologic understanding has supported the use of colloids for volume expansion and resuscitation since they are more easily retained in the intravascular space secondary to oncotic pressure [33]. However, a number of studies, summarized in a 2012 Cochrane Review, [34] have demonstrated that colloids do not offer any benefits over crystalloids with respect to mortality, safety or effectiveness. Furthermore, colloids are more expensive than crystalloids and impractical to administer in some settings. However, crystalloids must still be administered with caution and close monitoring. In general, crystalloids may cause interstitial edema, and normal saline, when used in excess, may lead to hyperchloremic metabolic acidosis and acute kidney injury. Balanced salt solutions have been supported as an appropriate alternative to normal saline, but data are not sufficient at this time to make conclusions [22]. The safety of hypertonic saline has not been established for resuscitation of patients with sepsis and septic shock, though basic science experiments suggest that inflammation is altered significantly by changes in tonicity.

SSC guidelines currently endorse crystalloids as the initial fluid of choice in the resuscitation of patients with sepsis and septic shock [9]. Albumin may be used in adjunct for fluid resuscitation of patients with sepsis and septic shock who require substantial amounts of resuscitation fluids. Trauma and more specifically patients with head injury should not receive albumin resuscitation. The initial fluid challenge in patients with sepsis-induced tissue hypoperfusion with concern for hypovolemia is a minimum of 30 mL/kg of crystalloid; a portion of this initial challenge may be albumin. The fluid challenge technique should be applied continuously, provided there is hemodynamic improvement based on dynamic (e.g., change in pulse pressure, stroke volume variation) or static (e.g., heart rate, arterial pressure) variables.

The SSC recommendations are based on a number of studies examining the use of crystalloid versus colloid for resuscitation of critically ill patients. In 2004, the results of a randomized controlled trial completed in Australia and New Zealand known as the Saline versus Albumin Fluid Evaluation (SAFE) study were published [35]. These results demonstrated no difference in 28-day mortality outcomes or new organ failure among 6997 adult ICU patients randomized to normal saline or 4 % albumin. A subsequent systematic review and meta-analysis in 2011 demonstrated that use of albumin-containing solutions for resuscitation of patients with sepsis was associated with lower mortality than other fluid resuscitation regimens

[36]. The Colloids Versus Crystalloids for the Resuscitation of the Critically Ill (CRISTAL) trial is a randomized trial that demonstrated no difference in 28-day mortality among ICU patients treated with crystalloid versus colloid [37]. While there was lower 90-day mortality among patients treated with colloids, the authors did not make any conclusions about the efficacy of colloids based on these findings. The Albumin Italian Outcome Sepsis (ALBIOS) trial, a randomized controlled trial in 100 ICUs in Italy, demonstrated no differences in 28-day and 90-day mortality among patients with severe sepsis randomized to crystalloid and albumin resuscitation or crystalloid alone [38]. A 2014 systematic review and meta-analysis did not find any mortality benefit with the use of albumin, but confirmed that albumin was indeed safe for use as part of the resuscitation management of patients with sepsis [39]. Crystalloid continues to be the first-line choice of fluid for resuscitation of patients with severe sepsis, but albumin may be considered a safe adjunct for patients who require large volume resuscitation.

SSC guidelines recommend against the use of hydroxyethyl starches (HES) for resuscitation of patients with sepsis or septic shock [9]. Multiple randomized controlled trials have demonstrated increased morbidity with use of HES solutions including renal failure, and some studies have shown increased mortality. The CRYSTMAS study demonstrated no difference in mortality between normal saline and 6 % HES 130/0.4 resuscitation among patients with severe sepsis [40]. However, the major criticism of this study was that it was underpowered to detect the observed 6 % absolute difference in mortality. Crystalloid versus Hydroxyethyl Starch Trial (CHEST), a randomized controlled trial among 7000 ICU patients in Australia and New Zealand, randomized ICU patients to receive 6 % HES 130/0.4 or normal saline [41]. There was no difference in mortality at 90 days, but there was evidence for significantly increased adverse events with use of HES. Furthermore, the need for renal replacement therapy was higher in patients who received HES versus normal saline. The Scandinavian Starch for Severe Sepsis/Septic Shock trial (6S) demonstrated increased mortality at 90 days among patients with severe sepsis or septic shock treated with 6 % HES 130/0.42 versus Ringer's acetate [42]. Patients treated with HES more commonly required renal replacement therapy. Similarly, HES was associated with higher rates of renal failure and renal replacement therapy when compared with Ringer's lactate among patients with severe sepsis in the Efficacy of Volume Substitution and Insulin Therapy in Severe Sepsis (VISEP) study [43]. These studies support the recommendations to avoid HES in the resuscitation of patients with sepsis and septic shock. Table 3.2 summarizes major studies investigating outcomes related to resuscitation fluid selection.

Fluid Resuscitation Strategy and Goals

The SSC guidelines recommend initial quantitative resuscitation of patients with sepsis-induced tissue hypoperfusion [9]. Sepsis-induced tissue hypoperfusion may be defined as hypotension persisting after the initial fluid challenge of 30 mL/kg or

Table 3.2 Selection for sepsis: summary of major studies

Year	Trial	*N*, population	Intervention	Control	Outcomes of interest	Conclusion
2004	SAFE [32]	6997 ICU patients	4 % albumin	0.9 % saline	28-d mortality, new organ failure, RRT	No differences in mortality or morbidity
2008	VISEP [40]	537 ICU patients with severe sepsis or septic shock	10 % HES 200/0.5	Ringer's lactate	28-d and 90-d mortality, new organ failure, RRT	No differences in mortality. Higher rate renal failure and RRT with HES
2012	CHEST [38]	7000 ICU patients	6 % HES 130/0.4	0.9 % saline	90-d mortality, new organ failure, RRT	No differences in mortality. Higher rate renal failure and RRT with HES
2012	6S [39]	798 ICU patients with severe sepsis	6 % HES 130/0.42	Ringer's acetate	90-d mortality, RRT	Increased 90-d mortality and RRT with HES
2012	CRYSTMAS [37]	196 patients with severe sepsis	6 % HES 130/0.4	0.9 % saline	90-d mortality, RRT	No difference in mortality or morbidity
2013	CRISTAL [34]	2857 ICU patients with hypovolemic shock	Colloids (including HES, albumin)	Crystalloid	28-d and 90-d mortality, RRT	No difference in 28-d mortality. 90-d mortality lower in colloid group
2014	ALBIOS [35]	1818 ICU patients with severe sepsis	20 % albumin and crystalloid	Crystalloid	28-d and 90-d mortality, new organ failure	No differences in outcomes

Abbreviations: *d* day, *HES* hydroxyethyl starch, *ICU* intensive care unit, *LOS* length of stay, *RRT* renal replacement therapy a blood lactate concentration ≥4 mmol/L. The specific goals of resuscitation to be attained during the first 6 h after recognition of sepsis are central venous pressure (CVP) 8–12 mm Hg, MAP ≥65 mm Hg, urine output ≥0.5 mL/kg/h, central venous oxygen saturation ($ScvO_2$) of 70 % or mixed venous oxygen saturation (SvO_2) of 65 % and normalization of lactate.

These quantitative resuscitation goals represent current best practice, but these should not be considered gold standard. For example, MAP interpretation may be difficult in patients with chronic hypertension or those with lower blood pressures at baseline; other signs of tissue perfusion must be considered. While central and mixed venous oxygen saturations are helpful to assess the difference between oxygen delivery and consumption, these lab values are typically obtained via invasive monitors. Measurement of $ScvO_2$ generally requires placement of a central venous catheter, and a true SvO_2 is obtained by placement of a pulmonary artery catheter. CVP is not an accurate determination of volume status, particularly in mechanically ventilated patients, or those with preexisting decreased ventricular compliance or increased abdominal pressure. Other methods, such as the passive leg raise test, pulse pressure variation, and bedside ultrasound examination can assess intravascular volume status without necessitating the placement of a central venous catheter. Passive leg raise test is completed while the patient is supine; the legs are raised to 45°, effectively transferring a significant volume of fluid from the lower body and increasing venous return. Subsequent increase in cardiac output predicts fluid responsiveness [44]. Pulse pressure variation is determined by the maximum and minimum pulse pressure during the respiratory cycle; increasing variation predicts fluid responsiveness. Ultrasound may be used at the bedside by a trained provider to predict volume status; a highly collapsible inferior vena cava or an absolute diameter <2 cm may be associated with hypovolemia [45].

The 2012 SSC recommendations are still based in large part on the landmark study by Rivers et al. [10] published in 2001 this study demonstrated decreased mortality for patients with severe sepsis who were treated with an early-goal-directed-therapy (EGDT) protocol [10]. This single-center study randomized 263 patients presenting to the ED with severe sepsis or septic shock to 6 h of EGDT or usual care. The EGDT protocol employed intravenous crystalloids to achieve a CVP of 8–12 mm Hg. Vasopressors were then added if a MAP of 65 mm Hg could not be achieved with fluids alone. If the MAP was >90 mm Hg, vasodilators were used. If the $ScvO_2$ was <70 %, packed red blood cells were transfused to obtain a hematocrit of 30 %. Once CVP, MAP, and hematocrit were optimized, if $ScvO_2$ remained <70 %, dobutamine was given. This protocol essentially addressed preload, afterload and cardiac contractility to maximize oxygen delivery and tissue perfusion. In-hospital mortality among patients who were treated with EGDT was 30.5 % and mortality among patients treated with usual care was 46.5 % for a relative risk reduction of 42 %. This study, along with other nonrandomized studies, subsequently informed sepsis guidelines internationally.

Numerous studies, many of which were completed since the last SSC update, have failed to replicate the mortality benefit seen in the initial EGDT study.

ProCESS (Protocolized Care for Early Septic Shock) sought to determine whether EGDT is generalizable and whether all aspects of the protocol were necessary [12]. The study randomized 1341 patients with septic shock presenting to one of the 31 US EDs in a 1:1:1 ratio to one of the three groups. The treatment groups were (1) protocol-based EGDT per Rivers et al. [10] (2) protocol-based standard therapy, a less aggressive regimen with similar 6-h resuscitation goals, but without mandatory and protocolized use of a central line, inotropes, and transfusions, and (3) usual care at the discretion of the treating (nonstudy) physician. This study demonstrated no differences in 90-day or 1-year mortality and no differences in need for organ support among patients randomized to each of the three study groups. However, the 60-day in-hospital mortality was only 18.9 % in this study, much lower than the mortality rates reported in the initial EGDT trial. Furthermore, the patients in the initial EGDT trial had higher rates of preexisting heart and liver disease and higher initial lactate, although disease severity was similar among patients in both studies.

Two additional randomized controlled trials and a meta-analysis have found no benefit to EGDT. ARISE (Australasian Resuscitation in Sepsis Evaluation) enrolled 1600 patients at 51 centers in Australia and New Zealand [13]. The study randomized patients to receive EGDT for 6 h per Rivers et al. [10] or usual care. There was no mortality benefit to EGDT at 28 days or 90 days, and there was no difference in need for organ support. Overall incidence of mortality in this study was 18.8 %, similar to the ProCESS findings. ProMISe (Protocolized Management in Sepsis) enrolled 1260 patients at 56 hospitals in England [14]. Similar to the ARISE study, patients were randomized to 6 h of EGDT or usual care. Mortality at 90 days did not differ between the two groups, and EGDT was associated with higher health care costs. A 2015 systematic review and meta-analysis by Angus et al. [43] pooled 5 randomized clinical trials including ARISE, ProCESS, and ProMISe [46]. There was no difference in mortality between EGDT and usual care, and EGDT involved increased utilization of resources including ICU care and vasopressors. These findings highlight an important lesson as follows: single-center trials may report an inflated effect size that is not reproducible in multicenter trials. Table 3.3 summarizes findings from these trials.

Normalization of lactate was added as a resuscitation goal in the 2012 SSC guidelines [6]. This new guideline was based on two multicenter randomized controlled trials that used lactate normalization both as a single target for resuscitation and in combination with normalization of $ScvO_2$. The Emergency Medicine Shock Research Network (EMShockNet) was a noninferiority study that randomized 300 patients with severe sepsis to one of the two resuscitation goal strategies [47]. One group was resuscitated to normalize CVP, MAP and $ScvO_2$ to 70 % and the other group was resuscitated to normalize CVP, MAP and to achieve a lactate clearance of at least 10 %. There were no differences in in-hospital mortality or adverse effects between the two groups. The LACTATE study group published results demonstrating that ICU patients with hyperlactatemia have reduced hospital mortality when they are resuscitated to reduce lactate levels by 20 % or more per

Table 3.3 Resuscitation strategy in severe sepsis: summary of major studies

Year	Trial	*N*, Population	Intervention	Control	Outcomes of interest	Conclusion
2001	EGDT [7]	263 ED patients with severe sepsis or septic shock	EGDT	Usual Care	In-hospital mortality at 60 days	EGDT decreased in-hospital mortality
2014	ProCESS [9]	1341 ED patients with septic shock	1. EGDT or 2. protocol-based standard resuscitation	Usual Care	In-hospital mortality at 60 days	No difference in mortality
2014	ARISE [10]	1600 ED patients with septic shock	EGDT	Usual Care	Mortality at 90 days	No difference in mortality
2015	ProMISe [11]	1260 ED patients with severe sepsis	EGDT	Usual Care	Mortality at 90 days	No difference in mortality

2 h for an initial period of 8 h in the ICU [48]. These studies support normalization of lactate as an additional goal for resuscitation in patients with severe sepsis and septic shock.

Other Aspects of Management

Fluid resuscitation and supportive care remain the cornerstone of management for the patient with sepsis or septic shock. A number of other aspects of care are addressed by the SSC guidelines, [9] but an exhaustive review of these other topics is beyond the scope of this chapter. A brief review of infection issues, hemodynamic adjunctive support, and transfusion criteria are offered.

With respect to control of infection and treatment, blood cultures should be obtained before administration of combination broad-spectrum antibiotics if possible, and antibiotics should be administered within 1 h of recognition of sepsis or septic shock. Empiric antibiotics should not be administered for more than 3–5 days, and de-escalation to the most appropriate single therapy is warranted based on culture data. A specific anatomical diagnosis of infection should be sought. If intervention is warranted to obtain source control through surgical drainage or other intervention, this should be completed within 12 h of recognition.

Vasopressors may be used in conjunction with appropriate fluid resuscitation to maintain a MAP of 65 mm Hg. Norepinephrine is the first choice for vasopressor administration; epinephrine may be added or potentially substituted for norepinephrine should an additional agent be necessary. Vasopressin is not recommended as the first choice for a single initial vasopressor, but it may be added to norepinephrine to raise the MAP or decrease the amount of norepinephrine required. Dopamine may be used as an alternative to norepinephrine in highly selected patients with low risk of tachyarrhythmia and bradycardia. A trial of dobutamine is appropriate if there is evidence for myocardial dysfunction or ongoing hypoperfusion despite adequate MAP and intravascular volume.

Although the trial by Rivers et al. [10] endorsed transfusion of red blood cells to reach a hematocrit of 30 %, current SSC guidelines do not support routine use of blood transfusions for septic patients. In the absence of myocardial ischemia, severe hypoxemia, hemorrhage, or ischemic heart disease, red cell transfusion should only be administered if the hemoglobin level is <7.0 g/dL. The appropriate target hemoglobin concentration is 7.0 to 9.0 g/dL.

Conclusion

Sepsis and septic shock remain common diagnoses with incredibly complex pathophysiology and high rates of associated mortality. Resuscitation of the patient sepsis and septic shock remains an active area for research investigation, and evidence-based guidelines will continue to reflect advances in knowledge. Health care providers must critically evaluate the literature and update their practices to ensure optimization of patient outcomes and appropriate use and allocation of resources.

Clinical Scenario

Fifty-seven-year-old man returns to the SICU s/p R extended colectomy for cecal perforation—(Hx. Patient transferred from OSH est 24 h delay to OR) now in profound septic shock open abdomen. On vasopressin and norepinephrine, lactate 4.5 made very little urine intra-operatively.

Authors' Response to the Clinical Scenario:

This patient should be aggressively resuscitated with an initial fluid challenge of 30 mL/kg of lactated Ringer's or normal saline. Albumin is safe and may be used in addition to crystalloids. Resuscitation goals include a CVP of 8–12 (a higher CVP goal may be appropriate since this patient is mechanically ventilated), MAP ≥65 mm Hg, and urine output ≥0.5 mL/kg/h. A single CVP measurement, however, is not specific and at best a trend of values may be helpful. Further, measures of fluid responsiveness such as passive leg raising should guide the amount of fluid given. Other goals include achieving a central venous oxygen saturation of 70 % or a mixed venous oxygen saturation of 65 %. Normalization of lactate is an effective resuscitation target. Blood transfusion is only appropriate if the hemoglobin level is <7.0 g/dL. Use of norepinephrine is recommended if the patient continues to manifest signs of tissue hypoperfusion (lactate ≥4 mmol/L, oliguria) despite adequate fluid resuscitation. Vasopressin may be used as an adjunct, but not as a single agent. Antibiotics should be continued. While these are the current best practice recommendations, they are largely based on older clinical trials. Management should always be guided by the most current evidence or guidelines.

Key Questions

1. *What is the current indication for a pulmonary artery catheter?*
2. *What should be the resuscitation approach to the patient in either progressive acute renal injury/failure of the patient with end stage renal disease and on hemodialysis?*

References

1. Singer M, Deutschman CS, Seymour CW, et al. The Third International Consensus Definitions for Sepsis and Septic Shock (Sepsis-3). JAMA 2016;315(8):801-810.
2. Shankar-Hari M, Phillips GS, Levy ML, et al. Developing a New Definition and Assessing New Clinical Criteria for Septic Shock For the Third International Consensus Definitions for Sepsis and Septic Shock (Sepsis-3). JAMA 2016;315(8):775-787.
3. Seymour CW, Liu VX, Iwashyna TJ, et al. Assessment of Clinical Criteria for Sepsis For the Third International Consensus Definitions for Sepsis and Septic Shock (Sepsis-3). JAMA 2016;315(8):762-774.
4. Rangel-Frausto MS, Pittet D, Costigan M, Hwang T, Davis CS, Wenzel RP. The natural history of the systemic inflammatory response syndrome (SIRS): a prospective study. JAMA. 1995;273:117–23.
5. Funk DJ, Parrillo JE, Kumar A. Sepsis and septic shock: a history. Crit Care Clin. 2009;25:83–101.
6. Opal SM. The evolution of the understanding of sepsis, infection, and the host response: a brief history. Crit Care Clin. 2009;25:637–63.
7. Cerra FB. The systemic septic response: multiple systems organ failure. Crit Care Clin. 1985;1:591–607.
8. Beal AL, Cerra FB. Multiple organ failure syndrome in the 1990s: systemic inflammatory response and organ dysfunction. JAMA. 1994;271:26–233.
9. Dellinger RP, Levy MM, Rhodes A, et al. Surviving sepsis campaign: international guidelines for management of severe sepsis and septic shock. Crit Care Med. 2013;41(2):580–637.
10. Rivers E, Nguyen B, Havstad S, et al. Early goal-directed therapy in the treatment of severe sepsis and septic shock. N Engl J Med. 2001;345(19):1368–77.
11. Dellinger RP, Carlet JM, Masur H, et al. Surviving sepsis campaign guidelines for management of severe sepsis and septic shock. Crit Care Med. 2004;32(3):858–73.
12. Yealy DM, Kellum JA, Huang DT, ProCESS Investigators, et al. A randomized trial of protocol-based care for early septic shock. N Engl J Med. 2014;370(18):1683–93.
13. ARISE Investigators, ANZICS Clinical Trials Group. Goal-directed resuscitation for patients with early septic shock. N Engl J Med 2014;371:1496–506.
14. Mouncey PR, Osborn TM, Power GS, ProMISe Trial Investigators. Trial of early, goal-directed resuscitation for septic shock. N Engl J Med. 2015;372:1301–11.
15. Bone RC, Balk RA, Cerra FB, The ACCP-SCCM Consensus Conference Committee, et al. Definitions for sepsis and organ failure and guidelines for the use of innovative therapies in sepsis. Chest. 1992;101:1644–55.

16. Levy MM, Fink MP, Marshall JC, et al. International sepsis definitions conference. 2001 SSCM/ESICM/ACCP/ATS/SIS International sepsis definitions conference. Crit Care Med. 2003;31:1250–6.
17. Vincent JL, Opal SM, Marshall JC, Tracey KJ. Sepsis definitions: time for change. Lancet. 2013;381:774–5.
18. Sprung CL, Sakr Y, Vincent JL, et al. An evaluation of systemic inflammatory response syndrome signs in the sepsis occurrence in acutely ill patients (SOAP) study. Intensive Care Med. 2006;32(3):411–7.
19. Vincent JL. Dear SIRS, I'm sorry to say that I don't like you. Crit Care Med. 2007;25(2):372–4.
20. Kaukonen K, Bailey M, Pilcher D, Cooper DJ, Bellomo R. Systemic inflammatory response syndrome criteria in defining severe sepsis. N Engl J Med. 2015;372:1629–38.
21. Gaieski DF, Edwards JM, Kallan MJ, Carr BG. Benchmarking the incidence and mortality of severe sepsis in the United States. Crit Care Med. 2013;41:1167–74.
22. Angus DC, van der Poll T. Severe sepsis and septic shock. N Engl J Med. 2013;369(9): 840–51.
23. Angus DC, Linde-Zwirble WT, Lidicker J, et al. Epidemiology of severe sepsis in the United States: analysis of incidence, outcome, and associated costs of care. Crit Care Med. 2001;29:1303–10.
24. Brun-Buisson C, Meshaka P, Pinton P, Vallet B. EPISEPSIS: a reappraisal of the epidemiology and outcome of severe sepsis in French intensive care units. Intensive Care Med. 2004;30:580–8.
25. Kaukonen KM, Bailey M, Suzuki S, Pilcher D, Bellomo R. Mortality related to severe sepsis and septic shock among critically ill patients in Australia and New Zealand, 2000–2012. JAMA. 2014;311:1308–16.
26. Adhikari NK, Fowler RA, Bhagwanjee S, Rubenfeld GD. Critical care and the global burden of critical illness in adults. Lancet. 2010;376:1339–46.
27. Prescott HC, Dickson RP, Rogers MA, Langa KM, Iwashyna TJ. Hospitalization type predicts risk of subsequent severe sepsis. Am J Respir Crit Care Med. 2015 (in press). Available at http://www.atsjournals.org/doi/abs/10.1164/rccm.201503-0483OC#.Vaf4T5NViko. Accessed 16 July 2015.
28. Mayr FB, Yende S, Linde-Zwirble WT, et al. Infection rate and acute organ dysfunction risk as explanations for racial differences in severe sepsis. JAMA. 2010;303:2495–503.
29. Martin GS, Mannino DM, Eaton S, Moss M. The epidemiology of sepsis in the United States from 1979 through 2000. N Engl J Med. 2003;348:1546–54.
30. van der Poll T, Opal SM. Host-pathogen interactions in sepsis. Lancet Infect Dis. 2008;8: 32–43.
31. Cawcutt KA, Peters SG. Severe sepsis and septic shock: clinical overview and update on management. Mayo Clin Proc. 2014;89(11):1572–8.
32. Xiao W, Mindrinos MN, Seok J, et al. A genomic storm in critically injured humans. J Exp Med. 2011;208:2581–90.
33. Myburgh JA, Mythen MG. Resuscitation fluids. N Engl J Med. 2013;369(13):1243–51.
34. Perel P, Roberts I. Colloids versus crystalloids for fluid resuscitation in critically ill patients. Cochrane Database Syst Rev. 2012;6:CD000567.
35. Finfer S, Bellomo R, Boyce N, French J, Myburgh J, Norton R. SAFE study investigators. A comparison of albumin and saline for fluid resuscitation in the intensive care unit. N Engl J Med. 2004;350(22):2247–56.
36. Delaney AP, Dan A, McCaffrey J, Finfer S. The role of albumin as a resuscitation fluid for patients with sepsis: a systematic review and metaanalysis. Crit Care Med. 2011;39:386–91.
37. Annane D, Siami S, Jaber S, CRISTAL Investigators, et al. Effects of fluid resuscitation with colloids vs crystalloids on mortality in critically ill patients presenting with hypovolemic shock: the CRISTAL randomized trial. JAMA. 2013;310(17):1809–17.
38. Caironi P, Tognoni G, Masson S, Fumagalli R, Pesenti A, Romero M, ALBIOS Study Investigators, et al. Albumin replacement in patients with severe sepsis or septic shock. N Engl J Med. 2014;370:1412–21.

39. Patel A, Laffan MA, Waheed U, Brett SJ. Randomised trials of human albumin for adults with sepsis: systematic review and meta-analysis with trial sequential analysis of all-cause mortality. BMJ. 2014;349:g4561.
40. Guidet B, Martinet O, Boulain T, et al. Assessment of hemodynamic efficacy and safety of 6 % hydroxyethyl starch 130/0.4 vs. 0.9 % NaCl fluid replacement in patients with severe sepsis: the CRYSTMAS study. Crit Care. 2012;16:R94.
41. Myburgh JA, Finfer S, Bellomo R, CHEST Investigators, et al. Hydroxyethyl starch or saline for fluid resuscitation in intensive care. N Engl J Med. 2012;367:1901–11.
42. Perner A, Haase N, Guttormsen AB, 6S Trial Group, et al. Hydroxyethyl starch 130/0.42 versus Ringer's acetate in severe sepsis. N Engl J Med. 2012;367:124–34.
43. Brunkhorst FM, Engel C, Bloos F, German Competence Network Sepsis (SepNet), et al. Intensive insulin therapy and pentastarch resuscitation in severe sepsis. N Engl J Med. 2008;358:125–39.
44. Monnet X, Teboul J. Assessment of volume responsiveness during mechanical ventilation: recent advances. Crit Care. 2013;17(2):217.
45. Prekker ME, Scott NL, Hart D, Sprenkle MD, Leatherman JW. Point-of-care ultrasound to estimate central venous pressure: a comparison of three techniques. Crit Care Med. 2013;41 (3):833–41.
46. Angus DC, Barnato AE, Bell D et al. A systematic review and meta-analysis of early goal-directed therapy for septic shock: the ARISE, ProCESS and ProMISe investigators. Intensive Care Med. 2015. Available at http://link.springer.com.ezp.welch.jhmi.edu/article/10.1007%2Fs00134-015-3822-1. Accessed 19 July 2015.
47. Jones AE, Shapiro NI, Trzeciak S, Emergency Medicine Shock Research Network (EMShockNet) Investigators, et al. Lactate clearance vs central venous oxygen saturation goals of early sepsis therapy: a randomized clinical trial. JAMA. 2010;303:739–46.
48. Jansen TC, van Bommel J, Schoonderbeek FJ, LACTATE Study Group, et al. Early lactate-guided therapy in intensive care unit patients: a multicenter, open-label, randomized controlled trial. Am J Respir Crit Care Med. 2010;182:752–61.

Chapter 4
Intra-peritoneal Resuscitation in Trauma and Sepsis: Management Options for the Open Abdomen

Glen A. Franklin, Nicole M. Garcia and Jason W. Smith

First described by Rotondo et al. [1], damage control surgery (DCS) has now become commonplace in the management of abdominal injuries. The combination of acidosis, hypothermia, and coagulopathy are well-known precedents to mortality and using an abbreviated surgical procedure with bleeding control and initial injury management followed by resuscitation, rewarming and correction of coagulopathy with delayed definitive surgery has been shown to improve patient outcomes [2, 3]. While, initially, DCS was limited to trauma patients, it is now being further utilized on patients with abdominal catastrophes such as sepsis, severe pancreatitis, and ruptured aneurysms. The development of abdominal compartment syndrome in post-resuscitation surgical patients and burn patients has also provided another category of complex patients with the open abdomen. The physiologic derangements that occur during these types of events lead to issues in fluid management, electrolyte restoration, tissue ischemia, and edema as well as enhanced inflammation. The ongoing resuscitation efforts frequently provide an opportunity for significant fluid shifts and tissue edema limiting the ability of the surgeon to primarily close the abdomen even after a few return trips to the operating room [4]. Patients with the open abdomen are quite ill and have a higher rate of postoperative complications even if they have primary closure. In a recent study by Bruns et al. [5], patient with non-trauma open abdomens had a 36 % six-month mortality with over two-thirds of the survivors requiring significant post-discharge medical care.

G.A. Franklin (✉) · N.M. Garcia · J.W. Smith
Department of Surgery, University of Louisville, 2nd Floor ACB, 550 S Jackson Street, Louisville, KY 40202, USA
e-mail: glen.a.franklin@gmail.com; glen.a.franklin@louisville.edu

N.M. Garcia
e-mail: nicole.garcia@louisville.edu

J.W. Smith
e-mail: jasonw.smith@louisville.edu

J.J. Diaz and D.T. Efron (eds.), *Complications in Acute Care Surgery*,
DOI 10.1007/978-3-319-42376-0_4

For those patients who are not able to achieve primary fascia closure, a variety of options remain to provide temporary or permanent closure. While no formal classification or grading system exists for these complex abdominal wall defects, many closure techniques have been attempted and studied [6]. Prosthetic closure alone offers the ease of closure but often the highest rate of fistula formation and failure. Various techniques including a fascia bridge, component separation, and minimally invasive component separation have all been utilized with/without synthetic and biologic mesh. The development of a patient specific plan is paramount to success as these are not "one-size-fits-all" types of operative repairs.

Providing primary fascial closure following DCS with an open abdomen clearly reduces the morbidity and mortality for the patient. Decreasing time to abdominal wall closure and number of operative take-backs has been shown to significantly reduce morbidity and mortality in DCS [7, 8]. Hatch et al. [9] have also shown that early fascial closure was an independent predictor of complications in DCS patients. What is clear despite advances in resuscitation is the need for early primary closure whenever possible for those patients with DCS and an open abdomen. We describe here two cases utilizing a novel resuscitation technique with peritoneal dialysis solution we have termed "direct peritoneal resuscitation" (DPR). Our group has extensive experience with this procedure and has shown a decrease in time to fascial closure and a reduction in post-DCS complications when DPR is combined with DCS. The proposed physiologic mechanism of action is related to the osmolality of the dialysis solution. It triggers fluid shifts that enhance mesenteric blood flow, improve liver blood flow, and potentially influence the post-injury inflammatory response. The cases are to demonstrate the possibilities for use in both the trauma and the non-trauma emergency surgery patients. Each case represents a common use of DPR in our practice environment.

Case 1—The trauma team was called to the trauma bay to evaluate a patient brought in by emergency medical services. The patient was an 18-year-old male, gunshot victim, which had been shot just to the right of the umbilicus with a 9 mm round, no other wounds noted. The patient was found to be hypotensive (systolic blood pressure 80 s mm Hg) and tachycardic (heart rate 130 s). After performing a primary survey and administering two units of packed red blood cells (PRBC), the patient was taken to the operating room for an exploratory laparotomy. The institutional massive transfusion protocol was activated. Upon entering the abdomen, approximately 700 cc of blood was encountered. The abdomen was packed in all four quadrants and anesthesia continued to resuscitate the patient. At exploration, the patient was found to have multiple small bowel injuries as well as a through and through liver laceration. There were no major vascular injuries noted. The three small bowel injuries were resected via stapler to contain the contamination. The liver lacerations were reapproximated to control the bleeding with suture to provide compression. At this point, the patient continued to require blood products for ongoing resuscitation. Anesthesia notified us that the patient's temperature was 34 Å °C, and his base deficit on his most recent arterial gas was −15 (Table 4.1). We noted the patient had begun to ooze from multiple areas. Considering the patient was acidotic, hypothermic, and coagulopathic, we decided to finish the damage control operation by placing a Blake drain for direct peritoneal resuscitation (DPR) at the base of the mesentery and place a temporary vacuum closure system with plans to re-explore the patient was resuscitation was complete. In total, the patient was in the operating room for about 1.5 h. He was then transferred to the Surgical Intensive Care Unit (SICU).

Twenty-four hours later, the patient had received a total of 24 units PRBCs, 20 units fresh frozen plasma (FFP), and 4 packs of platelets as well as a unit of cryoprecipitate. The patient was normotensive with his most recent base deficit of −2. He had been receiving DPR for the past 24 h at 400 cc per hour. We elected to take the patient back to the operating room for a definitive closure. Upon re-exploration, we performed two small bowel primary anastomoses using a stapled side-to-side technique. The bowel wall was minimally edematous and appeared to be perfused adequately. The liver lacerations were hemostatic. The fascia was able to be reapproximated primarily without tension and was closed with running suture. The patient remained in the SICU for an additional 3 days and was transferred to a regular medical-surgical bed. He was discharged on post-injury day 8. Follow-up in clinic showed a healed wound with no evidence of fascial breakdown or hernia.

Case 2—The acute care surgery team was called to the emergency department to evaluate a 75-year-old woman who presented with a 24 h history of abdominal pain. The patient stated the pain had started approximately one day ago, described as crampy and colicky; accompanied by nausea, emesis, and obstipation. On presentation, the patient was obviously ill with a systolic blood pressure of 80 and a heart rate of 105. Physical examination demonstrated the patient's abdomen was distended and diffusely tender with rebound tenderness in the right lower quadrant. While the patient received fluid resuscitation, her laboratory data resulted with a bicarbonate of 17, blood urea nitrogen of 45, creatinine of 1.92, and white blood cell count of 26,000 (Table 4.1). After a nasogastric tube and Foley catheter were placed, a CT abdomen/pelvis was obtained that demonstrated dilated loops of small bowel proximally and a distended loop in the right lower quadrant concerning for an internal hernia. Her past surgical history was significant for an open appendectomy in the remote past. The patient was taken to the operating room for an exploration given her physical examination findings, laboratory data, and imaging. On exploration, the patient was found to have an internal hernia consisting of very edematous, maroon small bowel due to adhesions from her previous appendectomy.

Table 4.1 Physiologic parameters for patient case studies

	Case 1	Case 2
Blood pressure (mmHg)	86/56	80/48
Heart rate (bpm)	130	105
Temperature (Celsius)	34	37.2
WBC (10^9/L)	17	26
Blood urea nitrogen (mg/dL)	21	45
Creatinine (mg/dL)	0.97	1.92
Bicarbonate (mEq/dL)	11	17
Base deficit (mEq/dL)	−15	−9

The adhesion was released; however, the bowel continued to look inflamed and edematous with an ecchymotic area on the anti-mesenteric border of the distal ileum worrisome for ischemia. Anesthesia notified the surgeon that the patient was still hypotensive despite fluid resuscitation and was requiring increasing amounts of pressor agents. Considering the patient's ongoing hypotension, pressor requirement, and questionable viability of the distal ileum, a decision was made to place a Blake drain for DPR and a temporary abdominal closure. In total, the patient received 8 L of crystalloid and 500 cc of 5 % albumin solution during the operation. The patient was taken to the SICU for continued resuscitation with plans for a second-look laparotomy in 12–24 h.

After 16 h, the patient's vasopressor requirement was minimal, her urine output had increased, and bicarbonate had normalized. She received crystalloid resuscitation directed by standard physiologic parameters (i.e., central venous pressure, urine output, stroke volume variation, and base deficit). A decision was made to proceed with a second-look laparotomy. On re-exploration, the distal ileum looked viable including the previously described ecchymotic area. The small bowel was still a bit dilated, but the bowel wall edema had resolved. The patient's superior mesenteric artery was palpated and found to be patent and the patient had a good mesenteric and anti-mesenteric pulse. The patient was subsequently washed out, and her fascia was able to be reapproximated without tension. A running suture was used for fascia closure. The patient was successfully extubated following the case, and diet was advanced as her bowel function returned over the next 3 days. She remained in the SICU for 1-day post-op and was discharged home on postoperative day number 6. While standard practice may have been to wait 24–48 h for the second look, we felt that the addition of DPR allowed for a more rapid return to the operating room, a decrease in crystalloid resuscitation, and improved mesenteric blood flow in this elderly patient.

The temporary abdominal closure technique consists of a 19F silicone elastomer round Blake drain (Ethicon) placed in the left upper lateral quadrant and directed around the root of the mesentery along the left pericolic gutter and down into the pelvis. A sterile X-ray cassette cover is then fenestrated and placed over the abdominal contents but under the fascia. A sterile operating room towel is placed over the plastic cover and tucked under the fascia. Thoracostomy tubes are used for drains (32F) and placed on top of the towel with a "Y" connector. The abdomen is then covered with an occlusive dressing (typically an Ioban drape) and the chest tubes are placed to low-pressure suction. This creates a modified "Bogota Bag"-type closure [10, 11] with vacuum-assisted drainage. DPR patients receive dialysate instilled using the left upper quadrant drain, allowing a continuous lavage within the abdomen until suctioned out the top of the wound through the towel draining chest tubes. DPR was initiated using commercially available 2.5 % glucose-based peritoneal dialysis solution (Delflex; Fresenius, USA) within one hour of completion of damage control operation (Fig. 4.1). A bolus of 800 cc Delflex fluid was instilled over the first hour and followed at a rate of 400 cc/h until a repeat laparotomy was performed. Intravenous blood and crystalloid resuscitation were

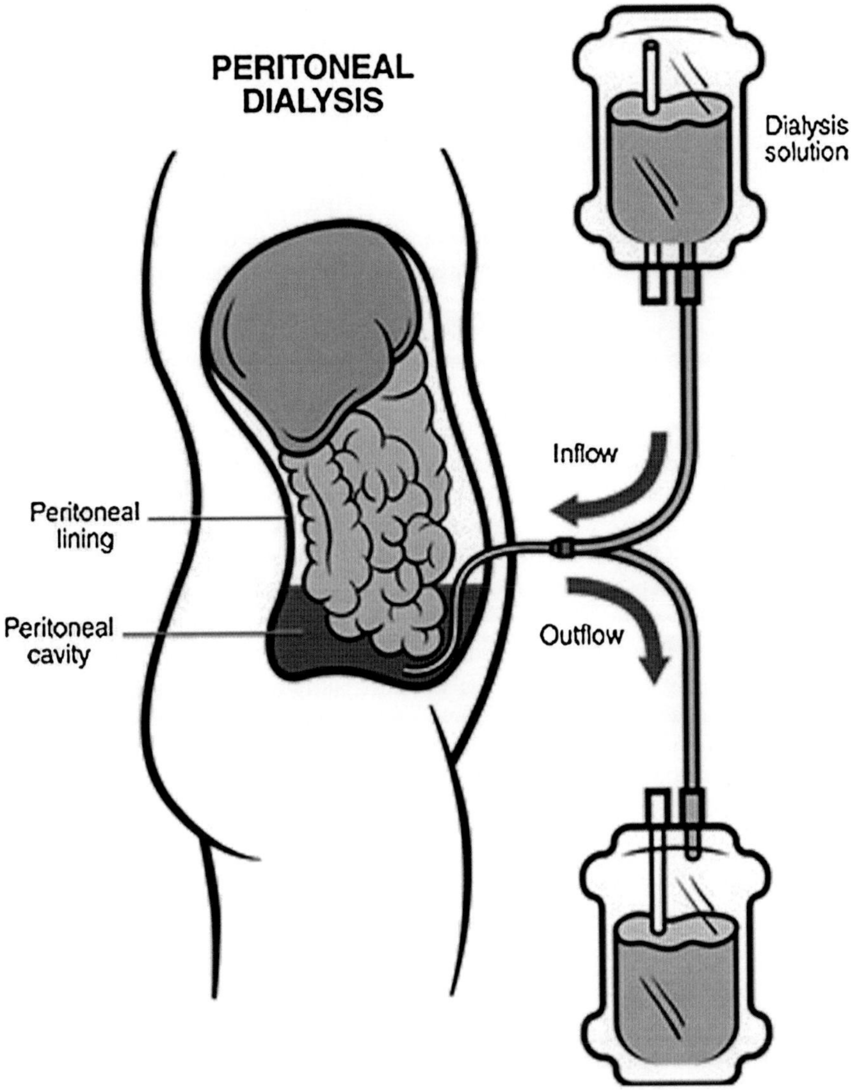

Fig. 4.1 Diagram for instillation setup for DPR. Deflex 2.5 % peritoneal dialysis solution is infused at 800 cc/h for the initial bolus within 1 h of DCS. The DPR is then maintained at 400 cc/h continuously until the next planned operation. Drainage is achieved via the vacuum-assisted dressing on the abdomen

administered at the discretion of the treating physicians, with an aim toward rapid restoration of hemodynamics and resuscitative parameters (goal-directed therapy).

We have previously demonstrated that instilling a hypertonic glucose-based peritoneal dialysis fluid to the peritoneal cavity (DPR) can improve microvascular perfusion and reduce tissue injury following hemorrhagic shock in a rodent laboratory model [12–14]. DPR also has been demonstrated to improve portal venous blood flow and help mitigate obesity-induced hepatic dysfunction following trauma [15]. Clinical studies in trauma patients showed that the use of DPR as an adjunct to resuscitation was associated with less tissue edema, decreased abdominal complications as well as decreased time to definitive abdominal closure [16]. In this study, patients who received DPR were closed in 4.4 $\pm$ 1.7 days compared to 7.0 $\pm$ 3.4 days for those who did not receive DPR. The odds ratio for primary fascial closure was 10.7:1 for who had received DPR ($p = 0.01$). In a small subset of patients, DPR ($n = 19$) was compared to the Wittmann patch ($n = 8$) and also found to significantly improve time to closure 4.4 days versus 6.4 days ($p = 0.003$).

We have also utilized DPR in the non-traumatic acute care surgery patient undergoing DCS. We have compared emergency surgery patients who had undergone DCS with and without adjunctive resuscitation using DPR [17]. There were 118 patients identified during the study who were propensity matched into case cohorts of two groups of 44 patients each. Significant physiologic scoring responses were noted in those patients who had received DPR for 48 h following DCS compared to those who did not in the control group. This included decreases in APACHE-II, SOFA, and SAPS-II scores at 48 h. Serum laboratory markers for pH, oxygenation, hepatic function, renal function, and coagulation all improved for those in the DPR group. This study also showed a decrease in time to definitive closure and abdominal complications, as well as in increase in primary fascial closure rate (Table 4.2). Mortality was not different between the groups. Recently, we have used DPR in the management of brain-dead organ donors. DPR as a resuscitative adjunct improved the total number of organs transplanted per donor from 3.0 $\pm$ 1.5 to 3.7 $\pm$ 1.7 [18]. This was a significant improvement over traditional donor management protocols and was thought to be due impart to improved liver blood flow, decreased overall resuscitation volume, and reduced need for vasopressor agents.

DCS with the resultant open abdomen presents many complications for the surgeon. The timing for second operation and subsequent abdominal wall closure techniques are not well standardized and tend to be surgeon dependent. While several studies discuss the importance of early abdominal wall closure and the variety of techniques for managing the acute and chronic hernia, few reports have addressed the primary problem of decreasing bowel and abdominal wall edema such that primary closure can be achieved. While goal-directed transfusion therapy ratios have helped with this problem, massive transfusion still provides significant fluid shifts and tissue edema limiting options for primary closure. We have

Table 4.2 Propensity-matched abdominal wall outcomes

	Controls ($n = 44$)	DPR ($n = 44$)	*P* value
Time to definitive abdominal closure (days)	7.7 ± 4.1	5.9 ± 3.2	0.02
Primary fascial closure *n* (%)	19 (43 %)	29 (68 %)	0.03
# of abdominal complications	21 (47 %)	12 (27 %)	0.04

described our experience with a simple resuscitation adjunct using peritoneal dialysis solution delivered via an indwelling catheter to the open abdomen patient. DPR is cost-effective with the solution costing less than $200 per 3 L bag. We have used it in both trauma patients and acute care emergency surgery patients. Our published data have shown a decrease time to closure, increase rate in primary fascial closure, and a decrease in long-term morbidity from recurrent abdominal wall hernia. We would recommend this resuscitative adjunct in those patients requiring DCS with a resultant open abdomen and in patients who develop abdominal compartment syndrome requiring emergent decompressive laparotomy. It is a simple, safe technique with significant patient benefit.

Clinical Scenario

A 50 year old woman with presents with perforated diverticulitis and has now undergone a sigmoid colectomy and Hartman's procedure. She remains in septic shock with markedly distended bowel noted during the operation. A decision is made to limit the initial operation to damage control and with a planned delayed maturation of the colostomy once she is better resuscitated. Intra-operatively, you decide to place a temporary abdominal wall closure but have concerns about retraction of the fascia and musculature. Tentatively, the plan is to return to the operating room within 48 h for a second-look and definitive closure. What techniques are available to assist with the abdominal wall closure? This patient requires a fair amount of resuscitation; therefore, the bowel wall edema is likely to increase making primary closure much more difficult. Are there resuscitative techniques that can assist with management of the bowel wall edema, while still providing adequate resuscitation for the septic shock? This is a common patient presenting to our acute care surgical team. This chapter will describe alternate techniques for adjunctive resuscitation and closure of the abdomen in the patient with in intra-abdominal disaster. Through the application of direct peritoneal resuscitation, this patient was taken back to the operating room in 48 h and underwent primary fascial closure. The small bowel edema was resolved despite fairly large volume resuscitation for the sepsis. The colostomy was matured and the septic shock resolved. Oral diet was initiated on post-operative day 5 after a return of bowel function. There were no wound complications and she was discharged home on post-operative day 10.

Intraperitoneal resuscitation in Sepsis: 50 year old woman DM and HTN presents with Hinchey III, perforated diverticulitis. She is now s/p sigmoid colectomy and Hartman's procedure (options for intra-peritoneal resuscitation).

Response

Considering the patient's ongoing hypotension, pressor requirement and questionable viability of the distal ileum, a decision was made to place a Blake drain for DPR and a temporary abdominal closure. In total, the patient received 8 L of crystalloid and 500 cc of 5 % albumin solution during the operation.

While standard practice may have been to wait 24–48 h for the second look, we felt that the addition of DPR allowed for a more rapid return to the operating room, a decrease in crystalloid resuscitation and improved mesenteric blood flow in this elderly patient.

Key Questions

(1) *In the current era of damage control resuscitation (1:1:1) of the trauma patient what is the role of direct peritoneal resuscitation?*
(2) *How does one calculate and included the "volume dialyzed" from the patient during direct peritoneal resuscitation in their volume status?*

References

1. Rotondo MF, Schwab CW, McGonigal MD, et al. 'Damage control': an approach for improved survival in exsanguinating penetrating abdominal injury. J Trauma. 1993;35(3): 375–82; discussion 382–3.
2. Khan A, Hsee L, Mathur S, Civil I. Damage-control laparotomy in nontrauma patients: review of indications and outcomes. J Trauma Acute Care Surg. 2013;75(3):365–8.
3. Shapiro MB, Jenkins DH, Schwab CW, Rotondo MF. Damage control: collective review. J Trauma. 2000;249(5):969–78.
4. Foy H. Reinforced silicone elastomer sheeting, an improved method of temporary abdominal closure in damage control laparotomy. Am J Surg. 2003;185:498–501.
5. Bruns, BR, Ahmad, SA, O'Meara, L, et al. Non-trauma open abdomens: a prospective observational study. J Trauma Acute Care Surg. 2016; doi:10.1097/TA.0000000000000958
6. Diaz JJ, Cullinane DC, Khwaja KA, et al. Eastern association for the surgery of trauma: management of the open abdomen, part III—review of abdominal wall reconstruction. J Trauma Acute Care Surg. 2013;75(3):376–86.
7. Bradley MJ, Dubose JJ, Scalea TM, et al. Independent predictors of enteric fistula and abdominal sepsis after damage control laparotomy: results from the prospective AAST open abdomen registry. JAMA Surg. 2013;148(10):947–55.
8. Miller RS, Morris Jr JA, Diaz Jr JJ, Herring MB, May AK. Complications after 344 damage-control open celiotomies. J Trauma. 2005;59(6):1365–71; discussion 1371–4.
9. Hatch QM, Osterhout LM, Podbielski J, et al. Impact of closure at the first take back: complication burden and potential overutilization of damage control laparotomy. J Trauma. 2011;71(6):1503–11.
10. Fernandez L, Norwood S, Roettger R, Wilkins HE III. Temporary intravenous bag silo closure in severe abdominal trauma. J Trauma. 1996;40:258–60.
11. Fox VJ, Miller J, Nix AM. Temporary abdominal closure using an i.v. bag silo for severe trauma. AORN J. 1999;69:530–5.
12. el Zakaria R, et al. Generalized dilation of the visceral microvasculature by peritoneal dialysis solutions. Perit Dial Int. 2002;22(5):593–601.
13. Zakaria R, et al. Intraperitoneal resuscitation improves intestinal blood flow following hemorrhagic shock. Ann Surg. 2003;237(5):704–11; discussion 711–3.

14. Hurt RT, Matheson PJ, Smith JW, et al. Preservation of hepatic blood flow by direct peritoneal resuscitation improves survival and prevents hepatic inflammation following hemorrhagic shock. Am J Physiol Gastrointest Liver Physiol. 2012;303(10):G1144–52.
15. Matheson PJ, Franklin GA, Hurt RT, Downard CD, Smith JW, Garrison RN. Direct peritoneal resuscitation improves obesity-induced hepatic dysfunction after trauma. J Am Coll Surg. 2012;214(4):517–28; discussion 528–30.
16. Smith JW, Garrison RN, Matheson PJ, et al. Direct peritoneal resuscitation accelerates primary abdominal wall closure after damage control surgery. J Am Coll Surg. 2010;210(5):658–64.
17. Smith JW, Neal Garrison R, Matheson PJ, et al. Adjunctive treatment of abdominal catastrophes and sepsis with direct peritoneal resuscitation: indications for use in acute care surgery. J Trauma Acute Care Surg. 2014;77(3):393–8.
18. Smith JW, Matheson PJ, Morgan G, et al. Addition of direct peritoneal lavage to human cadaver organ donor resuscitation improves organ procurement. J Am Coll Surg. 2015;220:539–47.

Chapter 5
How to Feed the Open Abdomen

Katie M. Love and Bryan R. Collier

Introduction

Patients with hemorrhagic shock, severe sepsis, and necrotizing pancreatitis treated with damage control surgery develop a severe systemic inflammatory response characterized by release of pro-inflammatory mediators. Those with open abdomens represent the sickest, most inflamed, and most hypermetabolic cohort of surgical patients. The acute catabolic reaction associated with severe physiologic stress and inflammation results in muscle proteolysis with increased urinary nitrogen excretion and weight loss, compounded by an increased resting energy expenditure attributed to the large open wound. This severe catabolic pro-inflammatory cascade and physical loss of protein continues until the abdomen is closed. Enteral nutrition (EN) provided within 24–36 h after admission to the ICU has been advocated in critically ill surgical patients. This is thought to ameliorate immune suppression which is characterized by the cytokine-generated stress response at the level of the gut. EN is better than parenteral nutrition (PN). However, if PN is started there are fewer associated complications if it is started late, after 5–7 days post admission. In the open abdomen patient, higher protein and calorie requirements are usually present not only because of the hypermetabolic response, but also because of the physical loss of fluid and protein from the open abdomen and negative pressure

K.M. Love (✉)
Acute Care Surgery: Trauma, Surgical Critical Care, Emergency General Surgery, Virginia Tech Carilion School of Medicine, 1906 Belleview Avenue, Med. Ed. 3rd Floor Suite 304, Roanoke, VA 24014, USA
e-mail: klbower1@carilionclinic.org

B.R. Collier
Acute Care Surgery: Trauma, Surgical Critical Care, Emergency General Surgery, Virginia Tech Carilion School of Medicine, 1906 Belleview Avenue, Med. Ed. 3rd Floor Suite 301, Roanoke, VA 24014, USA
e-mail: brcollier@carilionclinic.org

J.J. Diaz and D.T. Efron (eds.), *Complications in Acute Care Surgery*,
DOI 10.1007/978-3-319-42376-0_5

dressing. Therefore, ongoing diligence regarding nutrition provision (EN, PN, or both) is essential for optimal outcomes in the open abdomen patient.

Admission

Upon entering this patient's abdomen, even the young surgeon knows that this patient is going to require multiple operative interventions and great attention to detail in all aspects of his critical care. His critical illness and hyperinflammatory or hypercatabolic state is compounded by the significant fluid, electrolyte, and protein losses from exposed viscera [1]. This immediate protein–calorie malnutrition develops with impairment of immune function, and subclinical multiple organ dysfunction will continue at least until his abdomen is closed [2].

Enteral nutrition (EN) provided within 24–36 h after ICU admission or initial operation is advocated. This early but lower than goal EN ameliorates the immune suppression and attenuates the systemic inflammatory response syndrome (Fig. 5.1). In addition, early EN with an open abdomen is associated with increased fascial closure rates, earlier fascial closure, reduced incidence of infectious complications, and a decrease in mortality, especially in patients without bowel injuries [3, 4]. Positive associations in the literature are inconsistent likely due to the heterogenous patient population studied, but there have been no reported adverse outcomes from EN with open abdomens.

After the debridement and full drainage of the patient's pancreas, full exploration of the health of the bowel must occur as ischemia of the small bowel and right and

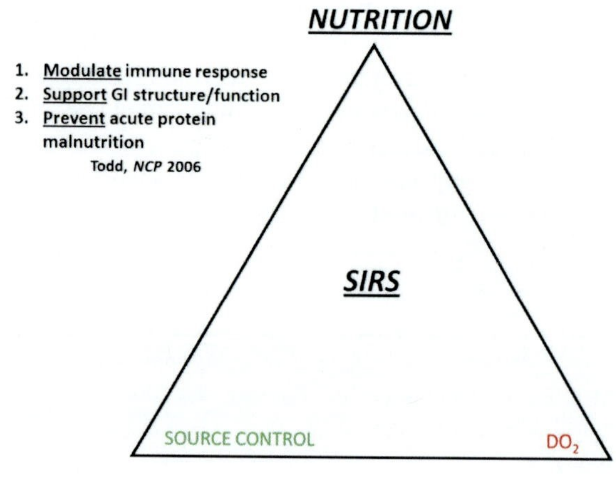

Fig. 5.1 The importance of early EN is less about the protein–calorie malnutrition and deficit, more about supporting the gastrointestinal immune structure and battling the systemic inflammatory response syndrome (SIRS) so common in patients with an open abdomen. In addition to nutrition, basic tenants of critical care such as source control and oxygen delivery address the SIRS response [5]

transverse colon is at times observed. Regardless, some type of nasoenteric feeding access is a must. At a minimum, a nasogastric or orogastric tube is required. We recommend if at all possible a nasojejunal tube and a nasogastric tube, one in each nostril. Either tube can be palpated at this point due to minimal bowel wall edema that is present day one. Commercial bridle systems can be used to prevent suturing to nasal septum and complications associated with tube securement. At this point, a negative pressure dressing is provided to the abdominal wall and the patient is ready for transport to the ICU.

EN is better than parenteral nutrition (PN), and if PN is started there are fewer associated complications if it is started late. PN should be considered if enteral nutrition is not providing at least 60–70 % of the calories and protein needed by the patient at the day 5–7 mark. Combined EN and PN nutrition support has a role in a selected group of patients [6].

Day 0

After damage control surgery, emphasis of management shifts from the operating room (OR) to the intensive care unit (ICU) where physiologic deficits are corrected in preparation for return to the OR. Goals of resuscitation are to restore physiologic reserve, tissue perfusion, normothermia, acid-base balance, and coagulation. Once euvolemia and hemodynamic stability ± vasopressor therapy are achieved and metabolic acidosis resolved, enteral feeds should be initiated.

Regarding enteric access at this point, a nasogastric or orogastric tube would be adequate. Traditional teaching is to feed post-pyloric, and nasojejunal tubes have been considered ideal feeding access with pancreatitis. However, clinical trials have demonstrated that feeding either the small bowel or stomach is well tolerated in severe pancreatitis [7]. In addition, the early (less than 24 h from admission) administration of EN is considered an active therapeutic intervention against severe pancreatitis. In general, post-pyloric feeding is preferred when feasible as there is evidence of a 30 % lower rate of pneumonia and an increase in the amount of nutrition delivered [8]. However, if it proves technically difficult, there is no reason to withhold pre-pyloric feeding. Tube feeding formula should be started at a low rate, ~20 mL/h or ~50 % of goal. If there is no evidence of gastroparesis, ileus, or mesenteric ischemia indicated by high residuals, emesis, or rising lactic acid levels, feeds can continue.

Achieving euvolemia with resuscitation is tantamount to the ability to close the abdomen. Hypervolemia causes bowel edema, increased protein losses, and ileus. Fluid resuscitation should cease when hourly urine output reaches 0.5–1 cc/kg/h in normal kidneys. More urine output is not better, and indicative of overresuscitation. There are a number of methods utilized to indirectly measure preload and vascular resistance as well; all are about equal in terms of reliability and accuracy. Direct peritoneal resuscitation can be helpful in terms of fluid balance in a patient with an open abdomen. It is a validated adjunct resuscitation strategy in patients with open abdominal wounds due to sepsis or hemorrhage. The practice consists of suffusing the peritoneal cavity with a 2.5 % glucose-based peritoneal dialysis solution (2.5 % Delflex: 25 g/L D-glucose, 0.567 g/L sodium chloride, 0.392 g/L sodium lactate 0.0257 g/L calcium chloride, 0.0152 g/L magnesium chloride at a pH of 6, osmolality of 486 mOsm/L) concurrent with intravenous resuscitation and negative pressure abdominal wound dressing. Though glucose is present, this would not be considered a part of nutrition provision. Direct peritoneal resuscitation causes microvascular vasodilation and increases visceral and hepatic blood flow, normalizes systemic water compartments [9], accelerates primary abdominal wall closure after damage control surgery, and prevents complications associated with an open abdomen [10, 11]. In addition to observed effects on microcirculation, it has marked ability to decrease visceral edema and normalize body water ratios, decreasing the incidence of ileus and improving enteric nutrition tolerance.

Day 1

Enteral nutrition continues. Usually by this point, EN has been initiated and calorie and protein goals are calculated, usually 35 kcal/kg/day and 2–2.5 g of protein/kg/day. Weight in kg is based on ideal body weight. If the patient demonstrates intolerance in terms of high residuals, emesis, or distension, or even ongoing SIRS, pushing rate to 100 % of goal is not necessary.

Day 1 is time to begin planning re-operation in terms of what needs to be accomplished prior to definitive closure. This includes further debridement if necessary, determining adequate drainage, planning reconstruction if necessary, and definitive feeding access. Even if a third exploration is necessary, surgical feeding access should be established as soon as intestinal continuity is restored. This helps avoid difficulty with positioning feeding tubes and iatrogenic injury related to inflammatory or edematous changes to the bowel wall. A gastrostomy tube is acceptable, but carries some risk of aspiration and pre-pyloric feeding intolerance. A gastrostomy and a jejunostomy tube can be placed to mitigate some of the risk associated with a gastrostomy tube alone, but the jejunostomy tube is traditionally fraught with complications including obstruction, dislodgement, volvulus, and leakage. Our favored approach is a single combination gastrojejunostomy tube, 22Fr soft silicone with retention balloon, inserted through a gastrostomy utilizing the Stamm technique. The distal lumen is guided and positioned toward the ligament of Treitz. Postoperative management is the same as a gastrostomy tube. It provides the option of simultaneous gastric decompression with concurrent post-pyloric feeding, without the additional enterotomy and risks associated with jejunostomy. We have used these tubes even in the presence of gastroduodenal pathology, such as perforated duodenal ulcers, with excellent results.

Day 2–5

Consideration must be given to how much nutrition is delivered versus what was ordered. Underfeeding has been demonstrated in multiple comparative clinical studies, with a fraction of required calories being delivered to critical care populations across multiple ICUs [12]. Several factors contribute to the suboptimal delivery of nutrition, including gastrointestinal intolerance, elective disruptions for transport, radiographic imaging, surgeries, complications related to delivery system, and lack of efficient protocol support for the timely advancement of enteral feeds to goal due to fear of feed-related morbidity (i.e., high gastric residuals, bloating, vomiting, aspiration, and diarrhea). The deleterious effects of underfeeding on outcomes for hospitalized patients have long been recognized. Hypocaloric feeding and negative energy balances have been linked to prolonged ICU length of stay, prolonged mechanical ventilation, increased risk for infectious complications, and higher mortality [6]. Feeding protocols can help mitigate underfeeding, by providing staff with adjustable rates to achieve a 24 h caloric goal [13]. There is no harm in feeding patients who have controlled airways through a trip to the OR, especially if the feeding tube is post-pyloric. Keeping an intubated patient "nil per os," or EN turned off for operative procedures is an archaic practice and potentially detrimental. During the time period from day 2 to 5, the patient should be improving. The systemic inflammation should be abating, resuscitation end points reached, vasopressor requirement diminishing, and overall the patient is preparing for extubation with the abdomen hopefully closed. During this time, patients should come closer to meeting full protein and calorie goal requirements. Not only should the physician-led team increase the order or delivery of the EN, but the patient will also demonstrate tolerance to this delivery.

Day 5 and Beyond

By hospital day 5 of an open abdomen patient, successful resuscitation is complete. Though the ventilator or vasopressors may still be required, the patient is certainly in a different place than when admitted. There should have been at least numerous attempts to provide enteral nutrition via the potential routes described above. In addition, goal feeds should have been attempted with distal feeds or gastric motility agents if true gastric intolerance is present. The patient is still likely in a systemic inflammatory state and hypermetabolic. With this in mind, attempts to decrease this catabolic state can be attempted with agents such as propranolol. Though no literature describing associations between open abdomens and the use of propranolol exists, burn literature utilizing propranolol to decrease the hypercatabolic state has been noted and may be beneficial in the open abdomen patient [14]. The same can be described for agents such as oxandrolone as an anabolic agent in the open abdomen patient [14].

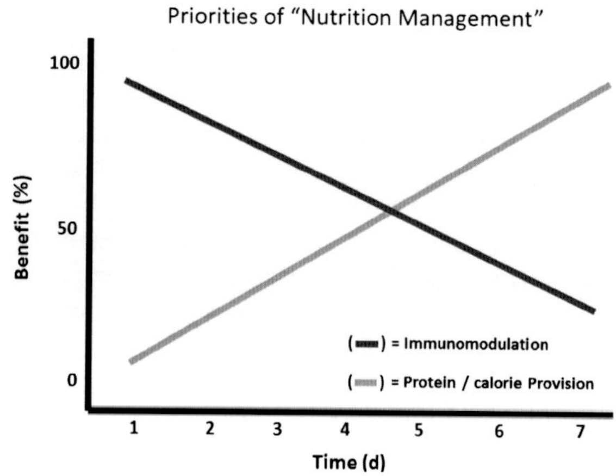

Fig. 5.2 Beyond the first 7 days, the immunomodulatory benefits of early EN have decreased to the point that the protein–calorie deficit is more pressing. This theory, supported in the clinical literature, is the basis of starting parenteral nutrition by post admission days 5–7

As illustrated in Fig. 5.2, at some point protein and calorie provision or deficit becomes a priority. Regardless of the reason, unsuccessful provision of enteral nutrition adds to the severe protein–calorie malnutrition that is associated with the critical illness present in patients with an open abdomen. Therefore, if enteral nutrition is not providing at least 60–70 % of the calories and protein needed by the patient at the day 5–7 mark, parenteral nutrition must be considered. In their landmark prospective randomized study examining early (within 48 h of admission to the ICU) vs late (>7 days after admission to ICU) PN in >4600 critically ill adults (89 % of whom were complex surgical patients), Casaer et al. found that patients in the late PN initiation group had fewer ICU infections, a lower incidence of cholestasis, decreased mechanical ventilation days, reduced duration of renal replacement therapy, a mean reduction in health care costs, and an increased likelihood of being discharged alive earlier from the ICU and from the hospital [15]. To specifically address trauma patients, Sena et al. studied trauma patients and examined the effects of early PN use (within first 7 days post-injury) to address caloric deficit. In those patients receiving early PN and a modest amount of EN during the first week (>1000 kcal/kg), there was an increased risk of nosocomial infection, late acute respiratory distress syndrome (ARDS), duration of mechanical ventilation, ICU length of stay, and mortality compared with those patients receiving EN alone. Supplemental PN to achieve nutrition goals within the first week after injury provided worse outcomes in trauma patients. The high risk for or presence of severe protein–calorie malnutrition related to critical illness is associated with poor outcomes; however, supplemental PN was associated with even worse outcomes [16].

In three other recent studies, early PN either demonstrated no change in outcomes or improvement in quality of post-ICU life, fewer ventilator days, fewer infections and less muscle and fat loss [17–19]. However, methodological issues, timing of PN, and ultimately interpretation of results still has not changed the overall message that a delay of 5+ days of PN in the open abdomen patient who presents well nourished is what is most accepted.

To start parenteral nutrition (PN), central access must be present. Options include internal jugular, subclavian, or peripherally inserted central catheters. The femoral vein location should not be used. The tip of the catheter should be located at the superior vena cava/atrial junction to prevent the hyperosmolar load of PN being caustic to smaller veins, thereby increasing the risk of thrombus. Once access is present, ordering the PN usually is performed through central pharmacy. It is imperative that the surgeon be directly involved in the process of PN ordering and administration. The surgeon will better understand the complexity of the pro-inflammatory open abdomen patient, and therefore the higher than expected protein and calorie needs. As noted previously, it is not uncommon to lose at least 30 g of protein per day just from the fluid that is suctioned off the negative pressure device or dressing that is required with the open abdomen patient [2].

Typically, 2.0 g/kg of dosing patient weight per day of protein should be ordered. If the patient is also undergoing continuous renal replacement therapy (CRRT), 2.5 g/kg/day should be ordered as this therapy will pull off protein as well. Carbohydrates in the form of dextrose should also be ordered but started at less than goal for the patient. Typically, 150–200 g of dextrose is a good starting point for the first 24 h. The key is for the patient not to become hyperglycemic beyond approximately 150 mg/dl. It is not uncommon for the open abdomen patient, especially with necrotizing pancreatitis/pancreatic necrosectomy, to be hyperglycemic and receiving an insulin drip via protocol. The PN should not exacerbate this process; therefore, the glucose should be increased to goal as the glucose levels allow. Lipids are typically held from the PN formula for the first seven or so days of initiating PN. Though the data is quite soft, lipid formulas that are currently available in the United States are soy based, have a higher omega-3 to omega-6 ratio, and have potential to be more pro-inflammatory. Therefore, lipids are held until the second week of PN. The potential deficiency of free fatty acids is so uncommon, and there is no significant harm to the patient withholding the lipids.

Every day of this patient's care should include a plan or an attempt to provide EN, just as every day of ventilator care should include a plan of potential extubation. If PN is needed, the key is providing it safely, as described. In addition, short- and long-term plans should be arranged to transition PN to EN or nutrition per os. The plans could include simply to treat gastroparesis pharmacologically and provide distal feeding access, or to arrange for fistula care and home PN until gastrointestinal reconstruction can be completed. Typically transitions to EN or per os and off of PN should occur when the enteral route reaches 70+ % of the patient's nutritional goals. In addition, transition off of EN can occur when the oral route provides 70+ % of the patient's nutritional goals.

Conclusion

In response to DCS and open abdominal decompression for management of ACS, patients being managed with an open abdomen have become increasingly more common in medical and surgical ICUs. Those patients with an open abdomen commonly represent one of the most critically ill patients in the ICU. These patients have a tremendous inflammatory response, are intensely hypermetabolic, and subsequently are at the highest risk for the development of malnutrition.

Only a handful of studies specifically address nutrition and the open abdomen; however, experience by numerous authors and the few studies dealing with this population have demonstrated safety with administration of enteral feeds. In addition, given the morbidity- and mortality-reducing benefits of EN, provision of appropriate and early goal-directed protein and caloric support should be considered an essential component in the management of the patient with an open abdomen. In fact, patients show benefit to early enteral nutrition (though not necessarily at goal) directly and indirectly related to their open abdomen. PN on the other hand should be held for the first 5–7 days of hospital care in most of these patients with an open abdomen, despite the difficulty of delivering EN. Regardless, patients with an open abdomen must have nutrition addressed daily, to ensure appropriate access and nutrition is available, considered, and adjusted as the need for specialized nutrition (EN and PN) will likely continue for weeks to months after the hospital admission.

Example of Nutrition Protocol Guidelines

Initial Nutrition Evaluation

- Resuscitation goals met?
  - No → Continue resuscitation. Do not start nutrition provision.
  - Yes → Consult nutrition support and start enteral nutrition (EN) (see below, enteral nutrition).

    All patients should have nutrition regimen within 36 h.
    EN is preferred over parenteral nutrition (PN) (see protocols below).

- Protocols
  - GI stress ulcer prophylaxis.
  - Lab protocol.

    Obtain pre-albumin and CRP levels at day 2 if anticipated ICU stay is >3 days.
    Repeat and re-assess every Monday/Thursday.

  - Glucose control <150 mg/dl, avoid hypoglycemia.
  - Wound healing protocol (for open abdomen, burns, large wounds, or fistulas).

Ascorbic acid (Vitamin C) 500 mg BID PO/PT/IV × 10 days.
Vitamin A 10,000 IU, PO/PT/IM × 10 days (Excluded in pregnancy).
Zinc 220 mg PO × 10 days PO or PT −50 mg/10 ml elemental oral solution (Excluded in pregnancy).

– Severe cachexia/malnourishment.

  Consider use of oxandrolone 10 mg po/pt twice daily.

Enteral Nutrition (EN)

- Initiation of EN
  - Start EN at 50 % of goal (~25–30 ml/h) within 24–48 h of admission, or when GI continuity restored.
  - Advance as tolerated to goal by day 5 with improvement of SIRS or critical illness.
  - If not at 60 % of goal after 5–7 days, consider PN supplementation (refer to protocol).
- Withhold EN if hemodynamically unstable, increase in pressors, or lactic acidosis.
- EN Access
  - Placement

    Begin with blind bedside nasogastric feeding tube.
    Consider bedside Cortrak ©, endoscopic, fluoroscopic, or intraoperative placement.
    OGT and NGT placement confirmed by physical exam and X-ray.
    Small-bore feeding tube placement confirmed by X-ray or Cortrak © placement.

  - Gastric access

    Short term: OGT, NGT, small-bore feeding tube.
    Long term (>30 days): PEG (initiate TF 4–6 h post PEG placement).

  - Post-pyloric access

    Short term: Consider blind/endoscopic/fluoroscopic/Cortrak©/intra-operative placement.
    Long term (>30 days): endoscopic placement of PEG/J.
    Indications

    - Gastroparesis with persistent high (500 ml) gastric residual volume (GRV) despite prokinetic agents or recurrent emesis.
    - Severe active pancreatitis (endoscopic placement for jejunal feeds).
    - Open abdomen.

Parenteral Nutrition (PN)

- If previously healthy, initiate PN only after the first 5–7 days of hospitalization if EN is not feasible.
- If severe protein–calorie malnutrition present and EN not feasible, start PN immediately after resuscitation.
- Weaning TPN when:
  - TFs tolerated at 60 % of goal.

    Decrease TPN by discontinuing lipids, decrease dextrose and continuing goal dose of amino acids/protein.
    Wean off TPN as TF rate advances to goal or per clinician judgment.

  - POs tolerated at 60 % of meals consumed.

    Decrease TPN by discontinuing lipids, decrease dextrose and continuing goal dose of amino acids/protein.
    Wean off TPN as TF rate advances to goal or per clinician judgment.

Nutritional Goals

- Dosing weight:
  - Use IBW for height if actual body weight is >IBW.
  - Hamwi method:

    Men:106# (48 kg)1st 5 ft, then add 6# (2.7 kg) per inch >5ft, ±10 %.
    Women: 100# (45 kg)1st 5 ft, then add 5# (2.3 kg) per inch >5ft, ±10 %.

  - Use actual body weight if weight is <IBW
- Caloric goals:
  - 25–35 kcal/kg dosing weight.
  - If BMI >30, use 22–25 kcal/kg IBW.
  - Consider the use of a metabolic cart if accessible every week for re-assessment.
- Protein needs:
  - General: 1.2–2.0 g/kg dosing weight.
  - Obesity

    BMI of 30–40, use >2 g/kg IBW.
    BMI >40, use >2.5 g/kg IBW.

  - Renal failure (HD/CRRT): 1.2–2.5 g/kg dosing weight.
  - Hepatic failure: 1.2–2.0 g/kg dosing weight.

- Fluid needs—1 ml/kcal baseline.
  - Cover additional losses—(i.e., fever, diarrhea, GI output, and tachypnea).
  - Fluid restriction–CHF, renal failure, hepatic failure with ascites, CNS injury, and electrolyte abnormality.

If LOS >7 days and pt has not consistently met near 100 % needs consider nutritional provision from a combination of PO/EN/PN route.

Clinical Scenario

Thirty-eight-year-old male status post pancreatic necrosectomy that was performed for 75 % pancreatic necrosis 2 weeks following initial presentation for severe alcohol associated pancreatitis. He has had two additional reoperations for debridement and hemostasis over the course of 5 days, and currently has an open abdomen.

Author Response: *NUTRITION MANAGEMENT IN AN OPEN ABDOMEN FOLLOWING NECROSECTOMY*: *Early enteral feeds.* Provide EN within 24–36 h of admission to ICU, ideally with nasojejunal feeding and concurrent naso- or orogastric decompression. If nasojejunal feeding is not possible, gastric feeding can safely be attempted. **Some is better than none**. If the patient cannot tolerate tube feeding formula at a rate consistent with caloric goals, feeding formula should be provided at a low rate. **Establish surgical feeding access** as soon as it is safe to do so. A gastrojejunostomy tube is a useful adjunct for mitigating complications in this type of patient. Consider using a **feeding protocol** to avoid underfeeding. By postoperative day 5, if attempts to provide EN have failed, **PN should be considered**. **Combination feeding** with EN and PN should also be considered at the outset if the patient presents in a malnourished state and it is projected that adequate caloric intake with EN will not be achieved by day 5–7.

Key Questions

1. *When do you feed the septic patient?*
2. *What formula should be selected, should we be focused on 24 h targets or hourly goals?*

References

1. Cheatham ML, Safcsak K, Llerena LE, Morrow CE, Jr., Block EF. Long-term physical, mental, and functional consequences of abdominal decompression. J Trauma. 2004;56 (2):237–41; Discussion. 41–2.
2. Cheatham ML, Safcsak K, Brzezinski SJ, Lube MW. Nitrogen balance, protein loss, and the open abdomen. Crit Care Med. 2007;35(1):127–31.

3. Burlew CC. The open abdomen: practical implications for the practicing surgeon. Am J Surg. 2012;204(6):826–35.
4. Burlew CC, Moore EE, Cuschieri J, Jurkovich GJ, Codner P, Nirula R, et al. Who should we feed? Western Trauma Association multi-institutional study of enteral nutrition in the open abdomen after injury. J Trauma Acute Care Surg. 2012;73(6):1380–7; Discussion. 7–8.
5. Todd SR1, Kozar RA, Moore FA. Nutrition support in adult trauma patients. Nutr Clin Pract. 2006 Oct;21(5):421–9.
6. Powell NJ, Collier B. Nutrition and the open abdomen. Nutrition in clinical practice: official publication of the American society for parenteral and enteral nutrition. 2012;27(4):499–506.
7. Marik PE. What is the best way to feed patients with pancreatitis? Curr Opin Crit Care. 2009;15(2):131–8.
8. Alkhawaja S, Martin C, Butler RJ, Gwadry-Sridhar F. Post-pyloric versus gastric tube feeding for preventing pneumonia and improving nutritional outcomes in critically ill adults. Cochrane Database Syst Rev. 2015;8:CD008875.
9. Zakaria el R, Matheson PJ, Flessner MF, Garrison RN. Hemorrhagic shock and resuscitation-mediated tissue water distribution is normalized by adjunctive peritoneal resuscitation. Journal of the American College of Surgeons. 2008;206(5):970–80; Discussion. 80–3.
10. Smith JW, Garrison RN, Matheson PJ, Franklin GA, Harbrecht BG, Richardson JD. Direct peritoneal resuscitation accelerates primary abdominal wall closure after damage control surgery. J Am Coll Surg. 2010;210(5):658–64, 64–7.
11. Smith JW, Neal Garrison R, Matheson PJ, Harbrecht BG, Benns MV, Franklin GA, et al. Adjunctive treatment of abdominal catastrophes and sepsis with direct peritoneal resuscitation: indications for use in acute care surgery. J Trauma Acute Care Surg. 2014;77(3):393–8; Discussion. 8–9.
12. McClave SA, Sexton LK, Spain DA, Adams JL, Owens NA, Sullins MB, et al. Enteral tube feeding in the intensive care unit: factors impeding adequate delivery. Crit Care Med. 1999;27(7):1252–6.
13. Heyland DK, Cahill NE, Dhaliwal R, Sun X, Day AG, McClave SA. Impact of enteral feeding protocols on enteral nutrition delivery: results of a multicenter observational study. JPEN J Parenter Enteral Nutr. 2010;34(6):675–84.
14. Gauglitz GG, Williams FN, Herndon DN, Jeschke MG. Burns: where are we standing with propranolol, oxandrolone, recombinant human growth hormone, and the new incretin analogs? Curr Opin Clin Nutr Metab Care. 2011;14(2):176–81.
15. Casaer MP, Mesotten D, Hermans G, Wouters PJ, Schetz M, Meyfroidt G, et al. Early versus late parenteral nutrition in critically ill adults. N Engl J Med. 2011;365(6):506–17.
16. Sena MJ, Utter GH, Cuschieri J, Maier RV, Tompkins RG, Harbrecht BG, et al. Early supplemental parenteral nutrition is associated with increased infectious complications in critically ill trauma patients. J Am Coll Surg. 2008;207(4):459–67.
17. Doig GS, Simpson F, Sweetman EA, Finfer SR, Cooper DJ, Heighes PT, et al. Early parenteral nutrition in critically ill patients with short-term relative contraindications to early enteral nutrition: a randomized controlled trial. JAMA. 2013;309(20):2130–8.
18. Harvey SE, Parrott F, Harrison DA, Bear DE, Segaran E, Beale R, et al. Trial of the route of early nutritional support in critically ill adults. N Engl J Med. 2014;371(18):1673–84.
19. Heidegger CP, Berger MM, Graf S, Zingg W, Darmon P, Costanza MC, et al. Optimisation of energy provision with supplemental parenteral nutrition in critically ill patients: a randomised controlled clinical trial. Lancet. 2013;381(9864):385–93.

Chapter 6
Intra-abdominal Hypertension and Abdominal Compartment Syndrome in Acute Care Surgery

Michael L. Cheatham and Karen Safcsak

"Abdominal compartment syndrome?" "But this isn't a trauma patient." Herein lies one of the great fallacies of surgery and the cause of many acute care surgery mortalities. IAH and ACS are actually more common and have a higher mortality rate among critically ill medical and general surgical patients than among trauma patients [10]. This is because IAH/ACS are widely recognized as complications of traumatic injury, but not so for other patient populations where the onset of organ dysfunction and failure is less dramatic and more insidious in onset. The acute care surgeon must be aware of this increased risk and be willing to apply the same damage-control principles to the general surgical patient as one would to a gunshot wound victim.

Definitions

Intra-abdominal pressure (IAP) is defined as the steady-state pressure within the abdominal cavity [7]. Most commonly measured as intravesicular or "bladder" pressure, it is expressed in mmHg and measured at end expiration in the supine position after ensuring that abdominal muscle contractions are absent and with the transducer zeroed at the level of the mid-axillary line. Analogous to cerebral perfusion pressure, abdominal perfusion pressure (APP) is calculated as mean arterial pressure minus IAP and has been demonstrated to be a sensitive predictor of IAP-induced malperfusion [5]. Intra-abdominal hypertension (IAH) is defined as a sustained or repeated pathological elevation in IAP ≥12 mmHg. Abdominal com-

M.L. Cheatham (✉) · K. Safcsak
Orlando Health Surgical Group, Orlando Regional Medical Center, Orlando, FL, USA
e-mail: michael.cheatham@orlandohealth.com

K. Safcsak
e-mail: karen.safcsak@orlandohealth.com

J.J. Diaz and D.T. Efron (eds.), *Complications in Acute Care Surgery*,
DOI 10.1007/978-3-319-42376-0_6

partment syndrome (ACS) is defined as a sustained IAP >20 mmHg (with or without an APP <60 mmHg) that is associated with new organ dysfunction or failure.

Primary IAH/ACS is a condition associated with injury or disease in the abdominopelvic region that requires surgical or angiographic intervention (damage-control laparotomy, bleeding pelvic fractures, massive retroperitoneal hematomas, failed non-operative management) or after elective abdominal surgery (secondary peritonitis, liver transplantation). This is the classic and well-known variant of ACS that is commonly dramatic and acute in onset. Secondary IAH/ACS represents the sequelae of shock resuscitation and interstitial edema formation. It typically develops due to conditions outside the abdomen (sepsis, capillary leak, major burns, or other conditions requiring increased fluid resuscitation). This under-recognized and arguably more common variant is typically gradual and insidious in its onset, occurring over the first day or two following emergent laparotomies. Recurrent IAH/ACS is a "second-hit" phenomenon after initial recovery from either primary or secondary ACS. The prevalence of IAH among critically ill surgical patients varies between 31 and 59 % with the incidence increasing with the length of ICU stay. Refractory ACS is present when the patient's organ dysfunction/failure continues to worsen despite interventions to reduce IAP, improve APP, and restore both systemic and regional perfusion and oxygenation.

Pathophysiology

IAP is determined by 3 factors: (1) abdominal organ volume, (2) the presence of space-occupying substances (such as blood, ascites, other fluid, air, or tumor), and (3) abdominal wall compliance. The normal adult IAP is less than 5 mmHg, but IAP in the post-laparotomy patient is typically 10–15 mmHg. In the critically ill patient with systemic hypoperfusion and shock, an IAP of 15–20 mmHg is common. Contrary to popular belief, IAP does not become zero once a patient's abdomen is open; IAH and ACS both may occur despite the presence of an open abdomen and temporary abdominal closure.

IAP, however, is only part of the equation. As a result of patient variability, there is no single threshold IAP value that can be globally applied to the decision making of all patients. IAP alone lacks sufficient sensitivity and specificity at the clinically appropriate thresholds of 10–25 mmHg to be useful as a resuscitation endpoint. APP assesses not only the severity of IAP, but also the adequacy of the patient's systemic and visceral perfusion. APP has been demonstrated to be superior to both IAP and global resuscitation endpoints, such as arterial pH, base deficit, and arterial lactate, in its ability to predict patient outcome. It represents an easily calculated parameter for guiding the resuscitation and management of the patient with IAH/ACS, having been demonstrated to exceed the clinical prediction of IAP alone in several clinical trials [5].

Clinical examination of IAP through abdominal palpation has a sensitivity of less than 50 % for determining the presence of elevated IAP. Therefore, if IAH is suspected to be present, IAP must be measured. Failure to identify IAH and/or ACS when present is associated with the reported mortality rates of up to 100 %. When recognized and appropriately treated, mortality is still 30–40 % in the best of centers. Serial determinations of IAP have been shown to reliably detect the development of IAH and facilitate early treatment of ACS, with significant reductions in patient morbidity and mortality. This is especially true in the patient with an open abdomen where IAP and APP become essential resuscitative parameters. Regrettably, studies demonstrate that many surgeons are reluctant to measure IAP in their patients at risk.

A morbidly obese patient with elevated IAP can present a difficult diagnostic situation. They are well-known to have elevated baseline IAP levels. As a result, the normal diagnostic IAP thresholds may not be clinically applicable in obese patients. There is currently insufficient evidence to identify different IAP thresholds for the bariatric population. The use of APP as a resuscitation endpoint, however, takes into account the potential baseline elevation in IAP and will ensure that visceral perfusion is adequate regardless of the patient's baseline IAP level.

Elevated IAP causes significant impairment of cardiac, pulmonary, renal, gastrointestinal, hepatic, central nervous system, and abdominal wall perfusion and function, with each organ demonstrating its own unique vulnerability. This differential response to IAP, coupled with the augmented susceptibility seen in the presence of hypovolemia and comorbid disease, further complicates the management of these complex patients. The detrimental effects of IAP on each of these organ systems are described in Table 6.1. The possibility of IAH should be considered in any patient who presents with one or more of the following: prolonged shock (acidosis, hypothermia, hemorrhage, coagulopathy), visceral ischemia/perforation, traumatic injury, sepsis, massive fluid resuscitation (>5 L in 24 h), ruptured abdominal aneurysm, retroperitoneal hemorrhage, abdominal neoplasm, liver dysfunction/ascites, pancreatitis, burns, or ileus/gastroparesis.

Finally, the severity of IAP is less important than the duration of IAH [8]. Prolonged elevations in IAP result in organ dysfunction and failure that can have a significant impact upon the patient morbidity and mortality. Every effort should be made to reduce the period of time that a patient's IAP exceeds 15 mmHg. The duration of IAH correlates significantly with the increased ICU and hospital length of stay, duration of mechanical ventilation, enteral nutrition intolerance, and mortality. For these reasons, primary fascial closure in the presence of marked visceral edema or abdominal contamination is rarely appropriate and only leads to the need for emergent abdominal decompression, prolonged critical illness, organ dysfunction, and increased healthcare costs.

Table 6.1 Pathophysiological implications of IAH/ACS

Organ system	Pathophysiologic effects	Clinical manifestations	Threshold IAP (mmHg)
Cardiovascular	Decreased preload/venous return Increased afterload Compression of inferior vena cava	Decreased cardiac output Increased susceptibility to hypovolemia	10
Pulmonary	Increased intrathoracic pressure Cephalad elevation of diaphragm Extrinsic compression of pulmonary parenchyma Alveolar atelectasis Increased airway resistance	Hypoxemia Hypercarbia Elevated airway pressures Increased intrapulmonary shunt Increased alveolar dead space	15
Renal	Decreased renal blood flow Renal vein compression Renal parenchymal compression	Oliguria Anuria Acute renal failure	15
Gastrointestinal	Decreased mesenteric blood flow Intestinal ischemia Bacterial translocation/sepsis	Increased susceptibility to hypovolemia Increased visceral edema/capillary leak Metabolic acidosis	10
Hepatic	Decreased hepatic vein blood flow Decreased portal vein blood flow	Hepatic dysfunction/failure Metabolic acidosis	10
Central nervous system	Increased intrathoracic pressure Decreased cerebral venous outflow	Increased intracranial pressure Decreased cerebral perfusion pressure	15
Abdominal wall	Decreased abdominal wall compliance Decreased rectus sheath blood flow	Fascial dehiscence	10

IAP intra-abdominal pressure, *IAH* intra-abdominal hypertension, *ACS* abdominal compartment syndrome

Prevention of IAH/ACS

When faced with a patient demonstrating risk factors for IAH/ACS, such as intestinal ischemia or abdominal sepsis, the acute care surgeon must decide intra-operatively whether to correct the patient's pathology through either a single, initial procedure or a staged approach. This decision is based upon the answers to three questions:

1. Is the patient too ill to tolerate a single procedure/definitive repair?
2. Can the patient tolerate the postoperative IAH that will accompany primary fascial closure without developing ACS?
3. Can the source of contamination be safely controlled using a single procedure?

The well-known principles of damage control, as applied to the traumatically injured, are directly applicable to the acute care surgery patient as well. As a result of delayed presentation, under-resuscitation, advanced organ dysfunction/failure, and pre-existing medical comorbidities, some patients are better served by a staged laparotomy approach with the maintenance of an "open abdomen" and temporary abdominal closure until their physiology has improved, and they can tolerate definitive repair. A "single-procedure" approach, in the presence of critical illness, is rarely the correct answer and frequently results in increased morbidity and mortality. The methods for performing such a staged approach are described below.

All patients with intestinal ischemia are at risk for postoperative IAH. Inappropriate primary fascial closure of those patients at significant risk will increase IAP through the mechanisms described in Table 6.1 and result in worsening end-organ dysfunction and failure. This commonly results in a vicious cycle of visceral edema, intestinal malperfusion, and increasing IAP that ultimately culminates in the development of ACS and need for emergent decompressive laparotomy. The keys to avoiding this runaway cascade of progressive shock and organ failure are appropriate end-organ resuscitation (described below) and staged laparotomy in patients at significant risk.

Abdominal sepsis and contamination are significant risk factors for visceral edema and subsequent IAH/ACS. Abdominal contamination initiates a pro-inflammatory cytokine cascade that promotes further visceral edema and elevated IAP. While early primary fascial closure places the patient at risk for IAH/ACS, staged laparotomy and evacuation of cytokine-rich fluid from the abdominal cavity through a temporary abdominal closure help to modulate and downgrade the pro-inflammatory response, improving organ dysfunction and patient survival (Fig. 6.1).

Management of IAH/ACS

While surgical decompression is widely and erroneously considered the only treatment for IAH/ACS, non-operative medical management strategies play a vital role in both the prevention and treatment of IAP-induced organ dysfunction and failure (Fig. 6.2) [7]. Appropriate management of IAH/ACS is based upon four general principles:

1. Serial monitoring of IAP
2. Optimization of systemic perfusion and end-organ function

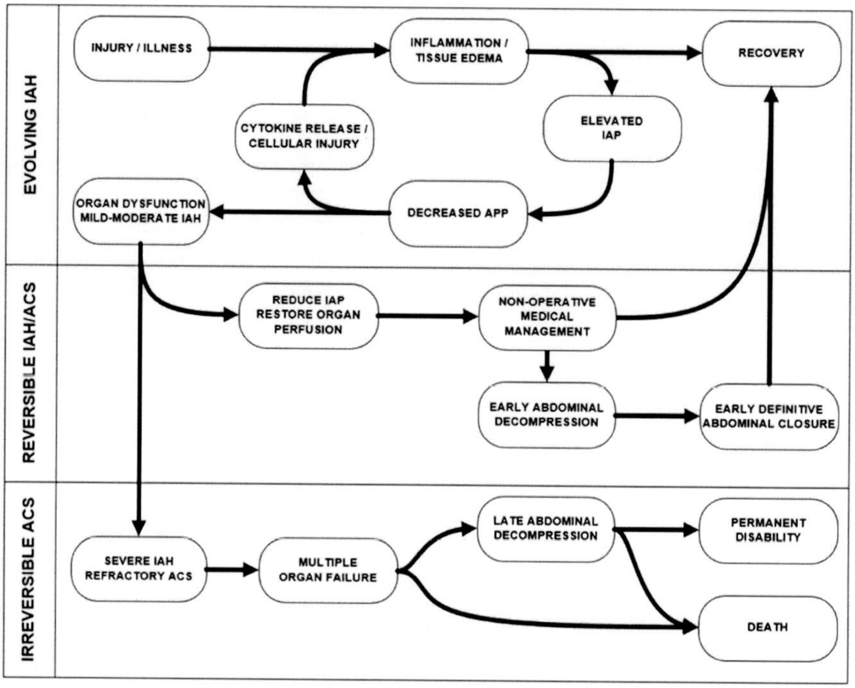

Fig. 6.1 The evolution of IAH/ACS: *IAP* intra-abdominal pressure; *APP* abdominal compartment syndrome; *IAH* intra-abdominal hypertension; *ACS* abdominal compartment syndrome

3. Institution of specific medical interventions to reduce IAP and the end-organ consequences of IAH/ACS
4. Prompt surgical decompression for refractory IAH/ACS.

Sedation and Analgesia

Pain, agitation, ventilator dyssynchrony, and use of accessory muscles during work of breathing may all lead to increased thoracoabdominal muscle tone and decreased abdominal wall compliance, resulting in elevated IAP. Appropriate patient sedation and analgesia can reduce muscle tone and potentially decrease IAP to less detrimental levels. In addition to ensuring patient comfort, adequate sedation and analgesia thus appear to play a useful therapeutic role in the patient with IAH. The goal should be to reduce IAP to less detrimental levels and raise APP above 60 mmHg to ensure adequate systemic perfusion. In patients with the significant elevations in IAP, sedation and analgesia to a level of general anesthesia may be necessary to overcome the increased abdominal wall tone.

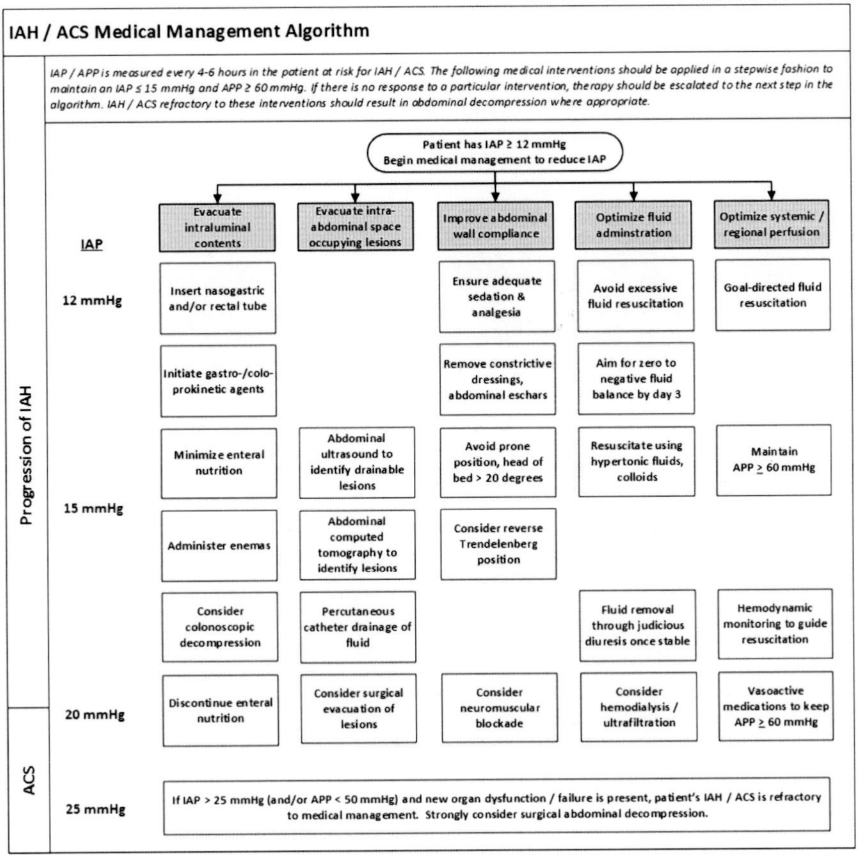

Fig. 6.2 Medical management of IAH/ACS: *IAP* intra-abdominal pressure; *APP* abdominal compartment syndrome; *IAH* intra-abdominal hypertension; *ACS* abdominal compartment syndrome

Nasogastric/Colonic Decompression, Prokinetic Motility Agents

Gastrointestinal ileus is common among patients who have had abdominal surgery, peritonitis, major trauma, significant fluid resuscitation, or electrolyte abnormalities, many of which are independent risk factors for IAH/ACS. Excessive air and fluid within the hollow viscera, as a space-occupying structure, can raise IAP and lead to organ dysfunction and failure. Nasogastric and/or rectal drainage, enemas, and even endoscopic decompression are relatively non-invasive methods for reducing IAP and treating mild-to-moderate IAH in patients with visceral distention. The administration of prokinetic motility agents such as erythromycin, metoclopromide, or neostigmine is also of use in evacuating the intraluminal contents and decreasing visceral volume. All patients with elevated IAP should undergo nasogastric decompression (with colonic decompression if clinically indicated). This simple maneuver, in our experience, can frequently reduce IAP, raise APP, and decrease the need for more aggressive interventions.

Fluid Resuscitation

Hypovolemia aggravates the pathophysiologic effects of elevated IAP, while hypervolemia (i.e., excessive volume resuscitation) is an independent predictor for the subsequent development of ACS. The fluid status of patients at risk for IAH/ACS should be carefully monitored to avoid over-resuscitation. Careful monitoring and maintenance of urinary output at no more than 0.5 mL/kg/h are appropriate. Avoidance of high-rate maintenance fluid infusions is essential as this tends to result in excessive fluid administration over time. When necessary, frequent, small volume as opposed to large-volume crystalloid boluses should be utilized to avoid over-resuscitation. Hypertonic crystalloid and colloid-based resuscitation have been demonstrated to reduce IAP and decrease the risk of subsequent secondary ACS. In critically ill patients, invasive hemodynamic monitoring using volumetric pulmonary artery catheters, arterial pulse contour analysis, or esophageal Doppler technologies may be necessary to assess intravascular volume status. Traditional pressure-based parameters such as pulmonary artery occlusion pressure and central venous pressure are inaccurate in the presence of elevated IAP and intrathoracic pressure and may lead to erroneous clinical decisions regarding fluid status.

Diuretics and Continuous Venovenous Hemofiltration/Ultrafiltration

Early intermittent hemodialysis or continuous hemofiltration/ultrafiltration may be more appropriate than continuing to volume load and increase the likelihood of secondary ACS with its attendant morbidity and mortality. Diuretic therapy, in combination with colloid, may also be considered to mobilize third-space edema once the patient is hemodynamically stable. These therapies must be utilized with caution, however, as they tend to decrease APP and may worsen the patient's systemic perfusion if not carefully monitored.

Neuromuscular Blockade (NMB)

Diminished abdominal wall compliance due to pain, tight abdominal closures, and third-space fluid can increase IAP to potentially detrimental levels. NMB has been reported anecdotally to be an effective method for reducing IAP in early IAH.

A brief trial of NMB for 24–48 h can be useful, in conjunction with other interventions, to reduce IAP and allow resolution of the patient's IAH, thus avoiding the need for decompressive laparotomy. NMB is not efficacious in the presence of advanced IAH or ACS, where delays in decompression will only serve to worsen the patient's end-organ failure. The potential benefits of NMB therapy must be balanced against the risks of prolonged paralysis.

Percutaneous Decompression

Percutaneous catheter drainage of free intra-abdominal fluid, air, abscess, or blood is an effective technique for reducing IAP and potentially correcting IAH-induced organ dysfunction. Performed under ultrasound or computed tomography guidance, percutaneous decompression can significantly reduce IAP and decrease the need for and morbidity of surgical decompression. This minimally invasive approach to IAH/ACS management is most effective in patients with secondary ACS due to excessive resuscitation, burns, acute pancreatitis, or ascites. Patients with IAH/ACS refractory to percutaneous catheter decompression should undergo urgent abdominal decompression.

Abdominal Decompression

Surgical decompression of the abdomen has long been the standard treatment for IAH/ACS [3, 6, 7]. It can be life saving when a patient's organ dysfunction and/or failure are refractory to the medical treatment. Delayed abdominal decompression and disregard of high IAP levels are associated with the significant increases in patient mortality [8]. "Prophylactic" decompression and creation of a "temporary abdominal closure" in patients at risk significantly reduce the subsequent development of IAH/ACS and improve survival. "Emergent" decompression, once ACS is present, may be performed either in the operating room or at the patient's bedside if cardiopulmonary instability precludes safe transport. While seemingly aggressive and potentially disabling, patients at risk for IAH/ACS who are treated with abdominal decompression demonstrate identical long-term physical and mental health function as well as resumption of gainful employment compared to similar patients who do not require an open abdomen. This potentially life-saving technique, therefore, should not be withheld from a patient who is demonstrating signs of ACS.

A variety of different methods ["vacuum pack closure," "Bogota bag" or silo, Velcro™ burr, absorbable mesh, and vacuum-assisted closure (VAC)] have been described for managing the "open abdomen." No one technique demonstrates superiority in all clinical situations, and the acute care surgeon must be familiar with the relative merits of each method. Increasing evidence suggests that active removal of cytokine-rich, pro-inflammatory peritoneal fluid using negative pressure wound therapy significantly improves renal and pulmonary dysfunction, facilitates primary fascial closure, and decreases patient mortality when compared with temporary abdominal closure techniques that allow such fluid to remain in the abdomen [1]. It is essential to recognize that recurrent ACS is possible with any technique, especially if applied in a fashion that does not allow continued visceral expansion during resuscitation. If recurrent ACS develops, the dressing should be immediately removed and reapplied so as to reduce IAP to an acceptable level.

Definitive Abdominal Closure

Following surgical decompression and resolution of the patient's ACS, the next therapeutic goal should be definitive closure of the patient's abdomen [2]. Most patients, if decompressed early prior to the development of significant organ failure, will tolerate primary fascial closure within five to seven days. Many centers that utilize the evidence-based medicine approach described herein report primary fascial closure rates of 80–90 % among patients who require abdominal decompression for IAH/ACS. Those patients who remain critically ill past this time period, with the significant loss of abdominal domain, will likely require either split-thickness skin grafting of the exposed viscera, with the subsequent fascial closure nine to twelve months later, or cutaneous advancement flap ("skin-only") closure, which allows definitive fascial closure after only three to six months. The acute care surgeon is frequently faced with the difficult decision of which closure to pursue. After considering the patient's age, severity of illness, and pre-existing comorbidities, it is frequently more prudent, life saving, and cost effective to perform a skin-only closure and proceed to rehabilitation rather than spending several weeks attempting to achieve primary fascial closure at the cost of organ failure and a prolonged hospital stay.

Based on state-of-the-art practices, a management algorithm for the patient with elevated IAP can be proposed (Fig. 6.3). First, serial IAP measurements are performed due to the significant incidence of IAH in the high-risk patient and its significant associated morbidity and mortality. Second, immediate abdominal decompression is performed in any patient who demonstrates evidence of ACS. This procedure is appropriate given that early decompression dramatically improves survival, the abdomen can generally be closed within the first week, and long-term outcome studies demonstrate no significant residual physical or mental health deficits. Third, in the patient with IAH, APP is maintained above 60 mmHg through a combination of volume resuscitation (based on volumetric resuscitation endpoints) and vasoactive medications as necessary. Fourth, inability to maintain an APP of at least 60 mmHg is an indication for decompressive laparotomy and maintenance of an open abdomen, using a temporary abdominal closure until the patient's clinical status improves. Post-decompression monitoring of IAP continues as, contrary to popular belief, IAH and ACS can recur despite an open abdomen.

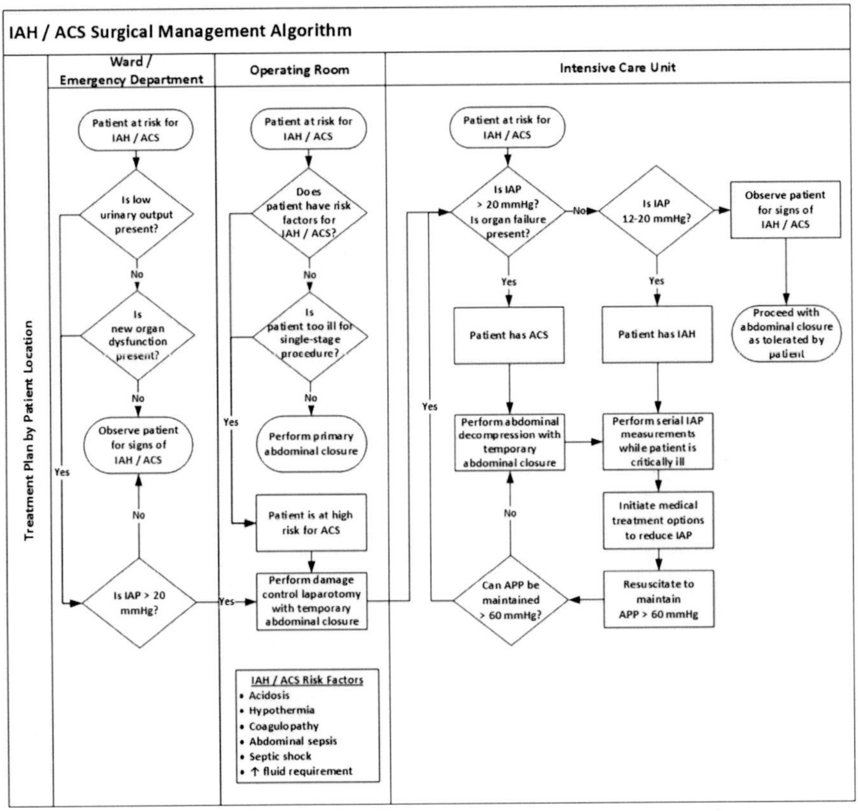

Fig. 6.3 Surgical management of IAH/ACS: *IAP* intra-abdominal pressure; *APP* abdominal compartment syndrome; *IAH* intra-abdominal hypertension; *ACS* abdominal compartment syndrome

Inability to maintain an adequate APP is an indication to decompress the abdomen further through either a larger laparotomy or a placement of a more compliant temporary abdominal closure. Fifth, attempts to close the patient's abdomen after decompression are guided by the patient's IAP and APP. APP can be used as a guide to determine when to perform a decompressive laparotomy as well as when and how to perform abdominal closure. While the same-admission primary fascial closure should always be the goal following decompressive laparotomy, persistent elevations in IAP with marginal APP calculations should lead to a surgical decision for either split-thickness skin grafting of the exposed viscera or skin-only closure, as opposed to attempts to tightly close the abdominal wall. Inappropriate fascial closure commonly results in recurrent ACS, decreased visceral perfusion, and a high mortality rate.

Clinical Scenario

A 45-year-old man undergoes emergent resection of a strangulated small bowel volvulus and primary repair of a complex ventral hernia. His intra-operative course is significant for an increasing fluid requirement and progressive metabolic acidosis. Postoperatively, he demonstrates abdominal distention, oliguria, ongoing acidosis and requires large-volume fluid resuscitation for persistent hypotension.

Unfortunately, this scenario is encountered all too often in acute care surgery. A patient presents, frequently in delayed fashion, with ischemic intestine as a result of a strangulated hernia, intestinal adhesions, or volvulus. The segment of malperfused or necrotic intestine initiates a pro-inflammatory cytokine cascade and the beginnings of abdominal sepsis. Bacterial translocation, progressive visceral edema, and systemic organ dysfunction occur placing the patient at a significant risk for septic shock, multi-system organ failure, and death if their IAH and ACS are not promptly recognized and appropriately treated.

Emergent laparotomy with resection of the ischemic small intestine is clearly indicated, and a segmental resection of the involved ischemic viscera is performed. Intra-operatively, the patient demonstrates an increased fluid requirement and an evidence of metabolic acidosis. These are both significant risk factors for IAH/ACS [7, 9, 10]. *The surgeon's next decision is arguably the most important of the patient's life.* Should the patient undergo a single procedure with primary fascial closure *OR* should the patient undergo a staged laparotomy with definitive abdominal closure once their critical illness has resolved?

In this scenario, the acute care surgeon elects to perform primary repair of the patient's ventral hernia despite the presence of significant risk factors for IAH/ACS. Not surprisingly, the patient develops ACS, organ failure, and severe shock requiring ongoing resuscitation rather than the desired uneventful postoperative recovery. Abundant clinical trials and experience suggest that this patient will develop progressive organ dysfunction and failure as a result of the surgeon's misguided decision, ultimately requiring emergent abdominal decompression, a prolonged intensive care unit (ICU), and hospital length of stay, a protracted course of mechanical ventilation, and exhibiting a mortality of 30–40 % [3, 4, 7, 9]. The decisions made during the patient's initial operative procedure thus have a significant impact upon the patient's subsequent hospital course and chances for survival.

Key Question

1. *In the bariatric patient do you have a different set of numbers for intra-abdominal hypertension/abdominal compartment syndrome?*

References

1. Cheatham ML, Demetriades D, Fabian TC, et al. Prospective study examining clinical outcomes associated with a negative pressure wound therapy system and Barker's vacuum packing technique. World J Surg. 2013;37:2018–30.
2. Cheatham ML, Safcsak K, Llerena LE, et al. Long-term physical, mental, and functional consequences of abdominal decompression. J Trauma. 2004;56:237–42.
3. Cheatham ML, Safcsak K. Is the evolving management of IAH/ACS improving survival? Crit Care Med. 2010;38(2):402–7.
4. Cheatham ML, Safcsak K. Longterm impact of abdominal decompression: a prospective comparative analysis. J Am Coll Surg. 2008;207:573–9.
5. Cheatham ML, White MW, Sagraves SG, et al. Abdominal perfusion pressure: a superior parameter in the assessment of intra-abdominal hypertension. J Trauma. 2000;49:621–7.
6. Coccolini F, Biffl W, Catena F, Ceresoli M, Chiara O, et al. The open abdomen, indications, management, and definitive closure. World J Emerg Surg. 2015;10:32.
7. Kirkpatrick AW, Roberts DJ, De Waele J, et al. Pediatric guidelines sub-committee for the World Society of the Abdominal Compartment Syndrome. intra-abdominal hypertension and the abdominal compartment syndrome: updated consensus definitions and clinical practice guidelines from the World Society of the Abdominal Compartment Syndrome. Intensive Care Med. 2013;39:1190–206.
8. Kyoung K, Hong S. The duration of intra-abdominal hypertension strongly predicts outcomes for the critically ill surgical patient: a prospective observational study. World J Emerg Surg. 2015;10:22.
9. Madigan MC, Kemp CD, Johnson JC, Cotton BA. Secondary abdominal compartment syndrome after severe extremity injury: are early, aggressive fluid resuscitation strategies to blame? J Trauma. 2008;64:280–5.
10. Malbrain ML, Chiumello D, Pelosi P, et al. Incidence and prognosis of intraabdominal hypertension in a mixed population of critically ill patients: a multiple-center epidemiological study. Crit Care Med. 2005;33:315–22.

Chapter 7
Empyema in the Acute Care Surgical Patient

Hunter B. Moore and Ernest E. Moore

Introduction

One of the most common indications for patient admission to the intensive care unit is respiratory failure. Endotracheal intubation is a major risk factor for developing pneumonia, and if inadequately treated can lead to progression to pleural space infection. Ventilator-associated pneumonias are more commonly due to multi-drug-resistant organisms [1]. This coincides with an increase incidence parapneumonic infections [2]. This has clinical significance, as infection of the pleural space is associated with a mortality rate that exceeds myocardial infarction [3]. These infections can develop in the absence of mechanical ventilation, most frequently from community-acquired pneumonia (CAP). The mortality rate of CAP triples in the presence of a parapneumonic process (5–15 %) and can reach over 25 % if it becomes a bilateral process [4]. Thus, prompt recognition and treatment of pleural space infections is essential for reducing morbidity and mortality. The disease can progress rapidly from a simple fluid collection amenable to pleural space drainage, to necrotizing empyema requiring thoracotomy, decortication, and open drainage. The keys to management of parapneumonic effusions are early diagnosis, appropriate therapeutic intervention, and recognition of failure of conservative management.

H.B. Moore (✉)
Department of Surgery, University of Colorado, 12631 E 17th Ave C302, Aurora, CO 80045, USA
e-mail: hunter.moore@ucdenver.edu

E.E. Moore
Department of Surgery, University of Colorado Denver, Suite 365, 655 Broadway, Denver, CO 80203, USA
e-mail: ernest.moore@dhha.org

J.J. Diaz and D.T. Efron (eds.), *Complications in Acute Care Surgery*,
DOI 10.1007/978-3-319-42376-0_7

Physiology of Pleural Space Fluid Shifts

Appreciation of the pleural space physiology helps conceptually understand the progression of pleural space disease. This is an active region of fluid exchange due to the leaky pleural membrane and negative pressure of the pleural space [5]. The fluid originates predominantly from the parietal capillaries because of hydrostatic pressure, augmented by the negative pressure of the pleural space. Less fluid is produced by the visceral pleura because the hydrostatic pressure is attenuated by pulmonary venous drainage. However, the visceral surface will add more pleural fluid with increased pulmonary interstitial pressure. A small volume of fluid is normal in the pleural space, but healthy individuals should have less than 4 mm of dependent pleural fluid on decubitus ultrasound [6].

Clearance of fluid from the pleural space is accomplished by lymphatic drainage. The visceral mesothelium of the pleural space is intricately connected to the lung parenchyma, whereas the parietal layer is more loosely connected to the thoracic structures separated by a variable fatty layer. The parietal pleura has specialized areas known as stoma, and an extensive lymphatic network exists underneath which is the predominant route of fluid resorption located at the dependent portion of the chest cavity [7]. Under normal conditions, it is estimated that each pleural cavity generates 0.2–0.4 mL/kg/h. The capacity for pleural fluid absorption is thought to exceed 500 mL of fluid from each cavity with an intact lymphatic system. Overall, the accumulation of pleural fluid is the result of a dynamic system of fluid production and absorption. Pathology of the pleural space tends to shift extra fluid into the region from increased oncotic drive due to increased particulate matter, increased permeability of the pleural membrane and decreased lymphatic clearance.

Evolution of Pleural Space Infection to Empyema

Complicated parapneumonic effusions, and ultimately empyema, develop in three conceptual phases [8, 9]. The early phase is a sterile effusion caused by parenchymal inflammation that activates mesothelial cells and enhances capillary permeability, termed exudative (days 2–5). This is thought to be driven by proinflammatory cytokines, including interleukin 8 and tumor necrosis factor-[alpha] [9]. Ultimately, the volume of fluid traversing into the pleural cavity exceeds the capacity to reabsorb the fluid and an effusion develops. The second phase is termed fibropurulent, which is initiated by bacterial infection (days 5–10). At this point, the immune system is activated and the once hypocoagulable environment is changed dramatically to hypercoagulable.

Bacterial and neutrophil activity acidify the fluid, consume glucose, increase protein content, and release lactate dehydrogenase (LDH) from cellular apoptosis and necrosis. The environment now becomes hypercoagulable because of the integrated responses of the innate immune and coagulation systems [10, 11]. These findings are directly relevant to the evolution of complicated effusions because the exuberant fibrin deposition is a concerted effort to control progressive infection. The final state of a complicated effusion is referred to as the organization phase (days 10–21). Fibroblasts migrate into the pleural space and create a dense fibrotic lining of the visceral and parietal surfaces. This phase is thought to be driven by regenerative cytokines, for example, transforming growth factor-[beta] and platelet-derived growth factor released primarily from activated mesothelial cells [12]. The net result is a progressive rind that encases the lung, reducing ventilatory capacity and sequestering bacteria.

Risk Factors and Bacteriology of Pleural Space Infection

There are over a million patients hospitalized for pneumonia a year, and 10 % of these patients will develop a pleural space infection [13]. Patients who present to the hospital with pneumonia have an increased risk for pleural space infection if they have a history of IV drug use and alcohol abuse [14], age less than 60 [15], and male gender [16]. Nosocomial pneumonia have a higher rate of pleural space infection and can require operative intervention in up to a third of patients [17]. The incidence of pleural infection in trauma patients with thoracic injuries is 3 % [18]. Risk factors for developing a post-traumatic empyema include multiple rib fractures, thoracostomy tube placed in the emergency department, and underlying pulmonary contusion. Another risk factor is tube placement by a non-surgical specialty. For example, it has been reported that 40 % of chest tubes placed by an emergency medicine resident are associated with a complication [19]. This has clinical significance as a retained post-traumatic hemothorax has the highest risk for empyema, with an infection rate of over 25 % [20].

A Gram stain and culture of the pleural fluid are often beneficial in directing management in pleural space infection, although 20–40 % of the time, there is no reported identifiable pathogen [15, 21, 22]. However, the patient's history is often helpful when directing empiric antibiotics while waiting for Gram stain and pleural cultures to finalize. In empyema associated with community-acquired pneumonia, the most common pathogen is *Streptococcus milleri* (32 %), whereas if hospital acquired, it is methicillin-resistant *Staphylococcus aureus* (28 %). Patient characteristics, including diabetes, alcoholism, age older than 60 years, and trauma, are associated with more anaerobic and resistant Gram-positive organisms [23]. Hospital-acquired empyema is reported to have a fourfold greater risk of death compared with community acquired [15]. *S. milleri is* also a common pathogen in patients who have undergone surgical intervention of the chest or upper digestive tract and often requires decortication [24]. Because of the differences in bacteriology of pleural space infections, an adequate history of patients with parapneumonic processes (community- vs. hospital-acquired pneumonia, vs. chest space intervention) is important for guiding early antibiotics [25]. Of note, although most antibiotics penetrate the pleura well, aminoglycosides may be inactivated at a lower pH [26].

Diagnosis of Pleural Space Infection

Radiographic identification of an effusion in a patient with a systemic inflammatory response syndrome (SIRS) does not necessarily correlate with a pleural space infection. Only 1 in 4 patients with an effusion associated with a CAP ultimately requires drainage of the pleural space [4]. The next step in management of an effusion is quantifying the volume of fluid. The standard method to estimate the amount of pleural fluid has been the lateral decubitus chest X-ray [27]. Recent comparative studies indicate that ultrasound is a more reliable method to quantitate a pleural effusion [27–29]. As previously mentioned, an effusion measured up to 4 mm is considered normal [6]. Earlier clinical studies by Light et al. [13] indicated that infections involving an effusion of less than 10 mm will resolve with antibiotics alone, and this has been supported by subsequent series [30, 31]. Therefore, patients with large effusions on upright films or CT images should proceed to drainage of the pleural space with a chest tube. Patient with smaller effusions should have a bedside estimate of the volume of fluid in their chest with ultrasound, and those with fluid levels greater than 10 mm in height should also have their pleural space tapped for evaluation of an infectious process.

If the decision is made to perform a thoracentesis of the pleural space, the fluid removed should undergo evaluation for an active infection. Gross purulence (empyema) at the time of thoracentesis is unusual but constitutes an indication for prompt video-assisted thoracoscopic surgery (VATS) decortication [8]. In all other circumstances, the pleural fluid should be submitted for laboratory analysis. The traditional technique to distinction an exudative versus transudative effusion is via Light's criteria: protein greater than 0.5 serum, LDH greater than 0.6 serum, or LDH greater than two-thirds normal serum [32]. However, the most cost-effective means to analyze this is to measure the pH of the pleural fluid using a standard blood gas analyzer, available in most intensive care units. A pH less than 7.2 is the threshold, although less than 7.3 is considered high risk [3, 33, 34]. An exception is a *Proteus* infection where the pH may exceed 7.4 because of ammonia production [9]. An alternative diagnostic criterion for infection is a pleural fluid glucose less than 60 mg/dL [9]. Because the evolution of an empyema may extend for days to weeks and the early phase is a sterile effusion, a repeat diagnostic thoracentesis should be done in any patient with a persistent unilateral pleural effusion and unexplained SIRS [8].

Early Management of Pleural Space Infection (Fig. 7.1)

Patients with fluid concerning for pleural infection require empiric antibiotic treatment to cover suspected pathogens in addition to tube thoracostomy drainage. The exception is patients with gross purulence aspirated from the pleural space that should under go prompt operative decortication. The optimal size of the chest tube

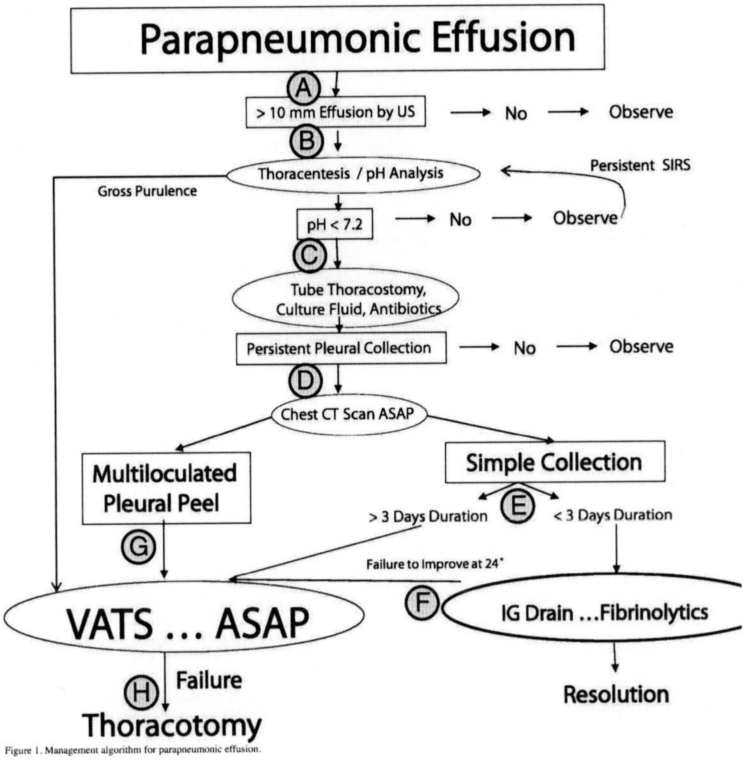

Fig. 7.1 A management algorithm for parapneumonic effusion. Reproduced with permission from Moore et al. [63, Fig. 1], with permission courtesy of Wolters Kluwer Health, Inc

remains debated [35, 36], but a guide wire inserted 18F seems effective in removing this hypercoagulable fluid. These smaller chest tubes are associated with less chest wall pain than blunt dissection-inserted tubes, without compromise in clinical outcome. The position of the chest tube, however, is important [36]. The tube should be placed in the posterior (dependent) pleural space and not within a pulmonary fissure. We have observed that the typical "trauma" chest tube introduced through the fifth intercostal space (ICS), at the mid-axillary line, favors fissure placement. Consequently, we recommend ultrasonography-guided tube insertion via the sixth intercostal space. A Gram stain and culture of the pleural fluid should be obtained at the time of tube thoracostomy to identify the offending organism, although as previously mentioned up to 40 % if the time no pathogen may be found. Most recent techniques such as countercurrent electrophoresis, latex agglutination, or bacterial DNA detection by polymerase chain reaction could improve pathogen identification, but are often not part of standard of care in the clinical setting [3].

After tube placement, vigilant follow-up of chest tube output and changes in radiographic appearance are critical. Pleural collections persisting for more than

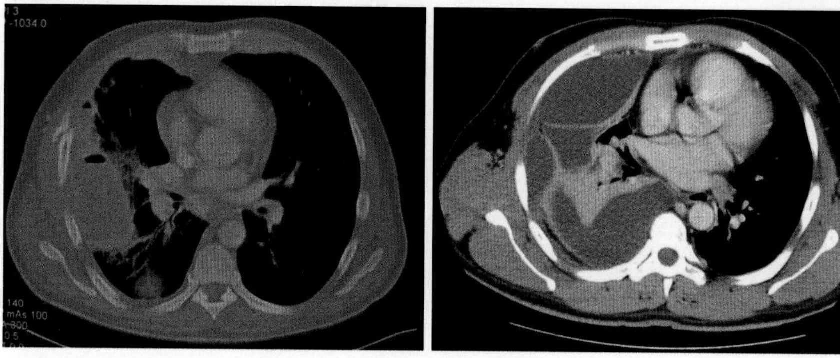

Fig. 7.2 CT imaging distinguishes a simple pleural collection (*left*) that may respond to fibrinolytic therapy versus a complex pleural collection that warrants prompt VATS. Reproduced with permission from Moore et al. [63, Fig. 2], with permission courtesy of Wolters Kluwer Health, Inc

24 h warrant prompt computed tomographic (CT) imaging for evaluation of the entire thoracic space [12, 32]. Delay in diagnosis of an undrained simple fluid collection allows progression to a complex multi-locular process and the final organization stage [37]. As Sahn and Light [31] stated in 1989, "the sun should never set on a parapneumonic effusion"; early diagnosis and treatment of complicated pleural infection is essential for optimal outcomes. CT images are crucial for the next step in the management of pleural space infections that have not resolved with tube drainage as this dictates operative versus fibrinolytic therapy (Fig. 7.2).

Fibrinolysis Therapy for Treating Pleural Space Infections

The rationale for obtaining a CT scan 24 h after failure for appropriate tube drainage of a pleural infection is for recognition of a persistent pleural collection trapped via thin fibrin septa. This fibrin deposition likely has an initial protective role. The prehistoric horseshoe crab uses a unique protease, Factor C, to initiate coagulation in the presence of endotoxin, trapping and killing pathogens [38]. This has been extrapolated to animal models, in which it has been demonstrated that antifibrinolysis is protective in Gram-negative infection [39]. However, excessive fibrin deposition maybe pathologic and impaired fibrinolysis recently been described ventilated patients [40]. It has become increasingly apparent that the majority of patients in sepsis [41] or sustaining significant injury [42] have resistance to fibrinolytic activity and prone to developing organ failure from what is believed to be microvascular fibrin deposition. This translates to the pleural space, where fibrin deposition is appreciated during inflammation and infection [43]. This early fibrin deposition may help contain the pathogen with impending progressive infection. Pathologic fibrin deposition occurs when the body is unable to clear the pathogen, and the septa become thickened, rendering chest tube drainage ineffective. The proposed therapeutic option enzymatically breaks down these fibrin depositions by up-regulating the fibrinolytic system.

The first report of fibrinolytic therapy in the pleural space was given by Tillett and Sherry [44] in 1949. They infused purified hemolytic streptococcal concentrates, presumed to contain streptokinase and deoxyribonuclease (DNase). Although apparently safe, there was no documented improvement in patient outcome during the ensuing 60 years. The first randomized trial, by Davies et al. [45] in 1997, demonstrated radiographic improvement in 24 patients but no discernible clinical benefit. This was followed by a number of underpowered randomized studies in Europe, suggesting that urokinase demonstrated a therapeutic value [46, 47]. These conflicting results led to the MIST I study [48] involving 52 hospitals in the UK with 412 randomized patients. The data indicated that 72 h of streptokinase treatment resulted in no improvement in mortality, rate of surgery, or length of stay and was associated with an increased rate of serious adverse events. This study was criticized for including a heterogeneous mix of patients with different comorbidities and different stages of pleural disease [49]. A subsequent Cochrane review in 2008 [50] noted that there was a discordance between earlier studies and the MIST I data and concluded that fibrinolytics should be used selectively because there has not been a proven benefit in high-quality trials; however, the authors acknowledged that there may be certain subgroups of patients who benefit from this therapy. Clinical studies in other arenas indicated that tissue plasminogen activator (tPA) was a more effective and safer agent than streptokinase or urokinase as a fibrinolytic agent [51]. Other studies suggested that the addition of DNase to streptokinase improves evacuation of an empyema [52, 53]. Subsequently, MIST II, using tPA with or without DNase, has been completed [54]. Unfortunately, this study (n = 210; four study groups) was only powered sufficiently to evaluate radiographic changes. But consistent with MIST I, tPA alone had no benefit over no fibrinolytic treatment. The combination of tPA and DNase, however, was beneficial in both the primary end point (radiographic clearance) and secondary end points (need for thoracotomy, hospital length of stay). The authors responsibly conclude, "Our study shows that combination intrapleural t-PA and DNAse therapy improves the drainage of pleural fluid in patients with pleural infection… This combined treatment may therefore be useful in patients in whom standard medical management has failed and thoracic surgery is not a treatment option. However, appropriate trials are needed to accurately define the treatment effects."

Thus, the debate continues regarding the role of fibrinolytics in the management of pleural collections. Most intensivists have observed effective eradication of early empyema in some patients, but agree that the appropriate population remains to be defined. On the basis of the pathophysiology of empyema and the morbidity of thoracotomy for delayed intervention, most intensivists believe that fibrinolytic treatment should be attempted for an early empyema with simple collections separated by thin septa documented by CT scan if tube thoracotomy drainage fails (Fig. 7.2). Image-guided direct infusion of fibrinolytics into the collection is superior to delivery via the failed chest tube. The precise agent, dosage, and timing of infusion remain to be determined, although the combination of tPA and DNase seems to be the most effective regimen at this time [54]. Large case series have emerged since the publication of MIST II. Piccolo et al. [55] reported a three-year experience using the MIST II protocol (5 mg DNase and 10 mg tPA BID for up to six doses) in 10 different centers. Inclusion criteria were patients with a pleural pH < 7.2 and clinical evidence of infection. The majority of these patients were male (69 %) had CAP (97 %), middle aged (median 56 years), and received 2 days of therapy. Of the 107 patients included in the analysis eight (93 %) had successful fibrinolytic/dnase therapy. Of note 23 % of patients had increased pain associated with infusion and required additional analgesic medication, which should be taken into consideration when starting therapy. A smaller case series from Mehta et al. [56] evaluating 55 patients using once-a-day therapy for 3 days had similarly positive results with 93 % of patients not requiring surgical intervention. They also appreciated that a decent number of patients (15 %) required additional analgesics during treatments.

Surgical Decortication

There are no randomized control trials evaluating VATs versus fibrinolytic therapy in adults. However, in adolescents a small trial demonstrated equal efficacy in fibrinolytic therapy and VATS in clearing infection, but the surgical intervention group has 3 fewer days with a chest tube and 3 fewer hospital days [57]. This is important to take into the context of the patient's physiologic status. There is a need to for a prospective randomized control trial to determine whether VATS or fibrinolytic therapy is the optimal treatment of patients with complicated parapneumonic effusions who are physically fit to undergo surgery. In addition, there are also patents who should proceed to decortication and avoid futile attempts at fibrinolysis therapy. Multi-loculated empyemas with an established pleural peel evident on CT scanning should undergo prompt VATS [50]. Although "medical" VATS using local anesthesia has been reported [58], the standard procedure is lateral decubitus positioning with dual lung ventilation to facilitate comprehensive evaluation of the involved pleural cavity and systematic decortication (Fig. 7.3). A key maneuver is to enter the pleural space without injuring the underlying lung because of extensive pleural adhesions. An initial incision in the upper thorax, where the empyema is least developed, is usually the safest strategy. In most of the cases, we have used the existing chest tube site to free the lung for placement of the initial port. With the thoracoscope in position and the lung at least partially deflated, additional working ports are added under direct vision. The sites for these ports are chosen to match the chest wall entrance of the chest tubes after VATS.

The objectives of VATS are to unroof all loculated collections, including those in the fissures, and to free the lung of the visceral pleural fibrous encasement. Usually, the decortication is initiated in the upper lobe, where the process is more limited, and ultimately, the fibrous debris is removed as much as possible from the

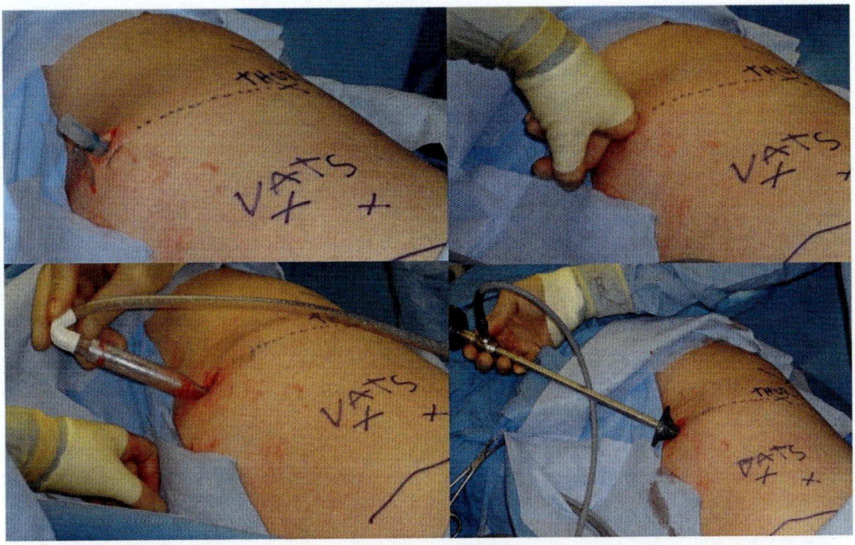

Fig. 7.3 In performing VATS, the thoracic cavity must be entered carefully to avoid tearing the lung because of firm adhesions. We prefer to use the existing chest tube site, digitally mobilizing the adherent lung and further opening a space for the thoracoscope with a large blunt suction tip. Reproduced with permission from Moore et al. [63, Fig. 3], courtesy of Wolters Kluwer Health, Inc

lung surface to enable reexpansion. Dissection must be done carefully on the mediastinal side to avoid injury to the phrenic nerve and pulmonary vasculature. Similarly, clearing the diaphragm must be done cautiously to avoid perforation. In fact, the diaphragm does not need to be systematically debrided as long as the lower lobe is freed. After extensive decortication, the thorax is usually drained with three relatively large chest tubes (28F) to facilitate removal of debris and blood associated with the procedure (Fig. 7.4). The most inferior tube is usually an angled tube positioned in the posterior-dependent recess of the chest.

In the event of a dense fibrous peel that precludes clearance via VATS, a limited lateral muscle-sparing thoracotomy ("mini thoracotomy") is performed to accomplish decortication. Transecting the posterior rib facilitates exposure of the fibrous cavity. Advanced empyemas often require scalpel incision to free the lung for reexpansion; inspection of the lung with periodic reinflation should be done to avoid extensive pulmonary parenchymal air leaks. In the unusual case of a chronic empyema, a standard posterolateral thoracotomy is required. Often, the safest approach is to develop an extrapleural plane and directly enter the empyema cavity before any further thoracic dissection is done. After these extensive decortications, the thorax is drained with three relatively large chest tubes (28F), and the most inferior tube is usually an angled tube positioned in the posterior-dependent recess of the chest. Occasionally, these tubes are simply transected to provide external drainage for outpatient management of extended processes.

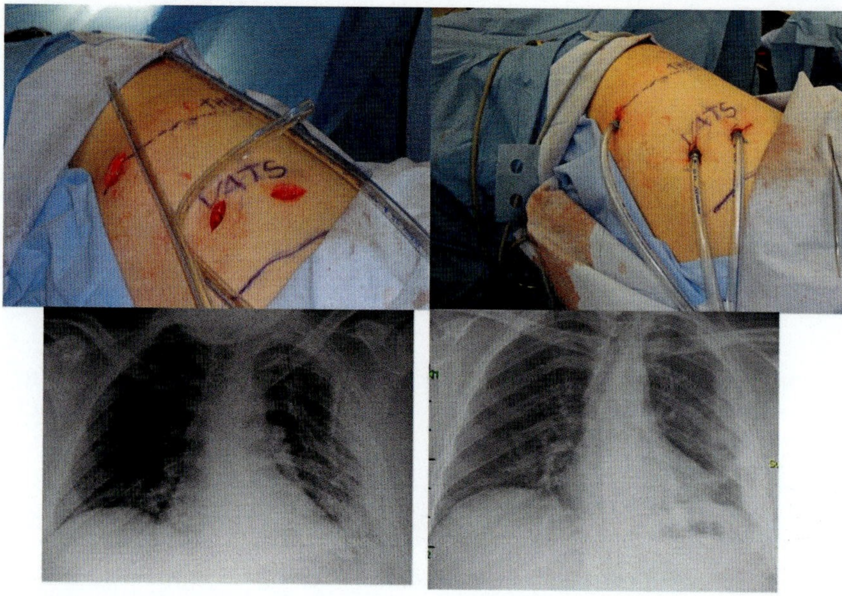

Fig. 7.4 With advanced empyemas, we usually place three relatively large chest tubes; 28F anterior, posterior, and angled above the diaphragm. The chest roentgenogram (*left*) illustrates the three tube thoracostomies and the follow-up examination at day 6 after sequential removal of the tubes. Reproduced with permission from Moore et al. [63, Fig. 5], with permission courtesy of Wolters Kluwer Health, Inc

Treatment of an advanced process caused by a necrotic infected lung with associated major air leaks in a severely immunocompromised patient warrants open thoracic drainage. The Eloesser flap, thoracic cavity marsupialization via segmental rib resection and suturing the skin to the underlying parietal surface, has been the standard for these complicated cases [59]. But recently, simple open drainage with suturing the skin margin to the chest wall, thoracostoma, and the application of a vacuum-assisted wound closure has been popularized [60, 61]. Ultimately, some of these wounds will heal by secondary intention, and the remaining can be closed with thoracomyoplasty [62].

Conclusion

Infection of the pleural space is a morbid condition requiring prompt intervention. The keys to optimal care in these patients are as follows: (1) early identification (2) antibiotics, and (3) clearance of infection from the pleural space. When a chest tube has incompletely drained the pleural space within 24 h, CT imaging to better characterize the pleural space is essential. Adjunctive techniques for drainage of these loculated persistent pleural infections favor small bore chest tubes with tPA/DNAse infusion for 3 days of therapy over surgery. However, there are certain patients who require urgent surgical decortication and bypassing the minimally invasive fibrinolytic approach. The Western Trauma Association has published a critical decision algorithm as recommendations for determining which patients should proceed to decortication versus fibrinolytic therapy [63]. It is important to note that there have been no randomized control trials in adults comparing early VATs to fibrinolytic therapy in patients who can tolerate surgery. Future studies are warranted to address this gap in knowledge, as pediatric literature supports early decortication may be more cost-effective and beneficial to the patient. Failure to appropriately treat pleural space infection resulting in empyema results in highly morbid open operations requiring prolonged hospitalization and lengthy recovery.

Clinical Scenario

Thirty year old woman s/p splenectomy for splenic abscess 3 weeks prior. Patient has been treated for LLL HAP for 2 weeks. She continues with daily fever spikes to 38.6 °C. Her recent CT scan demonstrates a large left thoracic pleural collection, which has pleural thickening and enhances on CT scan.

The next step in the management is a thoracostomy tube placement in the ICU with direct US visualization, which drains 200 cc of cloudy fluid. The fluid pH is found to be 7.1. The patient continues to be febrile, and WBC remains elevated over the next 24 h. AM CXR the following day demonstrates a persistent opacity in the left pleural space despite appropriate tube placement. A CT scan is performed the next day after the patient has failed to improve, which demonstrates a multi-loculated pleural collection in the chest confirming the diagnosis of a complicated parapneumonic effusion.

After a discussion of surgical VATS decortication versus fibrinolytic therapy including tPA and DNAse injections into the pleural space, the patient elects for the non-operative management. The patient receives three days of fibrinolytic therapy and despite increased drainage from her chest tube; she has a persistent fluid collection and remains febrile, now with purulent drainage.

The decision is made to take the patient to the operating room for VATS decortication, but due to extensive adhesions, the procedure is converted to an open thoracotomy. After meticulous dissection, loculated fluid collections and a thick rind are stripped from the pleural surfaces, the chest is irrigated, and three chest tubes are left in place.

Over the next 48 h, the patients fevers break, and WBC normalizes. Her chest tubes are sequentially removed, with no appreciable air leak in the post-operative period, and she is discharged from the hospital three days later.

Key Questions

1. *What are your triggers for a pleural tap for diagnosis?*
2. *What should be the time period to proceed to video-assisted thoracoscopic surgery (VATS) decortication if one is concerned for empyema?*

References

1. Kollef MH. Ventilator-associated complications, including infection-related complications: the way forward. Crit Care Clin. 2013;29(1):33–50.
2. Fletcher MA, Schmitt HJ, Syrochkina M, Sylvester G. Pneumococcal empyema and complicated pneumonias: global trends in incidence, prevalence, and serotype epidemiology. Eur J Clin Microbiol Infect Dis: Official Publ Eur Soc Clin Microbiol. 2014;33(6):879–910.
3. Davies HE, Davies RJ, Davies CW. Group BTSPDG. Management of pleural infection in adults: British Thoracic Society Pleural Disease Guideline 2010. Thorax. 2010;65(Suppl 2): ii41–53.
4. Hasley PB, Albaum MN, Li YH, et al. Do pulmonary radiographic findings at presentation predict mortality in patients with community-acquired pneumonia? Arch Intern Med. 1996;156(19):2206–12.
5. McCauley L, Dean N. Pneumonia and empyema: causal, casual or unknown. J Thorac Dis. 2015;7(6):992–8.
6. Kocijancic I, Kocijancic K, Cufer T. Imaging of pleural fluid in healthy individuals. Clin Radiol. 2004;59(9):826–9.
7. Mordant P, Arame A, Legras A, Le Pimpec Barthes F, Riquet M. Pleural lymphatics and effusions. Rev Pneumol Clin. 2013;69(3):175–80.
8. Christie NA. Management of pleural space: effusions and empyema. Surg Clin N A. 2010;90 (5):919–34.
9. Rahman NM, Chapman SJ, Davies RJ. The approach to the patient with a parapneumonic effusion. Clin Chest Med. 2006;27(2):253–66.
10. Delvaeye M, Conway EM. Coagulation and innate immune responses: can we view them separately? Blood. 2009;114(12):2367–74.
11. Massberg S, Grahl L, von Bruehl ML, et al. Reciprocal coupling of coagulation and innate immunity via neutrophil serine proteases. Nat Med. 2010;16(8):887–96.
12. Koegelenberg CF, Diacon AH, Bolliger CT. Parapneumonic pleural effusion and empyema. Respiration. 2008;75(3):241–50.
13. Light RW, Girard WM, Jenkinson SG, George RB. Parapneumonic effusions. Am J Med. 1980;69(4):507–12.
14. Chalmers JD, Singanayagam A, Murray MP, Scally C, Fawzi A, Hill AT. Risk factors for complicated parapneumonic effusion and empyema on presentation to hospital with community-acquired pneumonia. Thorax. 2009;64(7):592–7.
15. Falguera M, Carratala J, Bielsa S, et al. Predictive factors, microbiology and outcome of patients with parapneumonic effusion. Eur Respir J. 2011;38(5):1173–9.
16. Zablockis R, Petruskeviciene R, Nargela RV. Causes and risk factors of pleural empyema and complicated parapneumonic pleural effusion. Medicina (Kaunas). 2010;46(2):113–9.
17. Behnia M, Logan SC, Fallen L, Catalano P. Nosocomial and ventilator-associated pneumonia in a community hospital intensive care unit: a retrospective review and analysis. BMC Res Notes. 2014;7:232.
18. Eren S, Esme H, Sehitogullari A, Durkan A. The risk factors and management of posttraumatic empyema in trauma patients. Injury. 2008;39(1):44–9.

19. Ball CG, Lord J, Laupland KB, et al. Chest tube complications: how well are we training our residents? Can J Surg J. 2007;50(6):450–8.
20. DuBose J, Inaba K, Okoye O, et al. Development of posttraumatic empyema in patients with retained hemothorax: results of a prospective, observational AAST study. J Trauma Acute Care Surg. 2012;73(3):752–7.
21. Tsang KY, Leung WS, Chan VL, Lin AW, Chu CM. Complicated parapneumonic effusion and empyema thoracis: microbiology and predictors of adverse outcomes. Hong Kong Med J. 2007;13(3):178–86.
22. Maskell NA, Batt S, Hedley EL, Davies CW, Gillespie SH, Davies RJ. The bacteriology of pleural infection by genetic and standard methods and its mortality significance. Am J Respir Crit Care Med. 2006;174(7):817–23.
23. Chen KY, Hsueh PR, Liaw YS, Yang PC, Luh KT. A 10-year experience with bacteriology of acute thoracic empyema: emphasis on *Klebsiella pneumoniae* in patients with diabetes mellitus. Chest. 2000;117(6):1685–9.
24. Porta G, Rodriguez-Carballeira M, Gomez L, et al. Thoracic infection caused by *Streptococcus milleri*. Eur Respir J. 1998;12(2):357–62.
25. Meyer CN, Rosenlund S, Nielsen J, Friis-Moller A. Bacteriological aetiology and antimicrobial treatment of pleural empyema. Scand J Infect Dis. 2011;43(3):165–9.
26. Vaudaux P, Waldvogel FA. Gentamicin inactivation in purulent exudates: role of cell lysis. J Infect Dis. 1980;142(4):586–93.
27. Brixey AG, Luo Y, Skouras V, Awdankiewicz A, Light RW. The efficacy of chest radiographs in detecting parapneumonic effusions. Respirology. 2011;16(6):1000–4.
28. Heffner JE, Klein JS, Hampson C. Diagnostic utility and clinical application of imaging for pleural space infections. Chest. 2010;137(2):467–79.
29. Vignon P, Chastagner C, Berkane V, et al. Quantitative assessment of pleural effusion in critically ill patients by means of ultrasonography. Crit Care Med. 2005;33(8):1757–63.
30. Kocijancic I, Tercelj M, Vidmar K, Jereb M. The value of inspiratory-expiratory lateral decubitus views in the diagnosis of small pleural effusions. Clin Radiol. 1999;54(9):595–7.
31. Sahn SA, Light RW. The sun should never set on a parapneumonic effusion. Chest. 1989;95 (5):945–7.
32. Light RW. Clinical practice. Pleural effusion. New Engl J Med. 2002;346(25):1971–7.
33. Porcel JM. Pleural fluid tests to identify complicated parapneumonic effusions. Curr Opin Pulm Med. 2010;16(4):357–61.
34. Potts DE, Levin DC, Sahn SA. Pleural fluid pH in parapneumonic effusions. Chest. 1976;70 (03):328–31.
35. Rahman NM, Maskell NA, Davies CW, et al. The relationship between chest tube size and clinical outcome in pleural infection. Chest. 2010;137(3):536–43.
36. Fysh ET, Smith NA, Lee YC. Optimal chest drain size: the rise of the small-bore pleural catheter. Semin Respir Crit Care Med. 2010;31(6):760–8.
37. Sahn SA. Diagnosis and management of parapneumonic effusions and empyema. Clin Infect Dis: Official Publ Inf Dis Soc Am. 2007;45(11):1480–6.
38. Ding JL, Ho B. Endotoxin detection–from limulus amebocyte lysate to recombinant factor C. Subcell Biochem. 2010;53:187–208.
39. Luo D, Szaba FM, Kummer LW, et al. Protective roles for fibrin, tissue factor, plasminogen activator inhibitor-1, and thrombin activatable fibrinolysis inhibitor, but not factor XI, during defense against the gram-negative bacterium *Yersinia enterocolitica*. J Immunol. 2011;187 (4):1866–76.
40. El Solh AA, Schultz M. Decreased alveolar fibrinolysis in patients with ventilator-associated pneumonia: a species-specific event. Anesthesiology. 2007;107(4):677.
41. Panigada M, Zacchetti L, L'Acqua C, et al. Assessment of fibrinolysis in sepsis patients with urokinase modified thromboelastography. PLoS ONE. 2015;10(8):e0136463.
42. Moore HB, Moore EE, Gonzalez E, et al. Hyperfibrinolysis, physiologic fibrinolysis, and fibrinolysis shutdown: the spectrum of postinjury fibrinolysis and relevance to antifibrinolytic therapy. J Trauma Acute Care Surg. 2014 Dec;77(6):811–7; discussion 7.

43. Lin FC, Chen YC, Chen FJ, Chang SC. Cytokines and fibrinolytic enzymes in tuberculous and parapneumonic effusions. Clin Immunol. 2005;116(2):166–73.
44. Tillett WS, Sherry S. The effect in patients of streptococcal fibrinolysin (streptokinase) and streptococcal desoxyribonuclease on fibrinous, purulent, and sanguinous pleural exudations. J Clin Investig. 1949;28(1):173–90.
45. Davies RJ, Traill ZC, Gleeson FV. Randomised controlled trial of intrapleural streptokinase in community acquired pleural infection. Thorax. 1997;52(5):416–21.
46. Bouros D, Schiza S, Tzanakis N, Chalkiadakis G, Drositis J, Siafakas N. Intrapleural urokinase versus normal saline in the treatment of complicated parapneumonic effusions and empyema. A randomized, double-blind study. Am J Respir Crit Care Med. 1999;159(1):37–42.
47. Tuncozgur B, Ustunsoy H, Sivrikoz MC, et al. Intrapleural urokinase in the management of parapneumonic empyema: a randomised controlled trial. Int J Clin Pract. 2001;55(10):658–60.
48. Maskell NA, Davies CW, Nunn AJ, et al. U.K. controlled trial of intrapleural streptokinase for pleural infection. New Engl J Med. 2005;352(9):865–74.
49. Heffner JE. Multicenter trials of treatment for empyema–after all these years. The New Engl J Med. 2005;352(9):926–8.
50. Cameron R, Davies HR. Intra-pleural fibrinolytic therapy versus conservative management in the treatment of adult parapneumonic effusions and empyema. Cochrane Database Syst Rev. 2008(2):CD002312.
51. Gervais DA, Levis DA, Hahn PF, Uppot RN, Arellano RS, Mueller PR. Adjunctive intrapleural tissue plasminogen activator administered via chest tubes placed with imaging guidance: effectiveness and risk for hemorrhage. Radiology. 2008;246(3):956–63.
52. Simpson G, Roomes D, Heron M. Effects of streptokinase and deoxyribonuclease on viscosity of human surgical and empyema pus. Chest. 2000;117(6):1728–33.
53. Sherry S, Tillett WS, Christensen LR. Presence and significance of desoxyribose nucleoprotein in the purulent pleural exudates of patients. Proc Soc Exp Biol Med Soc Exp Biol Med. 1948;68(1):179–84.
54. Rahman NM, Maskell NA, West A, et al. Intrapleural use of tissue plasminogen activator and DNase in pleural infection. New Engl J Medicine. 2011;365(6):518–26.
55. Piccolo F, Pitman N, Bhatnagar R, et al. Intrapleural tissue plasminogen activator and deoxyribonuclease for pleural infection. An effective and safe alternative to surgery. Ann Am Thorac Soc. 2014 Nov;11(9):1419–25.
56. Mehta HJ, Biswas A, Penley AM, Cope J, Barnes M, Jantz MA. Management of intrapleural sepsis with once daily use of tissue plasminogen activator and deoxyribonuclease. Respiration. 2016 Jan;14.
57. Cobanoglu U, Sayir F, Bilici S, Melek M. Comparison of the methods of fibrinolysis by tube thoracostomy and thoracoscopic decortication in children with stage II and III empyema: a prospective randomized study. Pediatr Rep. 2011;3(4):e29.
58. Katlic MR, Facktor MA. Video-assisted thoracic surgery utilizing local anesthesia and sedation: 384 consecutive cases. Ann Thorac Surg. 2010;90(1):240–5.
59. Deslauriers J, Jacques LF, Gregoire J. Role of eloesser flap and thoracoplasty in the third millennium. Chest Surg Clin N Am. 2002;12(3):605–23.
60. Palmen M, van Breugel HN, Geskes GG, et al. Open window thoracostomy treatment of empyema is accelerated by vacuum-assisted closure. Ann Thorac Surg. 2009;88(4):1131–6.
61. Haghshenasskashani A, Rahnavardi M, Yan TD, McCaughan BC. Intrathoracic application of a vacuum-assisted closure device in managing pleural space infection after lung resection: is it an option? Interact CardioVasc Thorac Surg. 2011;13(2):168–74.
62. Walsh MD, Bruno AD, Onaitis MW, et al. The role of intrathoracic free flaps for chronic empyema. Ann Thorac Surg. 2011;91(3):865–8.
63. Moore HB, Moore EE, Burlew CC, et al. Western Trauma Association critical decisions in trauma: management of parapneumonic effusion. J Trauma Acute Care Surg. 2012;73(6):1372–9.

Chapter 8
Perforated peptic ulcer and the dislodged PEG

Charles A. Adams, Jr., William G. Cioffi, Carrie Valdez and Jose J. Diaz

The Dislodged PEG

Over 35 years ago, Gauderer et al. [1] described a technique to establish long-term enteral access without the need for laparotomy in a cohort of children with swallowing difficulties. The technique, percutaneous endoscopic gastrostomy (PEG), has become the preferred method to establish long-term enteral feeding access in patients with abnormal swallowing precluding medication or nutrition by mouth. Unlike the traditional surgical gastrostomy, PEG can be done at the bedside under local anesthesia and light sedation which makes it an attractive procedure for several reasons. Conservative estimates put the number of PEGs performed in the United States at well over 200,000 annually; thus, it is imperative that surgeons, intensivists, and all clinicians are familiar with the management of these devices and their complications [2]. Like most procedures, the complications of PEGs can

C.A. Adams Jr. (✉)
Division of Trauma and Surgical Critical Care, Rhode Island Hospital, Warren Alpert Medical School of Brown University, Providence, RI, USA
e-mail: Cadams1@lifespan.org

W.G. Cioffi
Department of Surgery, Rhode Island Hospital, Warren Alpert Medical School of Brown University, Providence, RI, USA
e-mail: wcioffi@lifespan.org

C. Valdez
R Adams Cowley Shock Trauma Center, University of Maryland Medical School, Baltimore, MD, USA
e-mail: carrievaldezmd@gmail.com

J.J. Diaz
Division of Acute Care Surgery, R Adams Cowley Shock Trauma Center, University of Maryland Medical Center, Baltimore, MD, USA
e-mail: jdiaz@umm.edu

J.J. Diaz and D.T. Efron (eds.), *Complications in Acute Care Surgery*,
DOI 10.1007/978-3-319-42376-0_8

be broadly grouped into minor and major complications. The minor complications include such things as tube fracture or blockage, leakage or minor peristomal infections that are easily addressed by bedside care; however, the major complications frequently require surgical intervention and include entities such as necrotizing fasciitis, peritonitis, hemorrhage, and early tube dislodgement [3]. Although the major complications are severe and life-threatening, their management is rather straightforward; however, this is not the case with early dislodgement of a PEG which requires a great deal of clinical judgment to successfully manage the patient.

Unlike an open Stamm gastrostomy where the gastric wall is sutured to the parietal peritoneum of the anterior abdominal wall, the apposition of the gastric wall to the abdominal wall following PEG is accomplished solely by the bumper of the PEG in the gastric lumen and the crosspiece on the tubing externally. By design, the PEG bumper is soft enough so that when the tubing is placed on sufficient tension, the bumper will deform and the tube can be removed when it is no longer needed. Unfortunately, any excess tension placed on the tube either by pulling on the tubing intentionally or accidentally can result in dislodgement of the PEG. In the early post-PEG period, there is insufficient time for adhesions and scar tissue to form between the abdominal wall and stomach so that removal of the PEG will result in the stomach "falling" away from the abdominal wall which may result in peritonitis and septic shock due to leakage from the site of gastric perforation. There are very little data available to suggest the length of this period, but PEGs removed within 7–10 days of placement are generally associated with falling of the stomach away from the abdominal wall and gastric leak. Sporadic case reports indicate that in certain populations such as patients with advanced malignancy, severe malnutrition, or intense immunosuppression, there may be a lack of effective adhesions securing the stomach to the abdominal wall for a month or longer [4].

A few days following PEG, there are some adhesions between the stomach and abdominal wall such that a nascent "tract" has begun to form. PEG removal occurring after 7–10 days may or may not result in the stomach falling away depending on the nature of these early adhesions; thus, the risk of gastric leakage and peritonitis is a function of the degree of adhesion formation between the two structures. Obviously, clinicians have no way of knowing the rate or degree these adhesions form so the management of patients with a dislodged PEG during this time period is fraught with unforeseen complications. Thus, it is important that clinicians maintain a high index of suspicion and vigilance following any PEG replacement since there is always a possibility that the tract has been disrupted or leaking and the patient is at risk for the development of intra-abdominal sepsis.

A long-standing PEG has a mature tract due to the presence of dense adhesions between the stomach and abdominal wall. PEGs that are removed during this time period rarely have any adverse consequences since that stomach is effectively held in place by scar. If desired, a tube may be reinserted into the gastric lumen with little risk of tract disruption but the decision to obtain confirmatory radiographic exams is an option should the clinician have concerns that the tract was disrupted or if the tube placement was difficult. The longer the PEG has been in place, the less likely that the tract will be disrupted and many ambulatory patients have their chronic PEGs changed in a physician's office or at a primary care clinic without the need for a confirmatory radiographic study. Again, the exact time period defining a matured PEG tract is unknown but most clinicians agree that a year is sufficient time to forego these studies; however, should there be any doubt or concern in the clinician's mind that the newly inserted tube is in the stomach, then it is advisable to obtain a contrast study.

It is apparent that the management of the dislodged PEG is greatly influenced by the time interval from its initial placement to its inadvertent removal. Since late removal is rarely a problem, we will focus our discussion on PEG dislodgement in the early period and the intricacies of managing patients during this period. It stands to reason that the need for the PEG and the indications for its placement are still valid in the early post-PEG period; thus, re-establishing enteral access is clearly indicated. In most patients, a tract has formed by day 10 and beyond so that a Foley catheter or balloon-tipped gastrostomy can be carefully inserted into the PEG site and proper intra-gastric placement confirmed with a water-soluble contrast radiograph [5]. Occasionally the confirmatory study demonstrates extravasation of contrast throughout the abdomen signifying that the tract has been disrupted and the tube is not in the gastric lumen. The clinician has several options in managing the patient in this condition ranging from laparotomy, washout of the abdomen removing contrast and gastric secretions, and creation of a Stamm gastrostomy to emergent repeat PEG placement and other temporizing maneuvers.

If there is suspicion that the tract may be tenuous or absent based on the patient's overall physiologic status, disease state or comorbidities, and the dislodgment was promptly recognized, a desirable course of action may be urgent repeat upper endoscopy to guide the insertion of a replacement tube instead of a blind attempt. At endoscopy, unsuccessful reinsertions can be immediately identified signifying that the stomach has fallen away from the anterior abdominal wall. In this setting, insertion of a new PEG adjacent to the site of the prior should be attempted [4, 6, 7]. If successful, the new PEG will bring the site of perforation up to the abdominal wall sealing the gastric perforation while at the same time re-establishing enteral access. Again, it is important to note that endoscopic replacement of the dislodged PEG should only be attempted if the dislodgement was promptly recognized since longer periods of perforation are associated with the development of peritonitis and sepsis. Similarly, laparoscopy may be undertaken in patient with a relatively recently discovered PEG dislodgment and affords not only the ability to re-establish enteral access but facilitates abdominal exploration and washout as well. Laparoscopy is not advisable in cases of established peritonitis or systemic sepsis due the adverse effects of insufflating the abdomen in a patient with capillary leak, ineffective circulating volumes, or those requiring vasopressors for septic shock.

Akin to the management of a patient with a perforated ulcer, the patient with a freshly dislodged PEG should be kept nil per os and a nasogastric tube inserted for gastric decompression. Intravenous crystalloids, acid reducing medications, and broad-spectrum antibiotics should be administered but the addition of antifungal for coverage of candida species is somewhat controversial [6]. This course of management has been embraced as a temporizing maneuver when repeat endoscopy is not available or in rare cases where endoscopy is ill-advised due to confounding patient factors or an adverse clinical scenario [7]. Occasionally, a patient with a freshly placed and dislodged PEG can be managed this way for several days and then undergo repeat endoscopy and PEG placement in a delayed fashion; however, it must be remembered that this course of management exposes the patient to a prolonged period without enteral access for medication and nutrition as well as the risk of developing intra-abdominal sepsis.

Patients who manifest diffuse peritonitis or signs of systemic sepsis following PEG dislodgment require formal abdominal exploration as these patients are beyond the window where less invasive measures such as endoscopy or laparoscopy are safe. A midline laparotomy should be done and the abdomen washed out evacuating any collections of pooled gastric secretions or tube feeds. If a tube was inserted into the tract but the contrast study showed extravasation, it is not uncommon to encounter water-soluble contrast throughout the abdomen upon abdominal exploration. If the PEG was placed in the antrum, it is advisable to freshen up the PEG site with sharp debridement of the gastric wall followed by a double-layer closure and a new gastrostomy should be placed in the gastric body utilizing a Stamm technique. For dislodged PEGs in the gastric body, it may be possible to place a gastrostomy utilizing the same gastric wall defect but this is generally ill-advised except in rare cases where inflammation of the gastric wall is minimal. Drainage of the peritoneal cavity is not required unless the dislodged PEG has been out for several days and a well-formed abscess cavity is encountered. Patients manifesting signs of diffuse peritonitis at laparotomy such as widespread fibrinous peel and hyperemia should be treated with a short course of broad-spectrum antibiotics otherwise one postoperative dose should be sufficient [8].

One other management option worth mentioning is the use of Natural Orifice Trans-luminal Endoscopic Surgery (NOTES) to explore the abdomen, remove gastric fluids, and facilitate placement of a new PEG. A recent case report [9] describes a failed attempt at a blind insertion of a freshly disrupted PEG discovered due to widespread extravasation of contrast on confirmatory radiography. An upper endoscopy was performed, and the site of the gastric perforation was identified and dilated with a balloon. This dilation allowed passage of the endoscope into the peritoneal cavity, and an endoscopic abdominal exploration was performed in order to suction out fluid and contrast from the peritoneal cavity. At the end of the exploration, a wire was passed through the skin defect in the abdominal wall, grabbed with the scope, and pulled into the stomach and out of the mouth so that a fresh PEG could be placed. The authors note that the patient was without peritonitis or signs of systemic sepsis since these would obviously preclude NOTES and indicate that a laparotomy was required [9]. The patient did well and did not develop an intra-abdominal abscess or other postoperative complication; however, it remains to be seen whether this technique will be widely embraced since NOTES is still in its early developmental stages.

It is often said that an ounce of prevention is worth a ton of cure, thus some gastroenterologists have advocated for T-fasteners to be placed at the same time the PEG is placed in order to prevent PEG dislodgment [10]. T-fasteners have proven effective in reducing the rate of PEG dislodgment but are associated with increased procedure times during PEG placement, added procedural difficulty as well as more abdominal pain and skin excoriations after the procedure. In some ways, the T-fasteners mimic the creation of a Stamm gastrostomy since the stomach is now affixed to the anterior abdominal wall. At the present time, there is a paucity of literature identifying which patients are at increased risk for PEG dislodgment but it is reasonable to assume that those with traumatic brain injury or other encephalopathies may benefit from T-fastener securing of their PEGs.

Perforated Peptic Ulcers

On January 1, 1979, the United States Food and Drug Administration approved Cimetidine, the prototypical H_2 receptor antagonist, which was highly effective in suppressing gastric acid secretion. Cimetidine was the first medication with annual sales exceeding $1 billion making it the first "blockbuster" drug in the pharmaceutical industry. For surgeons, the development of the H_2 antagonists had a profound effect on gastric surgery that is still evident in the present day. Prior to Cimetidine, gastric ulcer disease was rampant and gastric procedures treating peptic ulcer disease were commonplace; however, the widespread use of H2 antagonists resulted in a rapid decrease in the number of operations performed for peptic ulcer disease and ominously a pervasive unfamiliarity with the disease process itself developed among surgeons and surgical residents. The development of proton pump inhibitors and the discovery of the critical role that Helicobacter pylori (*H. pylori*) plays in peptic ulcer disease has further decreased the volume of elective gastric surgery as well as certain types of emergent gastric procedures. While the rate of peptic ulcer hemorrhage seems to have declined over the last few decades, the rate of perforation appears to be somewhat stable. Perforation remains a lethal development and nearly 70 % of all ulcer-related fatalities are due to perforation; thus, it is imperative that surgeons have a working fund of knowledge regarding perforated peptic ulcer (PPU) disease [11, 12].

The clinical presentation of a patient with a PPU often follows a similar course in that there is a sudden onset of intense abdominal pain that may awaken the patient from sleep, associated with nausea, occasional vomiting, and rapid-onset peritonitis. The presentation of PPU is so classic that nearly 200 years ago, the British physician Edward Crisp stated "The symptoms are so typical, I hardly believe it possible that anyone can fail to make correct diagnosis." On physical exam, the patient typically has board-like abdominal rigidity and obvious peritonitis with associated tachycardia. Fever and hypotension are very late findings in patients with PPU so their absence upon initial presentation should not be used to rule out this diagnosis. Upright chest radiograms classically demonstrate free intraperitoneal air under the hemi-diaphragms and further diagnostics studies are not indicated in cases of obvious peritonitis. The absence of free air on an upright chest radiogram does not rule out the possibility of a PPU since the sensitivity of this study is only about 75 %. Risk factors for PPU include medications such as aspirin or non-steroidal anti-inflammatory agents (NSAIDs), smoking, Helicobacter pylori infection, or an antecedent history of peptic ulcer disease although PPU may be the initial presentation in patients with undiagnosed peptic ulcer disease. About two-thirds PPU are juxta-pyloric with the remaining one-third of PPUs evenly distributed between the lesser curve of the stomach and the anterior wall of the gastric body [13]. Thankfully, perforations close to the gastroesophageal junction or posterior gastric perforations are rather rare since these are more difficult to treat surgically.

Similar to the temporizing maneuvers discussed previously when confronted with a freshly dislodged PEG tube, the patient with known or suspected PPU should be kept nil per os and a nasogastric tube inserted for gastric decompression. Intravenous crystalloid fluid resuscitation and broad-spectrum antibiotics should be administered along with acid reducing medications such as proton pump inhibitors [7]. In many ways, the approach to the patient with PPU is analogous to the approach of a patient with a freshly dislodged PEG in that the decision to operate or not is fairly nuanced and the clinician needs to create a plan of care considering the operative mortality and risk of complications associated with surgical exploration versus those of non-operative management. This decision is further complicated by estimates that 40–80 % of perforations seal spontaneously with omentum or viscera and that complication rates between operative and non-operative management are similar [11]. In order to help guide the decision process regarding the patient with PPU, several predictive models have been created to guide clinicians.

One of the earliest models to predict mortality and morbidity for patients with PPU undergoing surgery was described by Boey and is comprised of three factors: the patient's comorbidities, the presence of shock, and the duration of the perforation [14]. As would be expected, the more comorbidities the patient with PPU has, the worse they do following surgery. Likewise, delays from time of perforation to surgical repair and the presence of shock also portend a poor outcome. Other authors have described mortality risk predictive models for patients with PPU undergoing surgery such as the Hacettepe score, the Jabalpur score, and the Peptic Ulcer Perforation (PULP) score each encompassing their own patient variables derived from large retrospective series; however, none of these have been fully validated [15]. Of these three mortality predictive scoring systems, it appears the PULP score, which is derived from 8 clinical variables, has the best predictive value. While not specifically a mortality risk model, the American Society of Anesthesiologists (ASA) Score which classifies a patient's physical condition remains one of the simplest and most effective tools for stratifying risk in patients undergoing surgery. Recently, the American College of Surgeons has created a web-based risk calculator based on data gleamed from 1.5 million patient records; however, its utility in predicting mortality and morbidity for patients undergoing emergent surgery for PPU has yet to be validated. The real value of any predictive mortality model or scoring system is to identify moribund patients who are beyond salvage to avoid unnecessary operations. Fortunately few patients fall into this category since and the predictive power of all of these models is not discriminating enough.

Despite advances in diagnostic technology, operative management, and surgical critical care, PPU remains a lethal disease with mortality rates still as high as 27 % in some series [16]. As Boey initially showed, and others have confirmed, mortality is driven by delays in treatment, the development of shock and comorbidities, but it is important to consider the patient's age as well [14]. Advanced age is a consistent risk for operative mortality for individuals with PPU [11–13, 15, 16] which has fueled interest in non-operative management for patients considered to be at increased risk for adverse outcomes [17]. Non-operative management of PPU first described by Taylor in 1946 may be an effective way of managing PPU in select patients as well as a temporizing measure in patients with dislodged PEG or PPU awaiting definitive therapy. The key components of this method are NGT decompression, intravenous fluid resuscitation, anti-acid medications, and broad-spectrum antibiotics. If successful, the Taylor method can spare the patient, the added morbidity of general anesthesia, and surgical exploration; however, failures of this approach result in delays in source control and the development of sepsis and increased morbidity and mortality. Central to the successful non-operative management of a PPU is demonstration that the perforation has sealed with omentum or adjacent viscera by obtaining an upper gastrointestinal contrast study [17]. Non-operative management may be attempted in individuals with no evidence of leak on these studies, but those with contrast extravasation require surgical intervention. It is important to remember that even if non-operative management is "successful," the patient may still develop intra-abdominal abscesses, re-perforation, and in cases of gastric perforation may still be at risk for undiagnosed perforated carcinoma [18]. Additionally, length of stay may be longer in patients treated non-operatively compared to those operated on due to ileus, intra-abdominal abscess, and other complications.

Several studies, including two randomized control trials, have shown that non-operative management of PPU as first described nearly 75 years ago, is still a viable treatment option for patients with PPU [18, 19]. Review of this literature points to several factors that denote increased risk of failure of non-operative therapy such as age greater than 59–70, delays in initiating therapy greater than 12 h, the presence of large volumes of pneumoperitoneum on upright chest X-rays or signs of large volume pneumoperitoneum on physical exam such as abdominal distention, tympany on percussion, or signs of peritonitis such as tenderness on rectal exam or upon abdominal palpation [20]. Obviously, findings consistent with large volumes or ongoing pneumoperitoneum strongly suggest an unsealed PPU, and these patients are best managed operatively since obtaining an upper gastrointestinal contrast study to confirm what the clinician already knows only delays control of the perforation and invites poor outcomes. Clinicians should exhibit great caution when considering whether a perforation is sealed or not since there is a period following perforation where the pain and abdominal rigidity abate as the extravasated gastric contents are diluted out in the peritoneal cavity. Croft termed this period the "delusional state" since both the surgeon and the patient may be deluded into thinking the perforation has sealed when in fact gastric leakage is ongoing [18]. Established peritonitis, fever, hypotension, or other signs of shock denote a long-standing perforation, and these patients are beyond the window where non-operative management should be attempted. Accordingly, the ideal patient in whom non-operative management of a PPU should be attempted is a younger patient with a relatively recent onset of symptoms, a benign abdominal physical exam, and an absence of signs of systemic toxicity. Older patients, those with multiple medical comorbidities, long-standing perforations, or those with signs of ongoing peritoneal soilage or severe infection belong in the operating room. An exception to this would be the elderly patient who is at such extreme risk for perioperative mortality that surgical exploration is unwise and non-operative management is their only option. Non-operative invasive strategies such as endoscopic clips or sutures, biologic patches, or NOTES procedures at this point in time are still largely investigational and still require sedation and possible intubation which may still be too risky for patients with significant comorbidities.

In an attempt to minimize perioperative morbidities such as wound infection, pulmonary complications, and prolonged recovery periods, laparoscopic approaches for PPU are becoming increasingly popular [21]. Several studies have shown that laparoscopic patching of a PPU along with peritoneal washout is an acceptable alternative therapy to laparotomy. In the United States, laparoscopy for PPU is reserved for younger patients who are not manifesting systemic toxicity but surgeons in other countries have significantly pushed the envelope performing laparoscopy on patients with PPU despite established peritonitis or even septic shock [22, 23]. While this may acceptable as proof of concept, it is nonetheless ill-advised to attempt laparoscopy in such patients due to their tenuous hemodynamic state and propensity for complications. For some surgeons, the learning curve for laparoscopic surgery is steep and the placement of intracorporeal sutures tedious, both of which can result in longer operative times but over time results similar to open surgery are readily attainable [23]. Conversion from laparoscopy to open surgery for PPU is associated with increased postoperative leak rates and added complications, as are all laparoscopic PPU operations, but whether this is cause and effect or a marker of larger or more difficult perforations has not yet been clarified [24]. Overall, laparoscopy for PPU has reported success rate ranging from 81 to 92 % and a mortality rate lower but not statistically superior to open surgery although the anticipated reduction in pulmonary complications has not been realized [20]. The most consistent benefit of laparoscopy for PPU appears to be reduced postoperative pain and decreased need for narcotics.

In the past, multiple publications argued the risks and benefits of patching a PPU versus performing a definitive ulcer operation, but by and large, the development of potent anti-acid medications coupled with effective antibiotics against *H. Pylori* and an appreciation of its role in peptic ulcer disease has ended this vigorous debate. Simple suture closure when feasible or omental patching when not has been shown to be the procedures of choice compared to gastrectomy or pyloroplasty with or without vagotomy [25]. Primary closure of duodenal perforations should only be employed to close small defects since closing larger ones can lead to narrowing of the gastric outlet. While most surgeons refer to patching a PPU with omentum as

Graham's procedure, this is not technically correct. Patching a PPU with a pedicle of omentum affixed by overlying sutures was first described by Cellan-Jones while Graham's procedure involved a free omental plug sutured into the perforation [20]. Either way, omental patching of PPU has become the procedure of choice for both laparoscopic and open repairs and gastrectomy is reserved only for giant perforations not amenable to patching or when the perforation occurs in the setting of a gastric outlet obstruction or a severely scarred duodenum. The mortality rate for emergent gastrectomies approaches 20 % while the rate for omental patching procedures is less than half that [25]. It is worth mentioning that unlike duodenal perforations which are rarely if ever due to cancer, the risk of perforated gastric cancer is much higher; therefore, the edge of all gastric perforations should be biopsied. It is not desirable to perform a definitive oncologic resection in a patient with advanced peritonitis or sepsis so two-stage procedures may be required with control of the leak followed by formal resection in a few days when the peritonitis has resolved.

Abdominal washout is an integral component of PPU surgery, and it is important that the subphrenic spaces and the pouches of Douglas and Morrison be thoroughly irrigated. Although antibiotic containing lavage solutions have proved beneficial in animal models of peritonitis, their role in humans is less clear and most surgeons consider them unnecessary. The old adage, "the solution to pollution is dilution," suggests that there is a benefit to washing the abdomen with massive amounts of saline to reduce infection but this has never been substantiated [26]. Similarly, drains placed in the abdomen in the vicinity of the repair have not been shown to be helpful. Some surgeons leave a drain as a sentinel should the patch repair fails since it is anticipated that the character of the drain effluent will change from sero-sanguinous to bilious. Unfortunately, there is no evidence to support this practice and on the contrary drains may serve as a portal of infection and rarely can erode into vital structures so their routine usage is generally not advisable. Even the routine use of nasogastric tubes (NGTs) following repair of a PPU is not supported by the evidence, but specific studies looking at PPU operations have not been done, thus most surgeons leave a NGT in the hopes that this will diminish the rate of patch failure, prevent gastric distention, and limit nausea and vomiting [27]. In cases of long-standing perforation or if there is frank peritonitis with a dense fibrino-purulent peel on the viscera, a short course of antibiotics is warranted, otherwise a single postoperative dose should be given [8]. There is no literature to guide clinicians about the best time to feed a patient following treatment of a PPU, but most surgeons remove the NGT on day 1 or 2 and begin liquids thereafter. Routine upper gastrointestinal contrast studies are not required prior to feeding but it is important to be vigil for signs of re-perforation such as sever recurrent abdominal pain, tachycardia, or other signs of systemic toxicity.

The discovery of *H. Pylori* by Marshall and Warren in 1982 radically changed not only our understanding of the pathogenesis of peptic ulcer disease but its management as well, including its surgical management. Helicobacter pylori contribute to 90 % of duodenal ulcers and 80 % of peptic ulcer through chronic inflammation and the dysregulation of gastric digestive physiology promoting the development of gastritis and ulceration [11]. Previously, it was thought that *H.*

Pylori contributed more to gastritis and upper gastrointestinal hemorrhage but recent work shows it is intimately involved with perforation as well as re-perforation in patients in whom the organism is not eradicated [28]. Accordingly, it is now standard that all patients with peptic ulcer disease, including those with perforation or hemorrhage, receive empiric therapy aimed at clearing the organism from the patient's stomach. The Maastricht conference, a recurring symposium of experts dedicated to addressing the problem presented by *H. Pylori*, recommends triple therapy for regions where clarithromycin resistance is low and quadruple therapy for regions where resistance is high [29]. Several regimens have been tested but most combine the macrolide antibiotic clarithromycin with either amoxicillin or metronidazole along with high-dose proton pump inhibitors. As *H. Pylori* develops resistance to the components of this regimen, the dose and duration of its components have been altered with some temporary improvement with bismuth added to the quadruple regimens since there is no reported resistance to this agent [29]. All patients who have peptic ulcer disease including those who have perforations due to NSAID or aspirin use should be tested and treated for *H. pylori* since failure to do so is associated with complications [28]. Eradicating *H. Pylori* has proven so beneficial that it has rendered the argument for and against definitive ulcer surgery largely a moot point, and now simple patching followed by some iteration of the Maastricht consensus is considered standard therapy. Upper endoscopy and biopsy to document eradication of *H. Pylori* as well as to demonstrate healing and in cases of successful non-operative management to rule out cancer is indicated 6–8 weeks postoperatively since earlier endoscopy may result in patch disruption. Failure to eradicate *H. Pylori* warrants second tier therapies such as levofloxacin or tetracyclines and possibly bismuth [29].

In conclusion, PPU disease remains a highly lethal condition, and despite its typical presentation diagnosing, this entity may prove difficult, particularly in the elderly. Non-operative management may be attempted in younger patients with documented sealing of the perforation and limited signs of toxicity but older patients, those with peritonitis or systemic toxicity or ongoing gastric leak, require surgical intervention. Simple patching of the perforation is adequate and gastrectomy is to be discouraged unless absolutely necessary and treatment of *H. Pylori* with a cocktail of several agents is mandatory.

Incarcerated Paraesophageal Hernia

Hiatal hernias are classified into four types depending on the location of the gastroesophageal junction and the hernia sac [30]. In the acute setting with concern for incarceration or strangulation, a type IV hernia with gastric volvulus is the most common presentation (Fig. 8.1). Initial concern should focus on determining gastric viability that will determine the timing, approach, and extent of operative repair. The surgeon should maintain a high index of suspicion for operative intervention if the patient presents with a leukocytosis, fever, or hemodynamic instability.

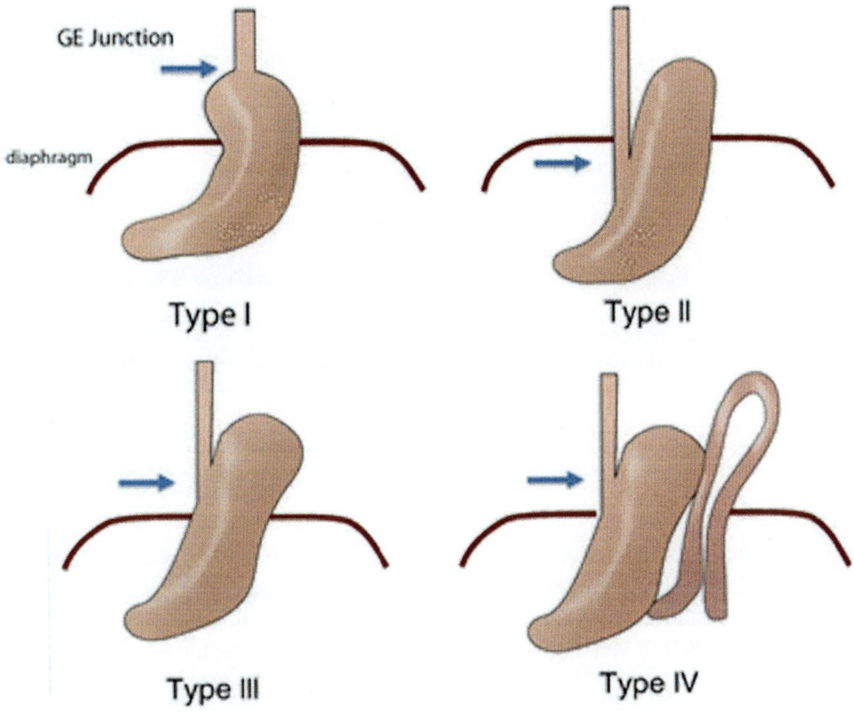

Fig. 8.1 Types of paraesophageal hernias. *Source* Schenarts et al. [46, Fig. 16.1], with permission of Springer

Diagnostics Evaluation

Patients experiencing acute paraesophageal incarceration/strangulation can present with variable symptoms. The clinical presentation was first described by Moritz Borchardt, who was a German surgeon in 1948, as upper abdominal pain, retching, and blockage against placement of a nasogastric tube. The classical Borchardt's triad in acute gastric volvulus is (1) minimal abdominal findings when the stomach is in the thorax, (2) a gas-filled viscus in the lower chest or upper abdomen shown by chest radiography, and (3) obstruction at the site of volvulus shown by emergency upper gastrointestinal series [31]. Symptoms can include retrosternal chest pain, epigastric pain, nausea, increased salivation with inability to swallow it, and retching with or without vomiting. If the stomach has incarcerated or volvulized, mucosal ischemia can lead to perforation and the patient may present in septic shock. The initial set of vital signs, a standard set of laboratories, and an upright chest X-ray are the appropriate first step to evaluate patient's acuity. An ECG and troponin level should eliminate concerns for a cardiac event.

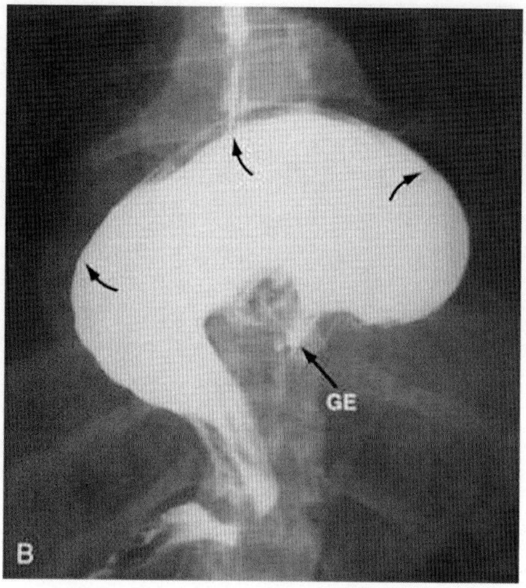

Fig. 8.2 Flouroscopic series with gastric volvulous. *Source* Jeyarajah and Harford [47, Fig. 24-7B], with kind permission from Clincal Gate (clinicalgate.com)

A significant paraesophageal hernia is often recognized on chest X-ray as a gastric bubble within the thorax. The X-ray or CT scan can also be helpful to determine perforation into the thorax by looking for a unilateral pleural effusion, typically on the left. It can also demonstrate intra-peritoneal perforation with free air under the diaphragm or CT scan (Fig. 8.2). If imaging demonstrates perforation, resuscitation and operative intervention should proceed without delay.

If the patient is hemodynamically stable without evidence of perforation, a nasogastric tube should be placed to decompress the stomach [32]. During placement, determine how easily the tube passes into the stomach. Gentle pressure may allow the nasogastric tube to pass, even with a gastric volvulus. The tube should be placed on low wall suction, and the evacuated content should be evaluated for blood. Gastric decompression may allow the stomach to untwist, thus reducing the risk of strangulation and turning an emergent/urgent scenario into a semi-elective one. If one cannot pass an NGT manually, it is mandatory to go to the OR for endoscopic placement in an urgent fashion.

Indications for Operative Intervention

If the NGT aspirate is non-bloody, the patient should be admitted and observed. The surgeon should complete a thorough workup and prepare for a semi-elective operative repair when possible [33, 34].

In the clinical scenario above, the patient is symptomatic, tachycardic, and has a leukocytosis concerning for sepsis which should make one concerned for a potential gastric perforation. This patient should be quickly resuscitated in preparation for urgent exploration. Once in the operating room, an esophagogastroduodenoscopy (EGD) should be performed first. Careful inspection of the esophagus, particularly the gastroesophageal (GE) junction, is critical. If there is evidence of necrosis, the EGD should be terminated and a laparotomy performed. However, if the esophageal mucosa is viable, gentle pneumatic pressure can be used to open up or untwist the GE junction. Once within the stomach, use caution not to over insufflate. Careful inspection of the mucosa should reveal mucosal ischemia if present. A NGT should remain in place.

Laparoscopic Approach

Initial inspection should quickly determine whether the case is going to stay laparoscopic. If no mucosal ischemia is present, a diagnostic laparoscopy with the assessment of gastric wall viability should follow. If the stomach is merely edematous, but not dead, reduce the stomach from the chest.

If there is no perforation or ischemia, one can proceed to definitive repair if there is minimal gastric edema. A laparoscopic paraesophageal repair has a low morbidity and mortality. This approach can offer the benefits of minimally invasive surgery in a group of patients that are often elderly and have multiple medical problems [35]. The majority of surgery occurs in the mediastinum, and laparoscopic port placement is critical. If ports are placed too inferior, there may be difficulty reaching the operative field.

The diaphragmatic defect is commonly on the left side of the esophageal opening in the diaphragm. If necessary, the defect can be widened directly lateral to avoid injury to the inferior phrenic vein. At this point, determine whether the patient is a candidate for definitive laparoscopic repair. Inspect the posterior stomach by making a window thru the gastrocolic ligament.

If your assessment remains that the stomach is edematous, but not ischemic, a staged laparoscopic procedure should be considered. One should terminate the surgery and resuscitate the patient. Return to the OR in a few days for definitive repair once the initial inflammation and edema has had time to resolve [36, 37]. This time period would allow for a more comprehensive evaluation of the esophagus and the patients comorbidities.

Not a Candidate for Repair

Occasionally, the patient may not be a surgical candidate for definitive repair of the diaphragm due to severe comorbidities. For the patient who has limited independence, chronic illness or is infirmed and would not tolerate a laparoscopic repair, an alternative would be a gastropexy with a laparoscopic or endoscopic gastrostomy tube. A laparoscopic approach is necessary to make sure the stomach is reduced and not volvulized. Either a laparoscopic gastrostomy tube or endoscopic approach can be used for gastric fixation to the anterior abdominal wall to prevent recurrence of a gastric volvulus. There are two options for gastric fixation: Two gastrostomy tubes can be placed or one gastrostomy tube and gastropexy of the falciform. The second fixation point should prevent recurrent herniation or volvulus [38].

Laparotomy

If there is mucosal ischemia demonstrated on EGD or evidence of ischemia or hemorrhagic fluid on laparoscopy suggesting gastric compromise, one should proceed to a laparotomy. An upper midline or chevron incision can be used to expose the upper abdomen. The surgeon should mobilize the left lobe of the liver to expose the esophageal hiatus and retract the liver to the right with a fixed retractor. Manual reduction of the stomach from the hernia with inferior retraction should proceed with caution. The diaphragmatic defect will commonly require widening laterally to allow for safe gentile reduction of the stomach. Commonly, there may be adhesions preventing complete reduction that can be taken sharply taking care to avoid entering the mediastinum or thoracic space.

At this point, the essential decision is to address either the stomach or the paraesophageal hernia. If there is perforation, ischemia, or any degree of gastric compromise, the procedure becomes primarily a gastric resection. If the stomach is healthy and completely viable, one can proceed to repair the paraesophageal hernia.

In the setting of gastric perforation, the mediastinum and the upper abdomen are contaminated. These patients are commonly in septic shock and may be hemodynamically unstable. At this point, the surgeon must make the decision to proceed with a "damage control surgery." The stomach is mobilized out of the chest. Typically, the greater omentum requires mobilization off the stomach. The goal would be to leave as much viable upper stomach for future reconstruction. The distal line of resection should be beyond the pylorus. A NGT is left in the gastric remnant, and the upper abdomen briskly irrigated. A temporary abdominal closure is placed.

The patient should be transferred to ICU for continued resuscitation and broad-spectrum antibiotic coverage. Once resuscitated, the patient can return to the operating room for definitive enteric reconstruction and diaphragmatic repair. Re-exploration should occur promptly as soon as the patient has been appropriately resuscitated. In the setting of a contaminated surgical field, the tissue will commonly be edematous during the re-operation for reconstruction. This will result in a more friable and edematous operative field.

Reconstruction

Paraesophageal hernias are a real hernia with a true hernia sac including the peritoneal layer [39]. Whether you are doing a reconstruction of the stomach or just a paraesophageal hernia repair, the hernia sac must be dissected free and completely remove from the mediastinum cavity. Care must be taken to avoid entering the thoracic pleura. Gross contamination from gastric perforation or ischemia increases concern for postoperative mediastinitis or empyema. If a hemi-thorax has been violated, it is mandatory to briskly irrigate it and place a thoracostomy tube for drainage.

- Stomach Reconstruction

The stomach should be reconstructed first. The esophageal hiatus should be determined to be below the diaphragm. It may be necessary to free the esophagus from the mediastinum to bring it down into the abdomen. This will be important during the paraesophageal repair. If sufficient amount of gastric pouch is viable, the reconstruction can be completed utilizing a Roux-en-Y reconstruction in standard fashion. A side-to-side gastroenteric (Bilroth II) anastomosis is commonly not possible nor recommended, as it will not reach up near the esophageal hiatus. In the rare occasion where the majority of the stomach is infracted and resected, an esophageal enteric anastomosis will need to be reconstructed. In this setting, a Roux-n-Y reconstruction is recommended with or without a reverse J pouch.

- Paraesophageal Hernia Repair

The next step is to encircle the esophagus with a soft drain (Penrose). Care must be taken to avoid injury to the Vagus nerves. The crural leaves of the diaphragm are identified. During the repair, a large gastric Bougie is placed crossing the GE junction to adequately size the closure. Permanent suture should be used and occasionally pledgets must be used as the tissues may be of poor quality. It is essential that the repair starts on the crux of the crura behind the esophagus and should be continued anteriorly. A few final esophageal pexy sutures can be placed to the diaphragm as this keeps the esophagus from migrating back into the chest [40].

There are limited indications for a gastric fundoplication in this setting as it can only be performed when no gastric resection has been done. Primarily, it would be to protect an injury to the esophagus during dissection. The type of fundoplication used is beyond the scope of this chapter. In this setting, primary repair of the diaphragmatic defect is adequate [41].

A drain should be placed into the mediastinum in all emergent/urgent cases as the rate of mediastinal abscess is high. Additional drains can be placed near the reconstruction and along the diaphragmatic hernia repair.

A nasogastric tube should be placed across the anastomosis or paraesophageal repair for decompression and to wait for resolution of an intestinal ileus. Most commonly, the repair may be studied with a Upper GI series in 3–5 postoperative days to assess for anastomotic leak or stricture of the paraesophageal repair. A feeding jejunostomy tube should be placed at the time of reconstruction for distal feeding in the setting of tenuous reconstructions.

Complications

After an acute paraesophageal herniation, the most common complication is an inadvertent pneumothorax. A chest X-ray should be completed prior to leaving the operating room. If the pneumothorax is small, and the patient is expected to be extubated after an uneventful semi-urgent/elective repair of a paraesophageal hernia, no intervention is needed and a follow-up chest X-ray should be obtained to confirm there is no worsening of the pneumothorax. If the pneumothorax is large, the patient is going to remain intubated or there is any difficulty with oxygenation, a thoracostomy tube should be placed.

A more worrisome thoracic complication is an empyema or effusion. Even without gross spillage, bacterial translocation in the setting of gastric ischemia may lead to intrathoracic infection. A simple effusion can be drained with a pigtail catheter. An empyema will commonly require operative video-assisted thoracic (VATS) drainage washout with apical and dependent chest tubes placed for drainage.

Anastomotic leak is a considerable risk in these patients. Drains should be placed prior to leaving the OR around, the gastric or esophageal anastomosis. If an anastomotic leak develops, a CT scan esophagogram should demonstrate the leak. A well-controlled leak with a well-placed drain can be managed non-operatively. If a patient develops sepsis due to uncontrolled leak, there are several surgical options each with increasing comorbidity. A limited leak needs only re-exploration with washout and placement of better localized drains. It is not recommended to explore the area to any degree as this could disrupt the anastomosis.

Abscess formation is a serious complication of this surgery, especially in the emergent setting. If the drains become purulent or the patient has an unexplained leukocytosis or fever a few days after closure, a CT of the torso may be necessary to look for undrained abscesses. Intra-abdominal abscesses can often be addressed with percutaneous drainage. Occasionally, mediastinal abscesses can be addressed percutaneously, but often they will require operative washout.

Outcomes

In an analysis of the National Surgical Quality Improvement Project database, Bahayani demonstrated there was no difference in mortality between patients undergoing surgical repair immediately or after resuscitation [42]. However, in patients with obstructed paraesophageal hernia, patients undergoing immediate repair had less postoperative sepsis and fewer days in the hospital. In patients without obstruction, Kohler observed the majority of patients with acute symptoms can be treated non-operatively [43]. The urgency of the situation depends on the acuity of your patient.

Clinical Scenario

A 52-year-old man with known history of hiatal hernia presents with upper abdominal discomfort. The patient has no distension and retching but no vomiting. WBC 18k. He is tachycardic to 118 bpm. CXR demonstrates a large intrathoracic gastric bubble. CT scan suggests a large paraesophageal hernia. EGD demonstrates black mucosa over most of the stomach delineated by the diaphragmatic lip.

At this point in the case, the critical issues and the proposed management are as follows;

- Patient presents septic and there is clear evidence of either partial or full thickness ischemia.
- A diagnostic laparoscopy could be considered if the patient is hemodynamically stable and sepsis is not yet a concern.
- In this patient, proceeding immediately to a laparotomy is indicated based on the mucosal ischemia seen on EGD as transmural necrosis must be ruled out.
- The order of the case should be to assess the degree of transmural gastric ischemia and determine the extent of gastric resection required for source control.
- The next step would be to determine whether the patient can proceed with definitive GI reconstruction and repair of the paraesophageal hernia.
- In the setting of full thickness ischemia or perforation, a "damage control surgery" should be considered.
- The actual staged GI reconstruction and hernia repair will be based on the remaining stomach.

Key Questions

1. *The best approach for isolation of the esophagus is from the left or the right?*
2. *When do you do a fundoplication vs. percutaneous endoscopic gastrostomy?*
3. *Should empiric treatment of H. pylori be the done in all peptic ulcer disease? What is your practice with nasogastric decompression?*

References

1. Gauderer MWL, Ponsky JL, Izant RJ Jr. Gastrostomy without laparotomy: a percutaneous endoscopic technique. J Pediatr Surg. 1980;15:872–5.
2. Gauderer MWL. Percutaneous endoscopic gastrostomy-20 years later: a historical perspective. J Pediatr Surg. 2001;36:217–9.
3. Schapiro GD, Edmundowicz SA. Complications of percutaneous endoscopic gastrostomy. Gastrointest Endosc Clin North Am. 1996; 6:409–422.

4. Schrag SP, Sharma R, Jaik NP, et al. Complications related to percutaneous endoscopic. Gastrostomy (PEG) tubes. A Comprehensive clinical review. J Gastrointest Liver Dis. 2007;16:407–418.
5. Rosenberger LH, Newhook T, Schirmer B, et al. Late accidental dislodgement of a percutaneous endoscopic gastrostomy tube: an underestimated burden on patients and the health care system. Surg Endosc. 2011;25:3307–11.
6. Marshall JB, Bodnarchuk G, Barthel JS. Early accidental dislodgement of PEG tubes. J Clin Gastroenterol. 1994;18:210–2.
7. Galat SA, Gerig KD, Porter JA, et al. Management of premature removal of the percutaneous gastrostomy. Am Surg. 1990;56(11):733–6.
8. Sandven P, Qvist H, Skovlund E, et al. Significance of Candida recovered from intraoperative specimens in patients with intra-abdominal perforations. Crit Care Med. 2002;30(3):541–7.
9. Mincheff TV. Early dislodgement of percutaneous and endoscopic gastrostomy tube. J S C Med Assoc. 2007;103(1):13–5.
10. Sawyer RG, Claridge JA, Nathens AB, et al. Trial of short-course antimicrobial therapy for intraabdominal infection. N Engl J Med. 2015;372:1996–2005.
11. Marks JM, Ponsky JL, Pearl JP, et al. PEG "Rescue": a practical NOTES technique. Surg Endosc. 2007;21:816–9.
12. Timratana P, El-Hayek K, Shimizu H, et al. Percutaneous endoscopic gastrostomy (PEG) with T-fasteners obviates the need for emergent replacement after early tube dislodgement. Surg Endosc. 2012;26:3541–7.
13. Bertleff MJOE, Lange JF. Perforated peptic ulcer disease: a review of history and treatment. Dig Surg. 2010;27:161–9.
14. Lau JY, Sung J, Hill C, et al. Systematic review of the epidemiology of complicated peptic ulcer disease: incidence, recurrence, risk factors and mortality. Digestion. 2011;84:102–13.
15. Thorsen K, Søreide JA, Terje Kvaløy J, et al. Epidemiology of perforated peptic ulcer: age- and gender adjusted analysis of incidence and mortality. World J Gastroenterol. 2013; 19(3):347–54.
16. Boey J, Wong J. Perforated duodenal ulcers. World J Surg. 1987;11(3):319–24.
17. Thorsen K, Søreide JA, Søreide K. Scoring systems for outcome prediction in patients with perforated peptic ulcer. Scand J Trauma, Resuscitation Emerg Med. 2013;21:25. doi:10.1186/1757-7241-21-25.
18. Thorsen K, Søreide JA, Søreide K. What is the best predictor of mortality in perforated peptic ulcer disease? A population-based, multivariable regression analysis including three clinical scoring systems. J Gastrointest Surg. 2014;18:1261–8.
19. Donovan AJ, Berne TV, Donovan JA. Perforated duodenal ulcer: an alternative therapeutic plan. Arch Surg. 1998;133:1166–71.
20. Crofts TJ, Park KGM, Steele RJC, et al. A randomized trial of non-operative management for perforated peptic ulcer. NEJM. 1989;32(15):970–3.
21. Songne B, Jean F, Foulatier O, et al. Non-operative treatment for perforated peptic ulcer: results of a prospective study. Ann Chir. 2004;129(10):578–82.
22. Moulya C, Chatib R, Scotté M, et al. Therapeutic management of perforated gastro-duodenal ulcer: literature review. J Visceral Surg. 2013;150:333–40.
23. Wright GP, Davis AT, Koehler TJ, et al. Cost-efficiency and outcomes in the treatment of perforated peptic ulcer disease: laparoscopic versus open approach. Surgery. 2014;156: 1003–8.
24. Schietroma M, Piccione F, Carlei F, et al. Peritonitis from perforated peptic ulcer and immune response. J Invest Surg. 2013;26:294–304.
25. Teoh AYB, Chiu PWY, Kok ASY, et al. The selective use of laparoscopic repair is safe in high-risk patients suffering from perforated peptic ulcer. World J Surg. 2015;39:740–5.
26. Kim JH, Chin HM, Bae YJ, et al. Risk factors associated with conversion of laparoscopic simple closure in perforated duodenal ulcer. Int J Surg. 2015;15:40–4.
27. Noguiera C, Silva AS, Santos JN, et al. Perforated peptic ulcer: main factors of morbidity and mortality. World J Surg. 2003;27(7):782–7.

28. Hunt JL. Generalized peritonitis. To irrigate or not to irrigate the abdominal cavity. Arch Surg. 1982;117(2):209–12.
29. Verma R, Nelson RL. Prophylactic nasogastric decompression after abdominal surgery. Cochrane Database Syst Rev. 2007;3:CD004929. doi:10.1002/14651858.CD004929.pub3.
30. Wong CS, Chia CF, Lee HC, et al. Eradication of helicobacter pylori for prevention of ulcer recurrence after simple closure of perforated peptic ulcer: a meta-analysis of randomized controlled trials. J Surg Res. 2013;182:219–26.
31. Malfertheiner P, Megraud F, O'Morain CA, et al. Management of helicobacter pylori infection —the Maastricht IV/Florence consensus report. Gut 2012; 61:646e664. doi:10.1136/gutjnl-2012-302084.
32. Dean C, et al. Hiatal hernias. Surg Radiol Anat. 2012;34(4):291–9.
33. Carter R, Brewer LA 3rd, Hinshaw DB. Acute gastric volvulus. A study of 25 cases. Am J Surg. 1980;140(1):99–106.
34. Polomsky M1, Jones CE, Sepesi B, O'Connor M, Matousek A, Hu R, Raymond DP, Litle VR, Watson TJ, Peters JH. Should elective repair of intrathoracic stomach be encouraged? J Gastrointest Surg. 2010;14(2):203–210.
35. Carrott PW1, Hong J, Kuppusamy M, Koehler RP, Low DE. Clinical ramifications of giant paraesophageal hernias are underappreciated: making the case for routine surgical repair. Ann Thorac Surg. 2012;94(2):421–426; discussion 426–428.
36. Carrott PW1, Hong J, Kuppusamy M, Kirtland S, Koehler RP, Low DE. Repair of giant paraesophageal hernias routinely produces improvement in respiratory function. J Thorac Cardiovasc Surg. 2012;143(2):398–404.
37. Bawahab M, et al. Management of acute paraesophageal hernia. Surg Endosc. 2009; 23(2):255–9.
38. Polomsky M1, Jones CE, Sepesi B, O'Connor M, Matousek A, Hu R, Raymond DP, Litle VR, Watson TJ, Peters JH. Should elective repair of intrathoracic stomach be encouraged? J Gastrointest Surg. 2010;14(2):203–210.
39. Köhler G, Koch OO, Antoniou SA, Emmanuel K, Pointner R. "Acute intrathoracic stomach!" How should we deal with complicated type IV paraesophageal hernias? Hernia. 2015;19 (4):627–33.
40. Ponsky J, et al. Anterior gastropexy may reduce the recurrence rate after laparoscopic paraesophageal hernia repair. Surg Endosc. 2003;17(7):1036–41.
41. Kaiser LR, Singhal S. Surgical foundations: essentials of thoracic surgery. 2004: Elsevier Mosby. Gulf Professional Publishing, Houston.
42. Houghton SG1, Deschamps C, Cassivi SD, Nichols FC, Allen MS, Pairolero PC. The influence of transabdominal gastroplasty: early outcomes of hiatal hernia repair. J Gastrointest Surg. 2007;11(1):101–106.
43. Pallabazzer G1, Santi S, Parise P, Solito B, Giusti P, Rossi M. Giant hiatal hernias: direct hiatus closure has an acceptable recurrence rate. Updates Surg. 2011;63(2):75–81.
44. Bhayani NH, et al. Wait only to resuscitate: early surgery for acutely presenting paraesophageal hernias yields better outcomes. Surg Endosc. 2013;27(1):267–71.
45. Kohler G, et al. "Acute intrathoracic stomach!" How should we deal with complicated type IV paraesophageal hernias? Hernia. 2015;19(4):627–33.
46. Schenarts PJ, Maness MR, Pender IV JR. Incarcerated Paraesophageal Hernia. In Common Problems in Acute Care Surgery. New York: Springer; 2013. p. 203–210. (05 Feb 2013)
47. Jeyarajah DR, Harford WV Jr. Abdominal hernias and gastric volvulus. New York: Springer; 2013.

Chapter 9
The Complicated Cholecystectomy and Management of Perforation Post-ERCP

Gregory R. English and Andrew B. Peitzman

The Complicated Cholecystectomy

With a difficult cholecystectomy, the collateral damage of a bile duct injury is never an acceptable outcome. Because of this, conversion to open cholecystectomy should not be considered a failure. The operation is safely performed and the anatomy to prevent this complication is clearly defined, whether laparoscopic or open. It is important to recognize and avoid pitfalls that could lead to bile duct injury as cholecystectomy is performed. We will discuss what we feel is a safe approach to the difficult gallbladder and techniques for avoiding trouble in this chapter.

Predicting the Difficult Cholecystectomy

Certain preoperative factors are predictive of the patient for whom cholecystectomy may be difficult and where a higher rate of conversion is anticipated. These include male patients, age >70 years, inflammation, duration of symptoms during both an acute episode and chronicity and duration of symptoms with recurrent disease, repeated bouts of cholecystitis, impacted stone, gallbladder wall thickness, pericholecystic fluid, elevated white blood cell count, previous upper abdominal surgery, or contracted gallbladder wall on imaging [1]. Acute inflammation compounding a contracted gallbladder may be the most dangerous of circumstances.

G.R. English
UPMC Hamot, Erie, PA, USA
e-mail: englishgr@upmc.edu

A.B. Peitzman (✉)
Department of Surgery, University of Pittsburgh Medical Center,
UPMC Presbyterian, Pittsburgh, PA 15213, USA
e-mail: peitzmanab@upmc.edu

J.J. Diaz and D.T. Efron (eds.), *Complications in Acute Care Surgery*,
DOI 10.1007/978-3-319-42376-0_9

Cholecystectomy: Performing It Safely

When performing difficult gallbladder surgery, one must adhere to key surgical basics to perform the procedure safely and to avoid pitfalls without risking collateral damage. The safest plane for dissection in a cholecystectomy, open or laparoscopic, is on the wall of the gallbladder. Dissection away from the wall of the gallbladder will lead to trouble and increase the risk of complication. It is far better to get into the gallbladder itself rather than risking injury to a surrounding structure.

The essentials for safe laparoscopic cholecystectomy begin using a high-definition angled laparoscope (30° or 45°) to take full advantage of visualizing the anatomy from different angles constantly throughout the operation. Hunter describes many of these key basic principles of safe laparoscopy in his classic article [2]. It is critical to follow these principles in the setting of severe inflammation or with uncertain anatomy. The image portrays and describes his laparoscopic technique below (Fig. 9.1) [2]. The key principles for safe laparoscopic cholecystectomy include the following [1, 2]:

1. 30° or 45° high-definition laparoscope
2. Cephalad traction on the dome of the gallbladder
3. Lateral traction on the infundibulum and finding the gallbladder wall and staying on it
4. Dissection from above down to the neck
5. Widely opening the hepatocystic triangle

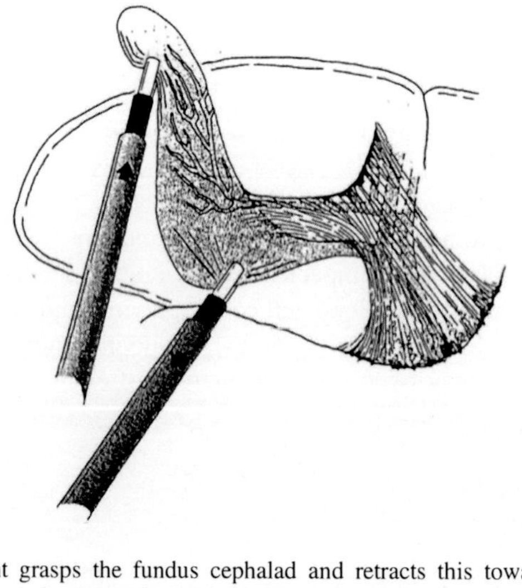

Fig. 9.1 The assistant grasps the fundus cephalad and retracts this toward the patient's right shoulder. This reduces redundancy in the infundibulum and exposes the cystic duct. A second grasper retracts the infundibulum laterally to make the cystic duct perpendicular to the common bile duct and again to separate the gallbladder from the common bile duct. From Hunter et al. [2, Fig. 1], with permission of Elsevier

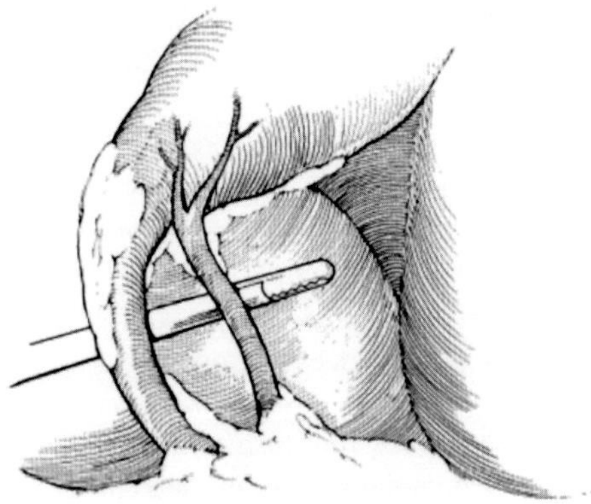

Fig. 9.2 The "critical view of safety." The triangle of Calot is dissected free of all tissues except for cystic duct and artery, and the base of the liver bed is exposed. At least one-third of the gallbladder should be dissected off the liver. When this view is achieved, the two structures entering the gallbladder can only be the cystic duct and artery. It is not mandatory to see the common bile duct. From Strasberg et al. [3, Fig. 2] with permission of Elsevier

6. Moving the infundibulum back and forth (wave the flag), repeatedly looking at both sides of the gallbladder
7. Critical view of safety
8. Dividing the cystic duct as close to the gallbladder as possible
9. Never dividing the cystic duct with any cauterizing instrument—if it turns out to be the common bile duct, the resulting ischemic injury will only lessen the chances for a good repair.

A safe technique for laparoscopic gallbladder surgery should ideally proceed with the critical view of safety prior to dividing any important anatomic structure (Fig. 9.2) [3]. Three criteria are required to achieve the critical view of safety:

(a) The triangle of Calot is cleared from fibrous tissue or fat
(b) The lower one-third of the gallbladder is separated from the liver to expose the proper view
(c) Only two structures should be seen entering the gallbladder (cystic duct and cystic artery).

Pitfalls Leading to Bile Duct Injury

Common factors include anatomic variation, acute inflammation, chronic scarring, misperception, and error traps that can lead to bile duct injury. Misperception by the surgeon of what he or she is seeing in the operative field is a common factor in the events leading to a duct injury. Bile duct injury occurs far more frequently from the common bile duct or right hepatic duct misidentified as the cystic duct (meaning normal anatomy) rather than an anatomic anomaly as the etiology of the bile duct injury. The surgeon sees what he or she believes and does not believe what he or she sees leading to injury [4].

Different dissection techniques have been described during laparoscopic cholecystectomy. Strasberg and colleagues [3, 5] discuss error traps when performing laparoscopic cholecystectomy. An error trap is an operative approach that works in most circumstances, but is prone to fail under certain circumstances. Because these techniques usually work, the surgeon develops confidence in them and fails to recognize when dangerous circumstances are present; it is important to recognize and avoid these error traps. Common dissection techniques for cholecystectomy include the infundibular, the fundus first (top-down) technique, and the semi-top-down approach 1. For an open cholecystectomy, the cholecystectomy is performed from the top-down—this is the safest approach to cholecystectomy. With the development of laparoscopic cholecystectomy, an infundibulum first approach was technically easier and thus promulgated. Thus, we apply an operation laparoscopically violating principles of safety for open cholecystectomy; this approach contributes to many of the complications with laparoscopic cholecystectomy. The semi-top-down approach and top-down approaches are safer approaches to the operation. When approaching the very difficult gallbladder, top-down is the preferred approach to cholecystectomy, whether open or laparoscopic.

The infundibular technique is a technique that works the majority of the time, but will fail in predictable circumstances, specifically anatomic variation or inflammation. This approach involves starting from the infundibulum and then working toward the fundus. In this technique, it is taught that the taper between infundibulum and cystic duct identifies the cystic duct. In a single view, this can be misleading, especially with any inflammation, short cystic duct, or a "parallel union" cystic duct. In these cases, the common duct can be mistakenly divided, believing it is the cystic duct ("infundibular view error trap") (Fig. 9.3) [3]. This produces the classic injury with resection of a portion of the common bile duct; concomitant right hepatic artery injury occurs in 25 % of these cases. The variability of the right posterior hepatic duct includes drainage into the cystic duct, gallbladder neck, or common hepatic duct (Fig. 9.4) [6]. With the infundibular approach to the gallbladder, injury to such an aberrant posterior right hepatic duct would be nearly unavoidable when present.

Conversion from laparoscopic to open cholecystectomy and a top-down approach still harbors danger, as conversion has generally occurred because of inflammation and obliteration of normal anatomic planes. The error trap with a top-down cholecystectomy again is caused by what is normally safe, applied in a dangerous situation. Strasberg states that the worst injuries occur in those patients who undergo conversion from laparoscopic to open cholecystectomy, performed top-down because of marked inflammation and difficult dissection. In the difficult gallbladder, the perceived safe operative plane coming down the medial wall of the gallbladder is obliterated by an inflammatory reaction, which incorporates the right-sided porta hepatis and the common bile duct. Thus, injury is commonly

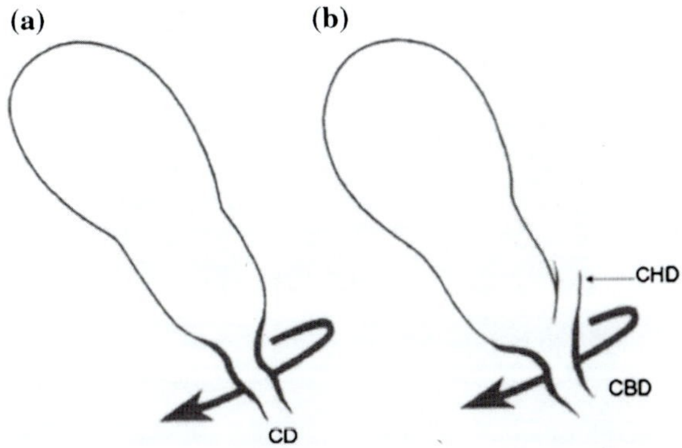

Fig. 9.3 The deception of the hidden cystic duct and the infundibular technique of laparoscopic cholecystectomy. *Left* appearance to surgeon when a duct appearing to be the cystic duct is dissected first. Note that the duct appears to flare (*heavy black line*), giving the appearance that the cystic duct has been followed onto the infundibulum. *Right* true anatomic situation in the case of some classical injuries. From Strasberg et al. [3, Fig. 3], with permission of Elsevier

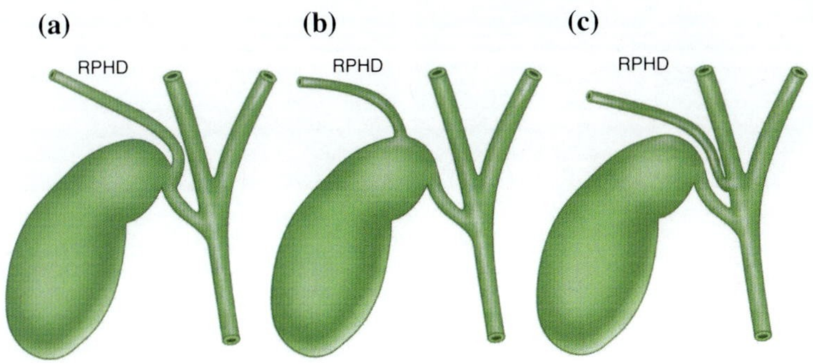

Fig. 9.4 Common anomalies of the posterior right hepatic duct [6, Fig. 4], with permission of Elsevier]

associated with major biliary and vascular injury, at times requiring liver resection for the ischemic injury [5].

The laparoscopic fundus first (top-down) technique mimics an open cholecystectomy. Certainly, with acute inflammation, this is the preferred approach. However, this can be awkward laparoscopically with a normal, particularly a large, gallbladder because of the floppiness of the gallbladder when it is fully detached from the liver. The semi-top-down technique of laparoscopic cholecystectomy combines the advantages of both approaches and minimizes the disadvantages [1]. Dissection is started higher on the gallbladder, above the infundibulum of the gallbladder (Fig. 9.5a–e). The peritoneum is scored circumferentially, lateral side first, coming across the peritoneum over the infundibulum of the gallbladder, and then opening the peritoneum coming up the medial side of the gallbladder, being

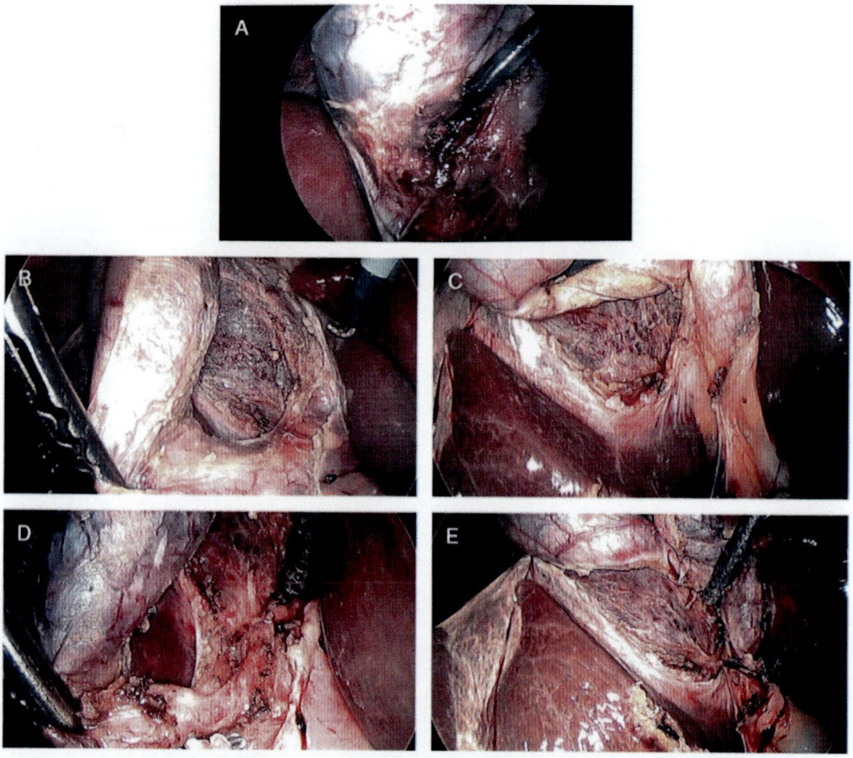

Fig. 9.5 Technique of semi-top-down laparoscopic cholecystectomy. **a** Dissection is started on the gallbladder, above the infundibulum of the gallbladder. The peritoneum is scored circumferentially, lateral side first, coming across the peritoneum over the infundibulum of the gallbladder, and then opening the peritoneum coming up the medial side of the gallbladder, being careful not to enter the cystic artery as you do so. Dissection of the gallbladder off the liver is being completed here on the lateral aspect of the gallbladder. **b** and **c** Then by rolling the gallbladder from the one side to the other, the gallbladder can be fully detached from the liver, leaving only the fundus attached, to provide full exposure. **d** At this point and only at this point is the infundibulum and its junction with the cystic duct approached, thus generating a top-down approach to the infundibulum, cystic duct, and cystic artery. When proceeding with the semi-top-down taking only tissues that you see through clearly, any structures that may be encountered such as an aberrant duct, right hepatic artery, or posterior cystic artery can be seen and avoided. **e** An exaggerated critical view of safety has resulted. The cystic artery has been divided, and the cystic duct is clearly defined and ready for clipping and division. From Peitzman et al. [1, Fig. 5], with permission of Wolters/Kluwer

careful not to enter the cystic artery as you do so. Then, by rolling the gallbladder back and forth, the gallbladder can be largely detached from the liver, leaving only the fundus attached to again provide easy retraction. At this point and only at this point is the infundibulum and its junction with the cystic duct approached, thus generating a top-down approach to the cystic duct and cystic artery. When proceeding with the semi-top-down taking only tissues that you see through clearly, any structures that may be encountered such as an aberrant duct, right hepatic artery, or posterior cystic artery can be seen and avoided. At this point in the operation, what you have generated is an exaggerated critical view of safety. It is now clear which structures are cystic artery and cystic duct; these structures can now be safely clipped and divided.

Operative Techniques for the Difficult Gallbladder

Operating on an acutely inflamed gallbladder for acute cholecystitis or hydrops is one of the most common challenges faced by an acute care surgeon. When seeing this laparoscopically and recognizing the need to open for safety, the surgeon must consider how sick the patient is, whether the patient can tolerate an open cholecystectomy, and whether the structures of the porta hepatis be safely avoided before proceeding. If it is clear that the patient is too ill or the anatomy is too hazardous from the inflammation, then cholecystostomy is the appropriate choice. However, when the decision is made to move forward with an open operation in the setting of significant inflammation, hydrops, or difficult anatomy, it should involve a paradigm shift in operative strategy as compared with the straightforward cholecystectomy. The strategy should now focus on the protection of the portal structures by knowing where to be and where not to be—staying only on the wall of the gallbladder (at times submucosa) at all times. The surgeon must know that in this setting, persistent attempts at obtaining the classical critical view of safety can lead to biliary or vascular injury; "no attempt is made to dissect the cystic duct or cystic artery when inflammation obscures the neck of the gallbladder" [7]. The key to the open operation in a difficult gallbladder is finding the wall and staying on/in the wall of the gallbladder. It is important to identify this correct plane and not drift outside of it into the liver bed as this can lead to significant bleeding and can increase the risk of ductal or vascular injury. The middle hepatic vein courses within millimeters of the gallbladder fossa normally with a branch of the middle hepatic vein within the fossa in 20 %. Particularly when performing cholecystectomy for acute cholecystitis, drifting off the wall of the gallbladder may result in life-threatening hemorrhage with injury to the middle hepatic vein.

A hydropic, acutely inflamed gallbladder is analogous to an onion with multiple peels of inflammatory tissue. These layers are carefully dissected to safely get onto the wall of the gallbladder (often the submucosa) and complete the dissection in this plane 1. This echos back to the fundamentals of gallbladder surgery—the safest plane for dissection, open or laparoscopic, is on the wall of the gallbladder.

Viewing the Gallbladder from Within

When difficult conditions such as severe inflammation exist in Calot's triangle, sometimes the safest and best approach is to view the anatomy from the inside of gallbladder where the surgeon knows it is safe. Hubert et al. [8] describes using this approach in patients with anomalous ductal structures, gangrenous cholecystitis, and scleroatrophic cholecystitis. The fundus of the gallbladder can be entered at a safe point, which provides decompression of the gallbladder and gives the surgeon the ability to visualize the infundibulum and cystic duct from within the gallbladder itself. This technique as it allows the ability to place a finger or probe into the gallbladder itself and provides the trajectory and course of the infundibulum and cystic duct, helping to guide the direction of dissection as the inflamed triangle is approached. This is especially helpful in the situation where the triangle itself is obliterated and has become a large phlegmonous mass. This approach is usually followed by subtotal (partial) cholecystectomy.

Partial or Subtotal Cholecystectomy

Partial cholecystectomy is a method to deal with the difficult open gallbladder without risking damage to the liver bed or structures near Calot's triangle in the setting of severe inflammation. The lateral, medial, and anterior walls of the gallbladder are excised using the electrocautery. The densely adherent posterior wall is left on the liver. The mucosa is fully cauterized to eliminate the mucus secreting cells. As you proceed proximally with this technique, you are now within the infundibulum of the gallbladder and visualizing infundibulum and cystic duct from within. Visible stones can be extracted at this time. The mucosa can then be oversewn from within the gallbladder with a purse string suture, being certain not to get to deep putting the portal structures at risk.

Another option, if the gallbladder can safely be taken off the liver but the infundibulum is markedly inflamed, is amputation of the gallbladder at the infundibulum [8]. Dissection can often be continued in a safe plane, separating peritoneum off the gallbladder wall until the point where the infundibulum is reached. The infundibulum is then transected rather than continuing dissection below this point into an area of severe inflammation. This, once again, allows the anatomy of the infundibulum and cystic duct to be identified from within the gallbladder itself.

At this point, the surgeon is left with a gallbladder trumpet, and the cystic duct mucosa can be oversewn from within using suture in a purse string fashion. Some surgeons would just elect to oversew the infundibular trumpet at this point. If too much infundibulum is left with a partial cholecystectomy, it puts the patient at a potential risk for recurrent symptoms by closing off this space and leaving an enclosed remnant portion of the gallbladder which most likely already has proximal cystic duct obstruction. If the infundibular itself cannot be closed safely ($\sim 12\ \%$ of these cases), a closed suction drain is simply left. In the setting of severe inflammation or hydrops, it is likely that the cystic duct is completely obstructed and therefore unlikely to cause a postoperative bile leak. Also, the infundibular tissue is often inflamed and unlikely to hold suture in the long term. In the setting where a bile leak was to develop in the postoperative setting, this area is already controlled with a surgical drain and can be managed with ERCP.

Adjuncts for Identification of Biliary Anatomy

Intraoperative cholangiography (IOC) is a useful tool during a difficult cholecystectomy. We selectively perform IOC for patients with a history suggestive of common duct stones, pancreatitis, jaundice, or any question of the biliary anatomy during the operation. The debate still continues as to whether all patients should have routine cholangiography. However, the results appear to be conflicting and are beyond the scope of this chapter. IOC is recommended, if not a necessity, in any situation where the biliary anatomy is unclear to help identify structures and prevent injury. Certainly, in any situation where there is a concern for possible bile duct injury, IOC remains a first-line approach for identification. Bile duct injury found early on IOC can lead to prompt diagnosis and treatment of these injuries.

Laparoscopic ultrasonography (LUS) is an alternative to IOC for the intraoperative assessment of biliary anatomy. LUS can delineate the common bile duct, cystic duct–common bile duct junction, and choledocholithiasis. It also allows the intraoperative identification of vascular structures such as the hepatic artery, portal vein, and anomalous vascular anatomy which IOC does not. However, there is a steep learning curve for the use of intraoperative ultrasonography. One must keep in mind for both IOC and LUS that the results are only as good as the surgeon's ability to identify and understand what he is looking at when using these adjuncts.

What to Do When a Bile Duct Injury Is Recognized

If recognized intraoperatively, the surgeon must assess his or her ability to repair the injury. The best result comes from early repair by a surgeon experienced in doing so; the first repair has the best outcome in skilled hands. Except in the very unusual circumstances, a duct-to-duct anastomosis is avoided. A tension-free Roux-en-Y should be performed. If the surgeon does not have an extensive experience with such a repair, the bile duct should be left alone. In this case, a drain is placed immediately next to the duct and the patient is transferred. The expertise of the surgeon dealing with this complication will impact outcome.

Management of Perforation Post-ERCP

Although endoscopic retrograde cholangiopancreatography is a commonly performed procedure, pancreaticobiliary and duodenal perforations are relatively rare complications. In three large retrospective studies, the perforation risk for ERCP was 0.45–0.6 % [9–11]. The need to operate for this complication is even less common. The majority of patients who suffer ERCP perforation can be treated non-operatively. In two larger studies, the successful non-operative management rate was 63 % [10] and 71 % [9] following ERCP perforation. Risk factors for ERCP perforation include sphincterotomy, previous ERCP, sphincter of Oddi dysfunction, Billroth II anatomy, and periampullary diverticulum. The major question regarding ERCP perforation is who needs an operation and who can be managed conservatively with the non-operative management.

Predictors of ERCP Perforation and Need for Surgical Intervention

As one would expect, patients undergoing ERCP for a therapeutic intervention are more likely to suffer perforation than those who are having a strictly diagnostic ERCP. The mechanism of ERCP perforation can result from passage of the guidewire (32 %), sphincterotomy (15 %), passage of the endoscope (11 %), cannulation of the bile duct (11 %), stent insertion (8 %), or stricture dilation (7 %) in one study with 12,427 patients [9]. The mechanism of injury and site of injury are indicative of the need for surgical intervention. Guidewire-related injuries are less likely to require surgical management, whereas injury caused by difficult passage of the endoscope or those caused by sphincterotomy are more likely to require surgical intervention. Perforations of the duodenum are more likely to require surgical intervention when compared to perforations of the bile duct (Table 9.1) [9, 10].

The indication for ERCP also appears to play a role in determining who will require operative management. Patients undergoing ERCP for sphincter of Oddi dysfunction are not only more likely to suffer perforation, but also more likely to require surgical repair in multiple studies. Patients who undergo ERCP for

Table 9.1 Perforation during ERCP (N = 75) (8)

	Laparotomy (n = 22)	Non-operative (n = 53)
Mechanism		
Guidewire (%)	14	41
Passing scope (%)	32	2
Cannulation (%)	9	11
Dilatation (%)	0	10
Sphincterotomy (%)	18	13
Stent placement (%)	9	10
Unknown (%)	18	13
Location		
Duodenum (%)	86	28
Bile duct (%)	10	60
Pancreatic duct (%)	4	0
Unknown (%)	0	12

jaundice/biliary stricture generally have guidewire-associated injuries and are more likely to succeed with the non-operative management. Patients requiring biliary stenting for multiple reasons are also more likely to be successfully managed with the non-operative management. Stenting may have a protective effect by diverting bile into the duodenum instead of the retroperitoneum or intraperitoneal space [9, 10].

Injury Classification

An injury classification system has been developed for post-ERCP perforation [11–14]. The type of injury is listed in descending order of severity and correlates with the mechanism of injury and the anatomic location of the damage. This can be used as a predictor of the need for surgical intervention as well in many instances. The locations of these injuries are detailed in Fig. 9.6. These types of injuries are described as types I–IV and are described as follows [11–14]:

(a) Type I injuries—these are caused by the endoscope passage and tend to occur along the lateral or medial duodenal wall. These perforations tend to be large and remote from the ampulla and often require immediate surgery.
(b) Type II injuries—these are peri-Vaterian injuries and vary in severity, but typically are smaller and less likely to require surgery than Type I injuries. These are often associated with sphincterotomy or associated periampullary diverticulum.

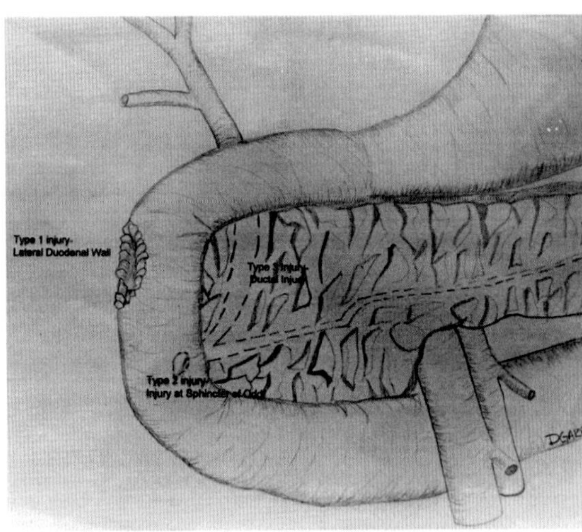

Fig. 9.6 Classification of post-ERCP perforations into types I through III based on anatomic location and mechanism of injury (type IV not shown). From Stapfer et al. [14, Fig. 1], with permission of Wolters/Kluwer

(c) Type III injuries—these represent injuries to the distal bile duct and are often related to wire instrumentation and are often small.
(d) Type IV injuries—these represent findings of retroperitoneal air alone and result from over-insufflation during ERCP. These are managed non-operatively.

Determining When to Operate

Certainly, the reason for ERCP, mechanism of endoscopic injury, and site of perforation help predict who will require surgical intervention. However, the most important decision for the acute care surgeon is to decide upon whom to operate and who to manage non-operatively. A 4-point scoring system was developed to help determine patients best managed by operative intervention using the easily available clinical data. One point was assigned for fever, tachycardia, guarding, and leukocytosis. By using this system, Knudson et al. reported that all patients with a score of 4 required operation. In the operative group, 83 % of patients scored 3 or 4. Conversely, 83 % of patients with a score of 0 or 1 were successfully managed non-operatively [10].

Imaging studies have been used to provide guidance in determining operative need. However, because of the use of insufflated air during endoscopy, the amount of free intraperitoneal or retroperitoneal air may not reliably correlate with patients who require an operation. The extent of retroperitoneal air relates more to the degree of manipulation and the amount of insufflation after an injury than to the type or size of the perforation [12, 13]. Contrast studies can be helpful to evaluate the size and location of perforation and appear to correlate with the need for surgery better than intraperitoneal or retroperitoneal gas. Consideration should be made for surgical intervention if there is an evidence of extensive contrast extravasation seen from the duodenum as these rarely resolve with the non-operative management.

Patients with lateral duodenal wall injuries or injuries identified as being remote from the papilla (Type I) will do best with immediate surgical exploration and repair. Many duodenal injuries represent large free tears into the peritoneal cavity and usually occur secondary to a difficult passage of the endoscope. If the tears are significant in size, these can often be recognized at the time of endoscopy and are often difficult to repair endoscopically. Delaying surgery in this group will lose the time window for primary repair for these injuries. Delaying surgery allows the inflammation and tissue damage secondary to a large duodenal leak to progress. Periampullary perforations (Type II) can often be managed non-operatively unless surgery is indicated for retained stones or progressing systemic toxicity. Likewise, the majority of ductal perforations (Type III) from guidewire injury can be managed non-operatively [8, 12, 14, 15].

Fatima utilizes a helpful algorithm for determining operative versus non-operative management when faced with post-ERCP perforation (Fig. 9.7) [9]. This clinical algorithm, combined with the previously described 4-point scoring system and injury classification system, can help direct the surgeon in determining those patients who will require surgical exploration.

Non-operative Management of ERCP Perforations

Non-operative management consists of systemic support with broad-spectrum antibiotics and intravenous fluids along with nasogastric or nasoduodenal decompression of the patient. Endoscopic management can play a role in non-operative management when perforation is recognized at the time of endoscopy. Patients with periampullary (Type II) or bile duct injuries (Type III) during ERCP can often be managed with the endoscopic biliary stent placement or placement of a nasobiliary drain. Endoscopic stent placement allows diversion of the bile into the duodenum and away from the intraperitoneal or retroperitoneal cavity in the face of perforation. A more controversial subject is endoscopic placement of clips for duodenal perforation (Type I). If a small injury to the duodenum is identified at the time of endoscopy and can be easily closed with clipping, this may be a feasible option. However, often Type I injuries are large in size and will not completely seal with clips alone. This makes endoscopic therapy intuitively unwise in this setting.

Using the criteria in the previous section of this chapter, it is important to assure that the right patient is selected for the non-operative management and that they do not meet criteria for immediate exploration. Certainly, if the patient fails non-operative therapy and clinically becomes toxic, operative intervention is indicated. Surgeons should have a low threshold to convert to surgical management in the setting of worsening abdominal pain, leukocytosis, continued fevers, or follow-up imaging studies, suggesting worsening contamination and lack of improvement with the non-operative treatment.

Operative Management of ERCP Perforation

Operative management after ERCP perforation should focus on three basic surgical principles. First, the injury is repaired when at all possible. Second, bile or GI contents are diverted away from the area of the repair when the strength or location of the repair is in question. Third, drains are placed for control of contamination.

We find the injury classification system to be a useful tool when considering the type of repair to perform following ERCP perforation. In many ways, management of these injuries is similar to the treatment of trauma to the duodenum or biliary tree. For Type I injuries, repair will be lateral or away from the ampulla itself. When these injuries are recognized early and are not extensive, primary duodenal repair is the option of choice. In the setting of a large duodenal perforation, or with delayed diagnosis and significant contamination, more extensive surgery is required for control. In this scenario, repair of the injury when possible combined with pyloric

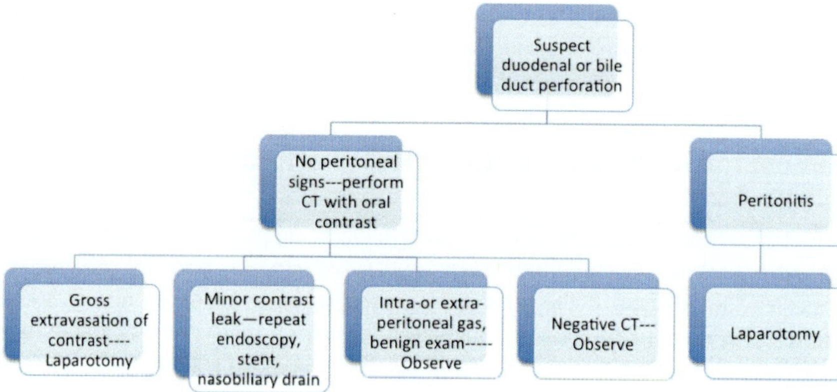

Fig. 9.7 Suspected perforation following ERCP (8)

exclusion and gastrojejunostomy is the appropriate option [16]. This allows diversion of enteric contents away from the site of perforation and should be combined with wide surgical drainage at all times.

Patients requiring Type II repair are particularly challenging given the periampullary location of injury. In these patients, achieving a repair is more complicated and often requires duodenal diversion. The difficulty is a combination of the location of injury and also the fact that often these patients are those who fail non-operative management. Because of this, contamination and inflammation are often extensive at the time of surgery, making a solid primary repair almost impossible. These injuries are often best managed using pyloric exclusion and gastrojejunostomy. Depending on the extent of the periampullary damage, and possible associated involvement of the adjacent bile duct, T-tube placement may be needed versus biliary bypass through hepaticojejunostomy to divert the bile flow away from this area. Often, if bile duct diversion is required, cholecystectomy is performed as well during the operation [11]. Once again, wide surgical drainage is a must.

Type III injuries are often treated successfully with the non-operative management with or without endoscopic biliary stent placement. However, if the patient does require operative intervention, the injury is to the bile duct in this scenario and does not involve the duodenum. Managing this injury consists of using a T-tube placement for control of small defects or biliary diversion with hepaticojejunostomy for larger injuries. Type IV injuries are those associated with over-insufflation and therefore, from a surgical prospective, do not truly represent an "injury" with regard to an area of perforation requiring surgical repair.

It is also important to mention that any primary underlying disease process causing biliary obstruction for which the patient initially underwent ERCP should also be dealt with at the time of surgical intervention. The caveat to this is if the obstruction was successfully alleviated prior to the perforation occurring. These may include common duct stones, masses, or strictures of the bile duct resulting in biliary obstruction. Patients may require common bile duct exploration, biliary bypass, or resection pending on the etiologies of the disease process causing the obstruction.

Clinical Scenario

28 yo woman 6 weeks post-partum presented with increased LFT, total bilirubin, normal amylase, and lipase. US demonstrated acute cholecystitis and CBD stones. Preoperative ERCP was performed, and stones were cleared from CBD. At laparoscopy the following day, peri-portal area with pneumatosis, bile staining of Morrison's pouch, and acute gangrenous cholecystitis were found.

Response:

Operating on an acutely inflamed gallbladder for acute cholecystitis or hydrops is one of the most common challenges faced by an acute care surgeon.

When seeing this laparoscopically and recognizing the need to open for safety, the surgeon must consider how sick the patient is, whether the patient can tolerate an open cholecystectomy, and whether the structures of the porta hepatis be safely avoided before proceeding.

The need to operate for this complication is even less common. The majority of patients who suffer ERCP perforation can be treated non-operatively.

Perforations of the duodenum are more likely to require surgical intervention when compared to perforations of the bile duct.

Key Questions

1. *What is role leaving the back wall of the gallbladder in place during resection?*
2. *What is the preferred method of identifying the cystic duct in the inflamed operative field?*

References

1. Peitzman AB, Watson GA, Marsh JW. Acute cholecystitis: when to operate and how to do it safely. J Trauma Acute Care Surg. 2015;78(1):1–12.
2. Hunter J. Avoidance of bile duct injury during laparoscopic cholecystectomy. Am J Surg 1991;162:71–6.
3. Strasberg SM, Eagon CJ, Drebin JA. The "hidden cystic duct" syndrome and the infundibular technique of laparoscopic cholecystectomy-the danger of the false infundibulum. J Am Coll Surg 2000;191:661–7.

4. Davidson AM, Pappas TN, Murray EA, Hilleren DJ, Johnson RD, Baker ME, Newman GE, Cotton PB, Meyers WC. Mechanisms of major biliary injury during laparoscopic cholecystectomy. Ann Surg 1992;215:196–202.
5. Strasberg SM, Gouma DJ. 'Extreme' vasculobiliary injuries: association with fundus-down cholecystectomy in severely inflamed gallbladders. HPB (Oxford). 2012;14:1–8.
6. Wojcicki M, Patkowski W, Chmurowicz T, Bialek A, Wiechowska-Kozlowska A, Stankiewicz R, Milkiewicz P, Krawczyk M. Isolated right posterior bile duct injury following cholecystectomy: report of two cases. World J Gastroenterol 2013;19:6118–21
7. Strasberg SM, Pucci MJ, Brunt LM, et al. Subtotal cholecystectomy-fenestrating vs reconstituting subtypes and the prevention of bile duct injury. J Am Coll Surg 2015. Available on-line, 9 Oct 2015.
8. Hubert C, Annet L, van Beers BE, Gigot JF. The "inside approach of the gallbladder" is an alternative to the classic Calot's triangle dissection for a safe operation in severe cholecystitis. Surg Endosc. 2010;24:2626–32.
9. Fatima J, Baron TH, Topazian MD, et al. Pancreaticobiliary and duodenal perforations after periampullary endoscopic procedures: diagnosis and management. Arch Surg. 2007;142: 448–54.
10. Knudson K, Raeburn C, McIntyre R, et al. Management of duodenal and pancreaticobiliary perforations associated with periampullary endoscopic procedures. Am J Surg. 2008;196: 975–82.
11. Preetha M, Chung YF, et al. Surgical management of endoscopic retrograde cholangiopancreatography-related perforations. ANZ J. Surg. 2003;73:1011–4.
12. Enns R, Eloubeidi MA, Mergener K, et al. ERCP-related perforations: risk factors and management. Endoscopy. 2002;34:293–8.
13. Kuhlman JE, Fishman EK, Milligan FD, et al. Complications of endoscopic retrograde sphincterotomy: computed tomographic evaluation. Gastrointest Radiol. 1989;14:127–32.
14. Stapfer M, Selby RR, Stain SC, et al. Management of duodenal perforation after endoscopic retrograde cholangiopancreatography and sphincterotomy. Ann Surg. 2000;232:191–8.
15. Howard TJ, Tan T, Lehman GA, et al. Classification and management of perforations complicating endoscopic sphincterotomy. Surgery 1999;126:658–63 (discussion: 664–5).
16. SCORE Website. Greenfield's surgery: scientific principles and practice, 5ed. Chapter 23. Abdominal Trauma.

Chapter 10
Acute Necrotizing Pancreatitis

Mayur Narayan and Jose J. Diaz

Introduction

Necrotizing pancreatitis can be seen in up to 20–30 % of all cases of pancreatitis leading to increased mortality. Studies have shown that acute pancreatitis results in greater than 200,000 admissions annually with an economic impact of greater than $2 billion [1]. Death usually occurs as a result of multisystem organ failure. The causes of necrotizing pancreatitis are similar to those that cause uncomplicated pancreatitis. These include, but are not limited to, alcohol, gallstones, hypertriglyceridemia, trauma, hypercalcemia, medications, certain viruses, and auto immune disorders [2]. Pancreatitis can occur in varying forms from mild to life threatening. It remains unclear why certain patients are prone to developing milder cases even with multiple episodes of pancreatitis while others can develop severe, life-threatening pancreatitis on their first episode [3].

Pathophysiology

The severity of acute necrotizing pancreatitis will depend on the degree of extravasation of pancreatic enzymes. It is important to remember that since the pancreas lacks a true capsule, extravasated enzymes are free to spread and may

---

M. Narayan (✉)
Division of Acute Care Surgery, Clements University Hospital,
UT-Southwestern Medical Center, Dallas, TX, USA
e-mail: mayur.narayan@utsouthwestern.edu

J.J. Diaz
Division of Acute Care Surgery, R Adams Cowley Shock Trauma Center,
University of Maryland Medical Center, Baltimore, USA
e-mail: jdiaz@umm.edu

J.J. Diaz and D.T. Efron (eds.), *Complications in Acute Care Surgery*,
DOI 10.1007/978-3-319-42376-0_10

cause damage involving various regions of the abdomen including the retroperitoneum, the small bowel, and transverse mesocolon, as well as the lesser sac [4].

Extravasation of these proteolytic pancreatic enzymes can also lead to significant complications beyond the pancreas. For example, arterial complications can occur as enzymes attack and weaken the arterial wall leading to pseudo aneurysm development. This injury can lead to massive intra-abdominal hemorrhage. Additionally, these enzymes can also act on the mesentery of the small bowel or colon. The resulting local inflammation in the vascular thrombosis can lead to bowel ischemia, necrosis, and/or perforation [5–8].

Diagnosis

Classically, the patient will present with varying degrees of abdominal pain, elevated pancreatic enzymes, and imaging findings consistent with acute pancreatitis. It is important to classify the severity of acute pancreatitis. In 1992, the Atlanta classification was developed to stratify severity as well as pancreatic complications based on clinical criteria [9]. A new, revised Atlanta classification (RAC) was developed in 2012 (Table 10.1) [10]. The RAC is an improvement over the previous Atlanta classification as it makes a clear distinction between clinical severity and morphologic severity based on CT imaging [11, 12].

The RAC has three categories of clinical severity: (1) mild acute pancreatitis defined as the absence of systemic or local complications, (2) moderately severe acute pancreatitis, a new category defined as the presence of transient organ failure,

Table 10.1 Initial assessment and stratification of risk

Severity in acute pancreatitis: original versus revised Atlanta classification	
1993	2013
Mild acute pancreatitis	*Mild acute pancreatitis*
Absence of organ failure	Absence of organ failure
Absence of local complications	Absence of local complications
	Moderately acute pancreatitis
	Local complications AND/OR
	Transient organ failure [>48 h]
Severe acute pancreatitis	*Severe acute pancreatitis*
Local complications AND/OR	Persistent organ failure >48 h[a]
Organ failure	
GI Bleed [>500 cc 24 h]	
Shock [SBP ≤ 90 mmHg]	
PaO_2 ≤ 60 %	
Creatinine ≥ 2 mg/dl	

Modified from [9, 10]

[a]Defines by modified Marshal score

deteriorating preexisting co-morbid disease and or the presence of local complications requiring prolonged stay or intervention, and (3) severe acute pancreatitis defined as persistent organ failure greater than 48 h [10–12].

In addition to this stratification, the RAC also differentiates the types of acute pancreatitis based on morphology. For example, while the pancreas will enhance normally on contrast enhanced CT in interstitial pancreatitis, there may be varying degrees of tissue necrosis in necrotizing pancreatitis [10–12].

The RAC further subdivides necrotizing pancreatitis into three major forms depending on whether the necrosis involves the pancreatic parenchyma, peri-pancreatic tissues, or combined necrosis of both the parenchyma and peri-pancreatic tissues. In addition, pancreatic collections in the early phase are classified as either acute peri-pancreatic fluid collections or acute necrotic collections. After a period of maturation, these can develop into either pseudo cysts or as walled off necrosis [10–12].

Scores for Organ Dysfunction

Necrotizing pancreatitis can be the inciting event leading to multisystem organ dysfunction. Over the past several years, there have been many attempts to quantify the severity of disease processes. Early scores such as Ranson's criteria were an attempt to predict clinical outcomes based on the severity of acute pancreatitis. Although historically significant, it is no longer routinely utilized. Newer scores such as the multiple organ dysfunction score [MODS] or the sequential failure assessment score (SOFA) have been developed to evaluate organ dysfunction in the intensive care units. The RAC adopted the modified Marshall score for their definition of organ failure [13] (Table 10.2).

Table 10.2 Modified Marshall scoring system for organ dysfunction[a]

Organ system	Score				
	0	1	2	3	4
Respiratory renal					
[PaO_2/FiO_2]	>400	301–400	201–300	101–200	≤101
Serum creatinine, μmol/L	≤134	134–169	170–310	311–439	>439
Serum creatinine, mg/dL	<1.4	1.4–1.8	1.9–3.6	3.6–4.9	>4.9
Cardiovascular[b]					
Systolic blood pressure, mmHg	>90	<90, fluid responsive	<90, not fluid responsive	<90, pH < 7.3	<90, pH < 7.2

Source Banks et al. [10, Table 1], with permission from BMJ Publishing Group Ltd.
[a]Score ≥ 2 *in any system* defines presence of organ failure
[b]Off inotropic support

Although previously routinely recommended to detect bacteria, percutaneous fine needle aspiration is no longer considered a mandatory requirement. Instead, clinical signs such as worsening or persistent fever or the presence of gas in peri-pancreatic collections are considered accurate predictors of infected necrosis in most patients [14].

Management

ICU Care

Patients with necrotizing pancreatitis should be admitted to the intensive care unit for aggressive fluid resuscitation and supportive care. The surgical team should work closely with surgical intensivists in monitoring the progress of these patients. Goal directed therapy should be based on both non-invasive and invasive clinical markers. These include heart rate, mean arterial blood pressure, and urinary output as well as stroke volume variation, echocardiograph examination, and laboratory assessments. Failure to aggressively fluid resuscitation these patients within the first 24 h of admissions is associated with increased rates of systemic inflammatory response syndrome and organ failure [4, 5, 7, 8]. Antibiotics are generally not recommended for prophylaxis of infected pancreatic necrosis. Several meta-analyses have shown that there are no significant differences in mortality, incidence of infected pancreatic necrosis, non-pancreatic infection, and surgical intervention. In fact, several studies have shown that there may even be an association with antibiotic use and pancreatic fungal infections. Therefore, the use of prophylactic antibiotics is not recommended. Antibiotics for treatment should be used for clinical suspicion for concurrent extra-pancreatic infection [15, 16].

Patients with acute severe pancreatitis are hypermetabolic with increased net protein catabolism, up to 40 g nitrogen/day. Enteral nutrition is an important mode of therapy in these critically ill patients and should be initiated within the first 72 hours of hospitalization. Multiple studies have shown that early nutritional support reduces catabolism and loss of lean body mass. Nutrition also helps modulate the acute phase response and may preserve visceral protein metabolism. In those patients with severe necrotizing pancreatitis that develop a prolonged paralytic ileus precluding complete enteral nutrition, it is still possible to administer small amounts of enteral nutrition. The route of nutrition delivery, either via the parenteral or enteral route, should be determined by patient tolerance. Enteral feeds are preferred and should be attempted in all patients. Nutritional markers should be monitored routinely. Some patients may require a combination of enteral and parenteral nutrition depending on their tolerance of enteral feeds. [17–20].

Abdominal Compartment Syndrome

Given the aggressive fluid resuscitation required for these patients, the acute care surgeon should always be concerned about the development of abdominal compartment syndrome. The clinical sequelae of this potentially fatal complication include abdominal distention, sustained elevated intra-abdominal pressure (greater than 25 mmHg measured by bladder pressure), decreased urine output, and increasing respiratory insufficiency. Paracentesis may be considered in the early stages to help with drainage of ascites that could be contributing to increased abdominal pressure. Should the concern for abdominal compartment syndrome persist, the definitive management is surgical decompression. A wound VAC is then placed for temporary abdominal closure [21].

Multidisciplinary Step-up Management

Clinical judgment should be used when considering pursuing pancreatic necrosectomy concomitant with abdominal decompression for compartment syndrome. It is advisable to delay surgical necrosectomy until pancreatic collections have become walled off to help delineate between viable and non-viable tissue [22, 23]. However, depending on the degree of necrosis, delayed operative management, despite wishful thinking, may not be possible. In this case, the patient can be expected to become sicker after exploration and debridement. All necrotic material should be debrided. Wide drainage of the pancreas including drains placed in the lesser sac, above the pancreatic bed, and below the level of the transverse mesocolon is encouraged [24].

The Step-Up Approach is another option for management of necrotizing pancreatitis [25, 26]. This approach utilizes a percutaneously placed drain [12 Fr] drain with assistance of interventional radiology through the left retroperitoneum. Proper positioning of this initial drain cannot be overstated, and the surgical team should have direct input into the exact location planned by interventional radiology (Fig. 10.1). A poorly placed drain will make it difficult to perform the video-assisted retroperitoneal debridement (VARDS) and potentially increase the chance of injury [27]. After placement of the initial drain, the patient is observed for clinical improvement as evidenced by drop in fever, WBC, and improvement of other physiologic parameters as well as resolution of fluid collections and inflammatory foci seen on CT scan. If no improvement is seen over the next 72 hours, upsizing of the drain should be considered. If this fails, the patient should proceed to VARDS [28–34] (Fig. 10.2).

Surgery is preferably postponed until at least 4 weeks from the onset of the disease [24]. This is considered essential as it allows for peri-pancreatic collections to sufficiently demarcate and the wall to mature, thus optimizing conditions for debridement. The VARDS technique we use is similar to that described by van

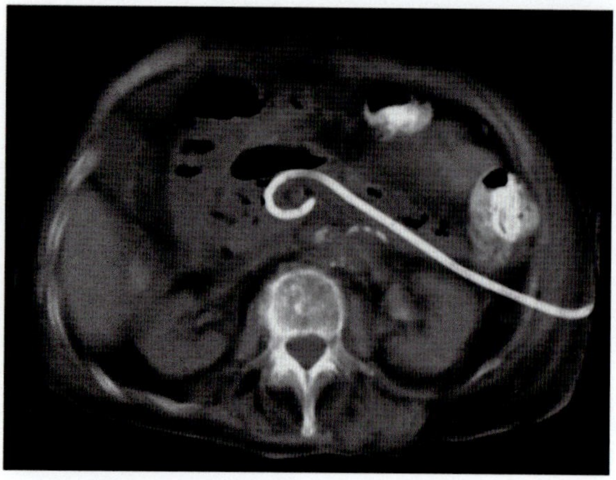

Fig. 10.1 Step-up approach: initial left-sided drain placement into retroperitoneum. From van Santvoort et al. [27, Fig. 1], with permission from Elsevier

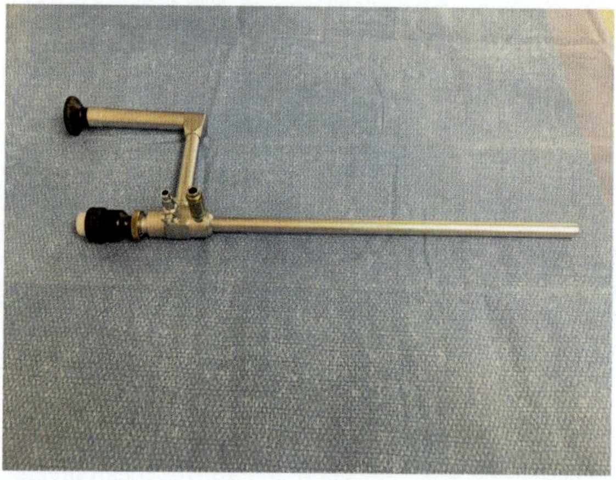

Fig. 10.2 Single port VARDS

Santvoort et al. The patient is placed in supine position with the left side elevated 30° to 40°. A subcostal incision approximately 5 cm in length is placed in the left flank at the mid-axillary line, close to the exit point of the percutaneous drain.

With the help of CT images and by using the in situ percutaneous drain as a guide into the peri-pancreatic collection, the fascia is dissected and the retroperitoneum is entered. The cavity is cleared of purulent material using a standard suction device. The first necrosis encountered is carefully removed with the use of long grasping forceps. Loose necrotic material is removed while periodic irrigation and continuous suction are performed to enhance vision as the percutaneous drain is followed as a road map deeper into the cavity (Fig. 10.3). When debridement can no longer be performed under direct vision, a single extra-long laparoscopic port is placed into the incision and a 0° videoscope is introduced. At this stage, CO_2 gas (10 L/min) can be infused through the percutaneous drain, still in position, to inflate the cavity, thereby facilitating inspection. Under videoscopic assistance, further debridement of retained

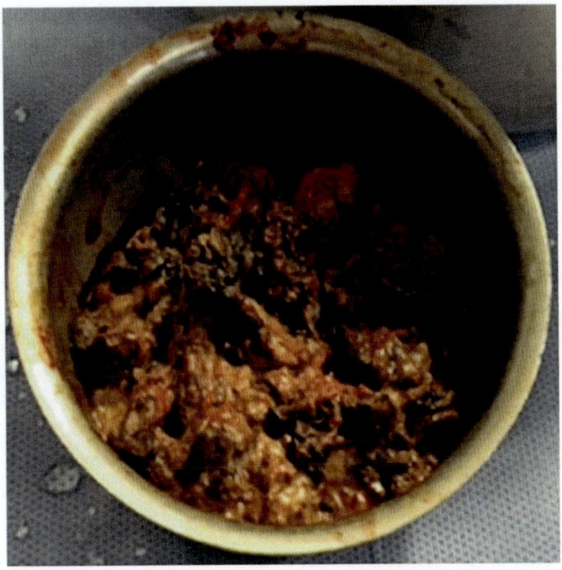

Fig. 10.3 Pancreatic necrosis after VARDS debridement

necrotic tissue is performed with laparoscopic forceps. Complete necrosectomy is not the ultimate aim of this procedure. Only loosely adherent pieces of necrosis are removed, thereby keeping the risk of tearing underlying blood vessels to a minimum. Overly aggressive necrosectomy of un-demarcated, necrotic tissue will increase the chance of injury and bleeding. The main complications of VARDS remain hemorrhage and colonic perforation. Significant retroperitoneal bleeding has a reported incidence of as high as 16–20 %. In the case of extensive bleeding, packing of the retroperitoneal cavity should be performed, either as definite treatment or as a bridge to laparotomy or angiographic coiling in the situation of persistent hemorrhage. When the bulk of necrosis is removed, the cavity is irrigated with saline until the fluid becomes clear. The percutaneous drain is removed, and two large-bore single-lumen drains are positioned in the cavity extending through the edges of the incision. Multiple large-bore drains are placed to allow for postoperative lavage. The fascia and skin are closed, and the drains are sutured to the skin. Continuous postoperative lavage is performed with 10 L of normal saline or dialysis fluid per 24 hours until the effluent is clear. One week after the procedure repeat CT is performed to evaluate resolution [35–38].

Pancreatic Necrosectomy

Emergency surgery in patients with necrotizing pancreatitis is associated with mortality rates as high as 40–80 % [39]. Complications can arise as a direct result of pancreatic enzyme extravasation resulting in hemorrhage, ischemia, perforation, or

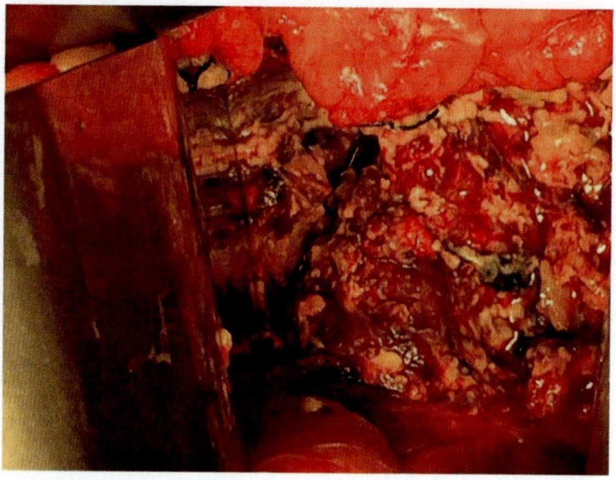

Fig. 10.4 Necrotic pancreas: open necrosectomy

fistula formation. In addition, iatrogenic injury while operating in areas with significant inflammation can also lead to complications that will directly impact morbidity and mortality [40–45] (Fig. 10.4).

Bleeding Complications

Pathophysiology/Diagnosis

Hemorrhage as a result of necrotizing paper has been estimated to occur in 1–6.2 % of patients [46]. Potential sites of bleeding include intra-luminally, frank hemorrhage into the peritoneal cavity, into fluid collections, or within the pancreatic parenchyma. The etiology is usually secondary to embarrassment of surrounding vessels as a result of pancreatic enzyme action. The resultant weakening of the vessel wall can lead to thrombus or pseudoaneurysm formation [47, 48]. Classic physical examination signs of retroperitoneal hemorrhage including Cullen's sign [peri-umbilical bruising], Grey-Turner's sign [bruising of the flanks], and Fox's sign [bruising of the inguinal region] may present in delayed fashion [48]. A sudden change in the patients hemodynamic profile with new onset hypotension, a drop in hemoglobin or hematocrit levels, or frank blood from previously paced drains should immediately raise the concern for massive hemorrhage and warrants prompt intervention.

Management Options

Initial management begins in the ICU with prompt recognition of the hemorrhaging patient. Aggressive resuscitation with initiation of surgical consultation and activation of massive transfusion protocol should be done immediately.

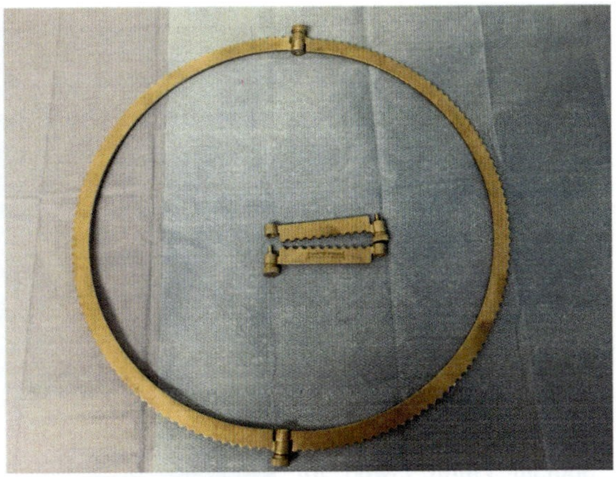

Fig. 10.5 Large ring measuring 12.5 "allowing for maximal exposure"

In minor bleeding cases and depending on the patient's hemodynamic profile as well as the status of the patient's abdomen, angiography with embolization can be considered as a first line management option [49]. Delays in setting up the interventional radiology suite may necessitate consideration of early surgical intervention.

Surgical intervention requires adequate exposure of the retroperitoneum. We prefer use of the large round retractor over the traditional oval shaped Bookwalter retractor (Fig. 10.5) for optimal exposure. Identifiable bleeding sources can be controlled with simple suture ligation. The more concerning problem arises when there is pooling of blood in the retroperitoneum with no identifiable source. Options in this setting include packing with a hemostatic dressing such as Combat Gauze and generous use of laparotomy pads, temporary wound VAC placement, and subsequent intervention radiology consultation. Identification and attempts of surgical control deep in the retroperitoneum may lead to significant blood loss and poor surgical outcomes. Discussion with anesthesia colleagues in the operating room is of paramount importance as communication will allow the team to direct resuscitation. This also allows the surgical team to hold manual pressure and gather their thoughts before any further attempts at surgical hemostasis are made [47].

The Resuscitative Endovascular Balloon Occlusion of the Aorta device (REBOA) can be considered should the surgical team encounter massive hemorrhage from the retroperitoneum. Our team has previously described the use of REBOA in a video-assisted retroperitoneal debridement for infected necrotizing pancreatitis [50]. The first step for proper placement is to expose the right common femoral artery (R CFA) via surgical cut down. This will make placement of the femoral sheaths easier. The R CFA is then accessed using open Seldinger technique using a 20 Fr hollow bore needle and a 0.035 guidewire. A 5 Fr sheath is then inserted to allow placement of a 0.035 Bentson wire (Cook Incorporated, Bloomington] into the thoracic aorta. The 5Fr sheath is subsequently removed and upsized to a 14Fr sheath. A 32 mm CODA balloon catheter (Fig. 10.6) is then inserted and deployed into the descending thoracic aorta. Prior to inflation, it is

described. Stent placement may lead to ductal stricture with prolonged placement and a risk of migration, occlusion, and perforation remains. Definitive management of a disputed duct remains a distal pancreatectomy with or without splenic preservation. Splenic preservation in the setting of significant retroperitoneal inflammation is unlikely, and the surgeon should be prepared for splenectomy from the outset [53].

Managing the Gall Bladder

The standard practice for patients who develop mild-to-moderate acute biliary pancreatitis has been to perform cholecystectomy during the index admission to reduce the risk of recurrent pancreatitis. For patients with severe pancreatitis, cholecystectomy is deferred for several weeks to avoid injury during either laparoscopic or open dissection and to minimize need for open conversion. The optimal timing of cholecystectomy in patients with severe necrotizing patients should depend on the status of the patient's abdomen and physiologic profile. If the abdomen has been explored for decompression or necrosectomy, we recommend cholecystectomy prior to abdominal closure. Single-stage cholecystectomy at the time of pancreatic necrosectomy has been well described and found to be safe in select patients. It is recommended if technically feasible to prevent future biliary complications and reduce the need for a subsequent separate operation [54].

Summary

Severe necrotizing pancreatitis has a high incidence of mortality when compared to mild pancreatitis. Aggressive resuscitation in the ICU, coupled with judicious antibiotic use, and early nutritional support in a multidisciplinary fashion are keys to successful outcomes in these patients. The acute care surgeon should maintain a high index of suspicion for complications as a result of pancreatic enzyme extravasation that may lead to ischemia, perforation, or hemorrhage. Prompt diagnosis and early intervention are keys to management.

Key Questions

1. *How does one decide to perform the initial "step-up" drain placement?*
2. *What are key decision points in planning of videoscopic assisted retroperitoneal debridement of pancreatic necrosis?*

References

1. Fagenholz PJ, Fernandez-del Castillo C, Harris NS, et al. Direct medical. costs of acute pancreatitis hospitalizations in the United States. Pancreas. 2007; 35:302–7.

2. Ahmed Ali U, Issa Y, Hagenaars JC, et al. Dutch pancreatitis study group. risk of recurrent pancreatitis and progression to chronic pancreatitis after a first episode of acute pancreatitis. Clin Gastroenterol Hepatol. 2016. pii: S1542-3565(16)00004-5.
3. Sabo A, Goussous N, Sardana N, et al. Necrotizing pancreatitis: a review of multidisciplinary management. JOP. 2015;16(2):125–35.
4. Isaji S, Takada T, Mayumi T, et al. Revised Japanese guidelines for the management of acute pancreatitis 2015: revised concepts and updated points. J Hepatobiliary Pancreat Sci. 2015;22 (6):433–45.
5. Yokoe M, Takada T, Mayumi T, et al. Japanese guidelines for the management of acute pancreatitis: Japanese guidelines 2015. J Hepatobiliary Pancreat Sci. 2015;22(6):405–32.
6. Sonbare DJ. Organ failure and infection in necrotizing pancreatitis: what are the predictors of mortality? Ann Surg. 2015. [Epub ahead of print].
7. Working Group IAP/APA Acute Pancreatitis Guidelines. IAP/APA evidence-based guidelines for the management of acute pancreatitis. Pancreatology. 2013;13(4 Suppl 2):e1–15.
8. Dua MM, Worhunsky DJ, Amin S, et al. Getting the dead out: modern treatment strategies for necrotizing pancreatitis. Dig Dis Sci. 2014;59(9):2069–75.
9. Bradley EL 3rd. A clinically based classification system for acute pancreatitis. Summary of the international symposium on acute pancreatitis, 1992. Arch Surg. 1993;128(5):586–90.
10. Banks PA, Bollen TL, Dervenis C, et al. Classification of acute pancreatitis—2012: revision of the Atlanta classification and definitions by international consensus. Gut. 2013;62(1):102–11.
11. Sarr MG, Banks PA, Bollen TL, et al. The new revised classification of acute pancreatitis 2012. Surg Clin North Am. 2013;93(3):549–62.
12. Choi JH, Kim MH, Oh D, et al. Clinical relevance of the revised Atlanta classification focusing on severity stratification system. Pancreatology. 2014;14(5):324–9.
13. Marshall JC, Cook DJ, Christou NV, et al. Multiple organ dysfunction score: a reliable descriptor of a complex clinical outcome. Crit Care Med. 1995;23:1638–52.
14. van Baal MC, Bollen TL, Bakker OJ, et al. Dutch pancreatitis study group. the role of routine fine-needle aspiration in the diagnosis of infected necrotizing pancreatitis. Surgery. 2014;155 (3):442–8.
15. Ukai T, Shikata S, Inoue M, et al. Early prophylactic antibiotics administration for acute necrotizing pancreatitis: a meta-analysis of randomized controlled trials. J Hepatobiliary Pancreat Sci. 2015;22(4):316–21.
16. Lim CL, Lee W, Liew YX, et al. Role of antibiotic prophylaxis in necrotizing pancreatitis: a meta-analysis. J Gastrointest Surg. 2015;19(3):480–91.
17. Dellinger RP, Levy MM, Rhodes A, et al. Surviving sepsis campaign: international guidelines for management of severe sepsis and septic shock: 2012. Crit Care Med. 2013;41(2):580–637.
18. Lodewijkx PJ, Besselink MG, Witteman BJ, et al. Nutrition in acute pancreatitis: a critical review. Expert Rev Gastroenterol Hepatol. 2016. [Epub ahead of print].
19. Bakker OJ, van Brunschot S, van Santvoort HC, et al. Dutch pancreatitis study group. early versus on-demand nasoenteric tube feeding in acute pancreatitis. N Engl J Med. 2014;371 (21):1983–93.
20. Bakker OJ, van Brunschot S, Farre A, et al. Timing of enteral nutrition in acute pancreatitis: meta-analysis of individuals using a single-arm of randomised trials. Pancreatology. 2014;14 (5):340–6.
21. Rosenberg A, Steensma EA, Napolitano LM. Necrotizing pancreatitis: new definitions and a new era in surgical management. Surg Infect (Larchmt). 2015;16(1):1–13.
22. Connor S, Raraty MG, Neoptolemos JP, et al. Does infected pancreatic necrosis require immediate or emergency debridement? Pancreas. 2006;33:128–34.
23. HartwigW, Maksan SM, Foitzik T, et al. Reduction in mortality with delayed surgical therapy of severe pancreatitis. J Gastrointest Surg. 2002;6:481–7.
24. Bugiantella W, Rondelli F, Boni M, et al. Necrotizing pancreatitis: a review of the interventions. Int J Surg. 2015. pii: S1743-9191(15)01423-5.

25. van Santvoort HC, Besselink MG, Bakker OJ, et al. Dutch pancreatitis study group, a step-up approach or open necrosectomy for necrotizing pancreatitis. N Engl J Med. 2010;362 (16):1491–502.
26. da Costa DW, Boerma D, van Santvoort HC, et al. Staged multidisciplinary step-up management for necrotizing pancreatitis. Br J Surg. 2014;101(1):e65–79.
27. van Santvoort HC, Besselink MG, Horvath KD, et al. Dutch Acute Pancreatis Study Group. Videoscopic assisted retroperitoneal debridement in infected necrotizing pancreatitis, HPB (Oxford). 2007;9(2) 156–9.
28. Hollemans RA, Bollen TL, van Brunschot S, et al. Dutch pancreatitis study group. predicting success of catheter drainage in infected necrotizing pancreatitis. Ann Surg. 2016;263(4): 787–92.
29. Sugimoto M, Sonntag DP, Flint GS, et al. Better outcomes if percutaneous drainage is used early and proactively in the course of necrotizing pancreatitis. J Vasc Interv Radiol. 2016;27 (3):418–25.
30. Guo Q, Li A, Hu W. Predictive factors for successful ultrasound-guided percutaneous drainage in necrotizing pancreatitis. Surg Endosc. 2015. [Epub ahead of print].
31. van Grinsven J, van Brunschot S, Bakker OJ, et al. Dutch pancreatitis study group. Diagnostic strategy and timing of intervention in infected necrotizing pancreatitis: an international expert survey and case vignette study. HPB (Oxford). 2015.
32. Sun J, Yang C, Liu W, Yang Y, Qi S, Chu Z, Xin S, Zhang X. Conservative treatment and percutaneous catheter drainage improve outcome of necrotizing pancreatitis. Hepatogastroenterology. 2015;62(137):195–9.
33. Bang JY, Holt BA, Hawes RH, et al. Outcomes after implementing a tailored endoscopic step-up approach to walled-off necrosis in acute pancreatitis. Br J Surg. 2014;101(13): 1729–38.
34. Terayama T, Hifumi T, Kiriu N, et al. A minimally invasive multiple percutaneous drainage technique for acute necrotizing pancreatitis. World J Emerg Med. 2014;5(4):310–2.
35. Souza LJ, Coelho AM, Sampietre SN, et al. Anti-inflammatory effects of peritoneal lavage in acute pancreatitis. Pancreas. 2010;39(8):1180–4.
36. Matsumoto K, Miyake Y, Nakatsu M, et al. Usefulness of early-phase peritoneal lavage for treating severe acute pancreatitis. Intern Med. 2014;53(1):1–6.
37. Dong Z, Petrov MS, Xu J, et al. Peritoneal lavage for severe acute pancreatitis: a systematic review of randomised trials. World J Surg. 2010;34(9):2103–8.
38. Caronna R, Benedetti M, Morelli A, et al. Clinical effects of laparotomy with perioperative continuous peritoneal lavage and postoperative hemofiltration in patients with severe acute pancreatitis. World J Emerg Surg. 2009;16(4):45.
39. Kokosis G, Perez A, Pappas TN. Surgical management of necrotizing pancreatitis: an overview. World J Gastroenterol. 2014;20(43):16106–12.
40. Martin RF, Hein AR. Operative management of acute pancreatitis. Surg Clin North Am. 2013;93(3):595–610.
41. Gou S, Xiong J, Wu H, et al. Five-year cohort study of open pancreatic necrosectomy for necotizing pancreatitis suggests it is a safe and effective operation. J Gastrointest Surg. 2013;17(9):1634–42.
42. Kiss L, Sarbu G, Bereanu A, et al. Surgical strategies in severe acute pancreatitis (SAP): indications, complications and surgical approaches. Chirurgia (Bucur). 2014;109(6):774–82.
43. Karakayali FY. Surgical and interventional management of complications caused by acute pancreatitis. World J Gastroenterol. 2014;20(37):13412–23.
44. Wormer BA, Swan RZ, Williams KB, et al. Outcomes of pancreatic debridement in acute pancreatitis: analysis of the nationwide inpatient sample from 1998 to 2010. Am J Surg. 2014;208(3):350–62.
45. Madenci AL, Michailidou M, Chiou G, et al. A contemporary series of patients undergoing open debridement for necrotizing pancreatitis. Am J Surg. 2014;208(3):324–31.

46. Rana SS, Sharma V, Bhasin DK, Sharma R, Gupta R, Chhabra P, Kang M. Gastrointestinal bleeding in acute pancreatitis: etiology, clinical features, risk factors and outcome. Trop Gastroenterol. 2015;36(1):31–5.
47. Zerem E. Treatment of severe acute pancreatitis and its complications. World J Gastroenterol. 2014;20(38):13879–92.
48. Andersson E, Ansari D, Andersson R. Major haemorrhagic complications of acute pancreatitis. Br J Surg. 2010;97:1379–84.
49. Fitzpatrick J, Bhat R, Young JA. Angiographic embolization is an effective treatment of severe hemorrhage in pancreatitis. Pancreas. 2014;43:436–9.
50. Weltz AS, Harris DG, O'Neill NA, et al. The use of resuscitative endovascular balloon occlusion of the aorta to control hemorrhagic shock during video-assisted retroperitoneal debridement or infected necrotizing pancreatitis. Int J Surg Case Rep. 2015;13:15–8.
51. Brenner ML, Moore LJ, DuBose JJ, et al. A clinical series of resuscitative endovascular balloon occlusion of the aorta for hemorrhage control and resuscitation. J Trauma Acute Care Surg. 2013;75(3):506–11.
52. Nagpal AP, Soni H, Haribhakti S. Severe colonic complications requiring sub-total colectomy in acute necrotizing pancreatitis—a retrospective study of 8 patients. Ind J Surg. 2015;77(1): 3–6.
53. Nadkarni NA, Kotwal V, Sarr MG, et al. Disconnected pancreatic duct syndrome: endoscopic stent or surgeon's knife? Pancreas. 2015;44(1):16–22.
54. Fong ZV, Peev M, Warshaw AL, et al. Single-stage cholecystectomy at the time of pancreatic necrosectomy is safe and prevents future biliary complications: a 20-year single institutional experience with 217 consecutive patients. J Gastrointest Surg. 2015;19(1):32–7; discussion 37–8.

Chapter 11
Small Bowel: The Problematic Duodenal Perforation

David V. Feliciano

Introduction

Acid-peptic Helicobacter ulcer disease is rarely discussed at academic conferences in the modern era. This is not surprising in light of the continuing decrease in operations performed for gastric and duodenal ulcers and their complications over the past 5 decades. This trend continues in the modern era with further decreases in admissions (40–50 %), hospital deaths, hospitalizations for perforations, and deaths per perforation [1]. Some epidemiologic series, however, have noted that the incidence of "peptic ulcer disease complicated by either bleeding or perforation has remained constant or even decreased" [2]. Lee and Sarosi note that this is related to the increased incidence of NSAID-related ulcer disease in elderly patients in the United States as the incidence of Helicobacter infections has decreased in younger patients [2].

Operative Management

The operative management of perforated ulcer disease has changed over the past 25 years, as well. Prior to the rediscovery of *Helicobacter pylori* by JR Warren and BJ Marshall in the early 1980s, perforated gastric and duodenal ulcers were considered to be life-threatening diseases to be treated aggressively in patients with a chronic (>3 months) history of ulcer disease [3–5]. Therefore, truncal vagotomy and antrectomy or hemigastrectomy were often performed in hemodynamically

D.V. Feliciano (✉)
IU Division of General Surgery, Indiana University Hospital,
Indiana University Medical Center, 545 Barnhill Drive, EH 509,
Indianapolis, IN 46202, USA
e-mail: davfelic@iupui.edu

J.J. Diaz and D.T. Efron (eds.), *Complications in Acute Care Surgery*,
DOI 10.1007/978-3-319-42376-0_11

stable patients [4, 5]. In contrast, patients with an acute (<3 month) history of ulcer disease and a perforation in the duodenum were treated with a modified Graham patch [4–6].

The patient described in the clinical scenario has already been brought to surgery. Patients with perforated duodenal ulcers usually have a 12- to 14-h delay from perforation to operation, though all series include stoic patients with delays in presentation over 48 h [7]. Free air is present in 80 % of patients on an admission chest X-ray, 10-min upright abdominal film, or the inevitable computed tomographic (CT) scan of the abdomen. With suspicion for a duodenal (or gastric) perforation in the remaining 20 %, an upper gastrointestinal or CT study with Gastrografin is performed.

Approximately 10 % of patients have some form of sepsis and will need preoperative resuscitation in the emergency department. All should have preoperative administration of a second- or third-generation cephalosporin antibiotic based on the modest bacterial content of the stomach and duodenum.

When obtaining a preoperative history from the patient, the following 4 areas should be discussed: (1) length of time since perforation, (2) known past diagnosis of "ulcer disease" mandating what type of medical or surgical treatment, (3) known prior diagnosis of *H. pylori* infection and success or failure of treatment, and (4) past medical and surgical history. Lee and Sarosi have noted that adverse prognostic factors increasing postoperative mortality such as age, American Society of Anesthesiologists' class, shock, hypoalbuminemia, increased serum creatinine, and a metabolic acidosis on presentation "are not modifiable" [2].

Exploratory Laparotomy

While an exploratory laparotomy has been the operative approach in the past, laparoscopic approaches are now preferred. The open approach, however, is indicated when the surgeon lacks advanced laparoscopic skills, when there is a history of extensive upper abdominal surgery, when there is extensive intra-abdominal contamination, or when a laparoscopic repair cannot be completed.

The goals of an emergency operation for a perforated duodenal ulcer are to close the perforation, wash out contaminated fluid, and, on occasion, perform a definitive anti-ulcer operation.

In patients with a smaller (<1 cm) anterior perforation of the juxtapyloric area or duodenal bulb, Bertleff and Lange have summarized the four different "suture techniques" for closure [8]. These techniques are appropriate in patients with modest ulcer scarring, no history of failed anti-Helicobacter therapy, a delayed (>24–48 h) presentation, hemodynamic instability, and the presence of a classical cocaine-induced juxtapyloric perforation [9]. *Primary suture closure* can be performed much as in every other perforation of the gastrointestinal tract. A permanent or slowly absorbable suture such as PDS (Ethicon, Somerville, NJ) or Maxon (Covidien, Minneapolis, MN) placed in an interrupted fashion is appropriate.

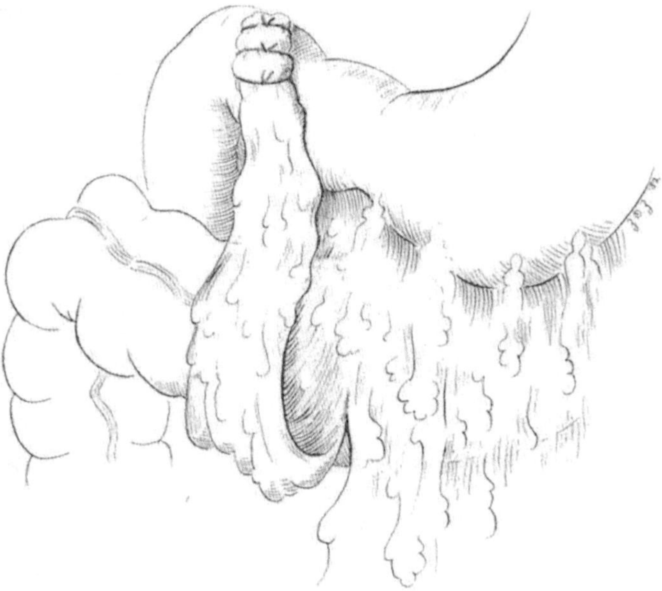

Fig. 11.1 Omental patch closure of anterior perforated duodenal ulcer

Primary closure cannot be completed in many patients because of the rigidity of the duodenal wall secondary to inflammation. Most surgeons performing a primary suture closure will "feel better" if a *pedicle of viable omentum* is added as a buttress. Graham's 1937 technique of *suturing a free omental plug* into the perforation is no longer used, but it worked well at the time and this would still be true. The "Graham patch" has been replaced by the *viable omental pedicle as a plug* described by Cellan-Jones in 1929 [10] (Fig. 11.1). The viable omental plug is created by dividing the gastrocolic omentum from the right side of the transverse colon, flipping it superiorly into the anterior duodenal perforation, and fixating it in place with sutures. With smaller softer perforations, 3–4 sutures can be passed full thickness around the perforation and tied down onto the omental plug. A thicker area of inflammation around the perforation prompts some surgeons to place a seromuscular in-and-out suture bite on either side of the perforation and then tie the 3–4 sutures down.

While impossible for the laparoscopic surgeon, the open surgeon has the opportunity to palpate the posterior duodenal wall before performing a primary anterior closure. The presence of a simultaneous posterior penetrating ulcer would indicate that the patient has "kissing ulcers." The concern in patients with this uncommon condition is that the extent of inflammation and the addition of an anterior omental plug may cause a gastric outlet obstruction. If this complication is a possibility, a more definitive ulcer operation should be performed (see below).

Saline solution containing antibiotics (bacitracin or a cephalosporin) is used to irrigate the entire abdomen after simple closure of anterior perforation. The primary subhepatic site of contamination and the sites of peritoneal fluid flow—pelvis and both subdiaphragmatic areas—are particular areas of focus during irrigation. The value of postrepair irrigation, however, remains controversial [8, 11].

Postoperative care after primary suture or omental plug repair of a small anterior perforation of the duodenum has changed considerably. Rather than the old 5–7 days of a nasogastric tube and NPO status, Enhanced Recovery After Surgery (ERAS) pathways are now used in many centers. Gonec et at described a pathway in which no postoperative narcotic analgesics are used, tramadol and diclofenac are substituted, a liquid diet is started on postoperative day one, and the patient is discharged when bowel sounds are present [12, 13].

The 2-cm anterior duodenal perforation with 1-cm thickened edges described in the clinical scenario precludes a primary or omental plug closure in the minds of most general or acute care surgeons. There is a much greater risk of prolapse of the omental plug into the lumen causing a postoperative duodenal destruction. A postoperative leak is more likely, as well, as many omental plugs are quite thin and epithelization of the underside of the plug will be prolonged.

There are two operative options in such a patient or in any patient needing a definitive operation for a complex perforation or scenario as previously described. The first is a Judd-Weinberg pyloroplasty with or without the addition of a truncal vagotomy. E. Starr Judd from the Mayo Clinic described an operation where the large anterior perforation was excised and duodenal closure performed [14]. If done transversely, this resembles a standard pyloroplasty. Joseph Weinberg from UCLA and the Long Beach Veterans Administration Hospital popularized the one-layer transverse closure (instead of the two-layer closure described by Heineke and Mikulicz) of pyloroplasties. The goal of the operation in the patient described would be to first excise the large anterior perforation and surrounding inflammation in either a transverse or longitudinal direction. A transverse direction would be preferred as it might eliminate the need for a Kocher maneuver before closure. If a longitudinal excision is performed, a Kocher maneuver would be mandatory to avoid tension on the transverse suture closure of the duodenum. Silk, Maxon, or PDS suture can be used for the transverse closure, while the historic technique of burying the suture knots has never made much sense to this author. The tips of a DeBakey tissue forceps are then placed between sutures of the transverse closure to see whether any defects remain that need closure. A viable omental pedicle can be sutured as a buttress over the transverse suture line if desired. While this operation is performed uncommonly in the modern era, it is quite simple if a transverse excision has been performed.

The second option is to perform a gastric antrectomy and a partial duodenectomy encompassing the large perforation. The addition of a truncal vagotomy would depend on whether the patient has failed prior anti-Helicobacter therapy, the experience of the surgeon, the patient's intraoperative hemodynamic status, and whether severe peritonitis is present (truncal vagotomy mandates opening into the posterior mediastinum). The antrectomy is performed up to the "crow's foot" division of the anterior nerve of Latarjet, while the partial duodenectomy should be limited to just beyond the area of inflammation distal to the perforation. Also, the anterior wall of the duodenum should be where the longest area of the excision is performed to avoid the medially based pancreatic duct of Santorini.

An end-to-end gastroduodenostomy is not commonly performed after the resection because of the inflammation in the subhepatic space. When inflammation is modest and the duodenectomy has been limited, it is a reasonable choice. The first step would be to excise a portion of the lesser curve of the stomach using a suture or staple closure (Schoemaker modification). This should narrow the gastric outlet to a size larger (by at least 1–2 cm) than that of the duodenal lumen. A Kocher maneuver is then performed to avoid tension on the 2-layer handsewn end-to-end gastroduodenostomy. The oversizing of the gastric end avoids narrowing of the anastomosis.

More commonly, an antecolic end-to-side gastrojejunostomy is performed with sutures or staples away from the area of subhepatic inflammation. There is no need to perform a Hofmeister modification to narrow the gastric outlet. The disadvantage of this approach is the need to add some type of closure of the duodenal stump. The four options when speaking about all closures of the duodenum for a variety of gastric diseases include the following: (1) routine closure, (2) Nissen closure (using the thickened edge of a penetrating posterior ulcer to pass sutures through), (3) Bancroft closure (preserving blood supply to pyloroantral area, coring out mucosa of pyloric channel and pyloric muscle ring, closing a long soft pyloroantral seromuscular cuff instead of a duodenal stump). Before a routine closure of a duodenal stump, it is worthwhile to remove the occluding clamp on the duodenum. Pulsatile arterial flow from the edges of the stump will almost guarantee a closure that will not leak in the postoperative period. Also, the original partial duodenectomy should have preserved a 1-cm cuff of posterior duodenal wall that can be lifted off the pancreas. Prior to closure, a Kocher maneuver may need to be performed to free up more of the anterior wall of the duodenum, especially if the posterior cuff is <1 cm in length. A continuous full-thickness 3-0 absorbable suture closure followed by an inverting seromuscular row of interrupted 3-0 silk sutures is performed. A closed suction drain is placed in the right subhepatic space inferior to the duodenal stump.

A tube duodenostomy is indicated when the stump is scarred and difficult to close in a watertight fashion. A #24-28 Fr. Pezzar or Malecot catheter is used as a tube and can be placed in the middle of the stump or in the superior or inferior corner. A purse string suture can be placed around the tube if the stump is narrow. Otherwise, the soft parts of the stump may be closed with one or two layers of sutures. The entrance site of the tube into the duodenum is wrapped with a viable omental pedicle that is sutured in place. Duodenostomy tubes are removed in the clinic 3 weeks after insertion, and the patient is warned about a transient leak of bile through the skin hole.

Laparoscopy

As previously noted, a laparoscopic suture or omental plug repair is preferred in the modern era and works well for small anterior perforations. Disadvantages have included a higher leak and abscess rate postoperatively in some series, presumably in nonroutine ulcers [15, 16]. When definitive operation is indicated for the reasons previously mentioned, a laparoscopic parietal cell vagotomy and anterior linear gastrectomy have been used [17].

Results

The overall mortality after surgery for a perforated duodenal ulcer has been 6–10 % for over 40 years, with almost all deaths occurring, as previously noted, in older patients with comorbidities, delays in treatment, or shock on admission [2, 4, 8]. With a combination of these factors, the mortality rate may be as high as 30 % [2].

Key Questions

1. *Is there a role for pyloric exclusion? If so, when?*
2. *When should a duodenostomy be the first choice?*

References

1. Wang YR, Richter JE, Dempsey DT. Trends and outcomes of hospitalizations for peptic ulcer disease in the United States, 1993 to 2006. Ann Surg. 2010;251:51–8.
2. Lee CW, Sarosi GA Jr. Emergency ulcer surgery. Surg Clin N Am. 2011;91:1001–13.
3. Marshall BJ, Warren JR. Unidentified curved bacilli in the stomach of patients with gastritis and peptic ulceration. Lancet. 1984;1:1311–5.
4. Feliciano DV. Surgical options and results of treatment of perforated ulcers. Probl Gen Surg. 1987;4:301–7.
5. Feliciano DV. Do perforated duodenal ulcers need an acid-decreasing surgical procedure now that omeprazole is available? Surg Clin N Am. 1992;72:369–80.
6. Graham RR. The treatment of perforated duodenal ulcers. Surg Gynecol Obstet. 1937;235–8.
7. Boey J, Wong J, Ong GB. A prospective study of operative risk factors in perforated duodenal ulcers. Ann Surg. 1982;195:265–9.
8. Bertleff MJOE, Lange JF. Perforated peptic ulcer disease: a review of history and treatment. Dig Surg. 2010;27:161–9.
9. Feliciano DV, Ojukwu JC, Rozycki GS, Ballard RB, Ingram WL, Salomone J, Namias N, Newman PG. The epidemic of cocaine-related juxtapyloric perforations. With a comment on the importance of testing for *Helicobacter pylori*. Ann Surg. 1999;229:801–6.
10. Cellan-Jones, CJ. A rapid method of treatment in perforated duodenal ulcers. BMJ. 1929;1076–1077.
11. Whiteside OJ, Tytherleigh MG, Thrush S, Farouk R, Galland RB. Intra-operative peritoneal lavage—who does it and why? Ann R Coll Surg Engl. 2005;87:255–8.

12. Gonec M, Dural AC, Celik F, Akarsu C, Kocatas A, Kalayci MU, Dogan Y, Alis H. Enhanced postoperative recovery pathways in emergency surgery: a randomized controlled clinical trial. Am J Surg. 2014;207:807–14.
13. Feliciano DV, Invited Commentary on Gonec M, Dural AC, Celik F, Akarsu C, Kocatas A, Kalayci MU, Dogan Y, Alis H. Enhanced postoperative recovery pathways in emergency surgery: a randomized controlled clinical trial. Am J Surg. 2014;207:815–6.
14. Judd ES, Hazeltine ME. The results of operations for excision of ulcer of the duodenum. Ann Surg. 1930;92:563–73.
15. Lunevicius R, Morkevicius M. Management strategies, early results, and risk factors of laparoscopic repair of perforated peptic ulcer. World J Surg. 2005;29:1299–310.
16. Thorsen K, Glomsaker TB, von Meer A, Soreide K, Soreide JA. Trends in diagnosis and surgical management of patients with perforated peptic ulcer. J Gastrointest Surg. 2011;15:1329–35.
17. Harbison SP, Dempsey DT. Peptic ulcer disease. Curr Probl Surg. 2005;42:346–454.

Chapter 12
Small Bowel: Aortoenteric Fistula

James H. Black, III and David T. Efron

Introduction

Aortoenteric fistula remains one of the most difficult acute care and vascular surgery challenges. It is an entity that often presents emergently, allowing limited time to plan, and requires complex surgical skill from two different specialties (GI and vascular surgery). Furthermore, these patients carry multiple comorbidities both chronic (athlerosclerotic disease) and acute (malnutrition) and the perioperative period often necessitates advanced critical care support and input from multiple subspecialties (e.g., infectious disease).

Etiology

An aortoenteric fistula may form between any level of the GI track that is able to be directly apposed to the vessel (or graft that has been placed). It is most common within the abdomen. The third and fourth portions of the duodenum are particularly at risk as this segment of the GI track drapes over the aorta as is courses along the retroperitoneum. Aneurysmal dilatation of the aorta displaces the duodenum anteriorly while also exerting pressure along its posterior wall. The virgin duodenum is fixed in the retroperitoneum at this point between its course posterior to the SMA/SMV and the ligament of Treitz. Similarly, the duodenum remains in this

J.H. Black III (✉)
Division of Vascular and Endovascular Surgery, Johns Hopkins University School of Medicine, Baltimore, MD, USA
e-mail: jhblack@jhmi.edu

D.T. Efron
Division of Acute Care Surgery, Johns Hopkins University School of Medicine, Baltimore, MD, USA

J.J. Diaz and D.T. Efron (eds.), *Complications in Acute Care Surgery*,
DOI 10.1007/978-3-319-42376-0_12

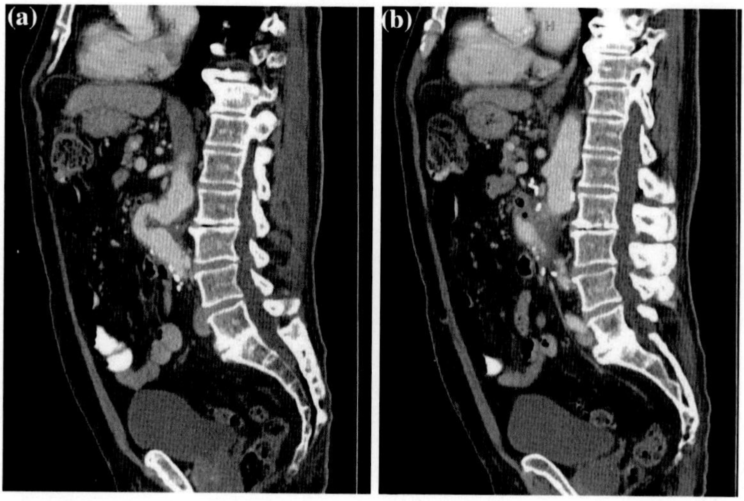

Fig. 12.1 **a** Anterior displacement of the duodenum by tortuous aortic graft placement resulting in aorto-duodenal fistula (**b**)

proximity once an aortic procedure is performed; the raw tissue from the dissection guaranteeing proximity of these tissues via adhesion formation. More distally, postoperative adhesions may draw both small and large bowels into proximity of the graft (both tube and limb grafts).

Fistulas may form to aortic grafts from open replacements, endovascular-stented aneurysms as well as primary aortic aneurysms [1]. As will be seen later in this chapter, this has significant effect on one's approach to the repair. The formation of the fistula may occur from several different inciting events. An infectious episode: For example, a diverticular abscess overlying the left iliac limb of an aorto-bi-iliac graft results in an aorto-colonic fistula. An iatrogenic event may occur such as catching bowel with a suture while closing the retroperitoneum following graft placement. Most frequently, in the case of aorto-duodenal fistula, simple tensioned apposition of the peristalsing duodenal segment over the foreign material of graft eventually leads to erosion of the back wall of the duodenum (Fig. 12.1).

The fistulas are usually all characterized structurally as being stuck to the aorta or graft with a full thickness violation of the bowel wall, the vessel, or graft essentially "patching" the defect. This pathologic structure is at the heart of the presentation of aortoenteric fistulas (Fig. 12.2).

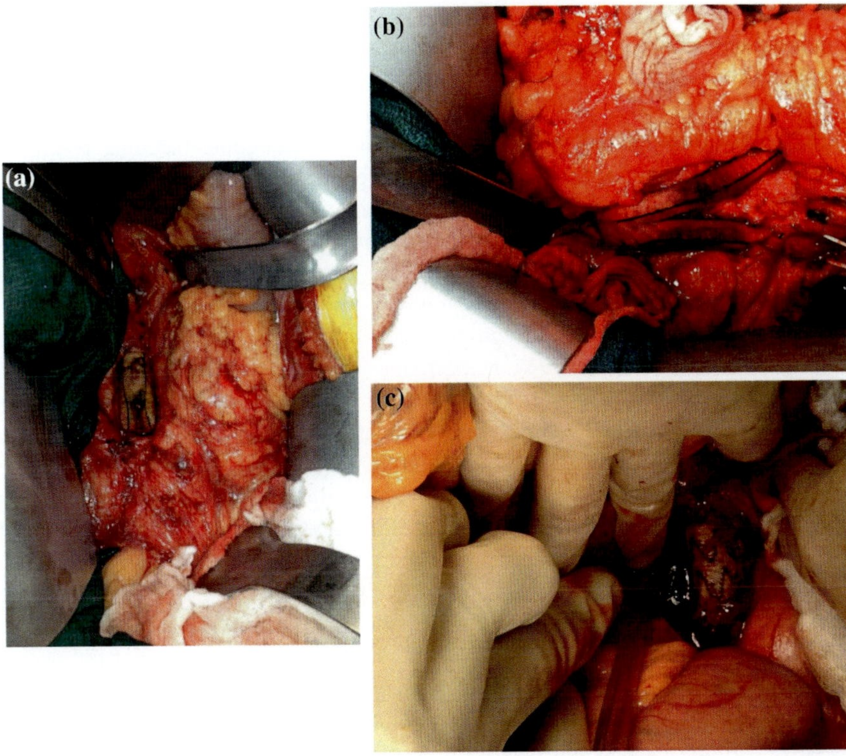

Fig. 12.2 **a** Exposed, stained aortic graft from an aorto-duodenal fistula (**b**) from a double fistula to both distal limbs of an aorto-bifemoral graft, the fistula from a segment of small bowel. **c** Fistula to exposed endostent

Presentation

Aortoenteric fistulae essentially demonstrate two distinctive patterns of presentation. The first is defined by sudden onset of an episode of massive gastrointestinal bleeding. This is painless, often with bright red blood per rectum and initially self-limited. In the setting of primary aneurysmal fistula, it can occur because of connection at any point along the aneurysmal sac. In the setting of prior graft replacement, the fistula usually has formed at one of the suture lines between the graft and the native aorta; at times, the infection of the graft can spread along its course, "un-incorporating" the Dacron material but bleeding still will occur from suture line failure (we have not seen dissolution of the graft material itself). As with other bleeds associated with infectious etiology, the first bleed is often known as a "heralding bleed," stopping from a combination of hypotension (reducing the pressure at the suture line) allowing acute coagulation. Aggressive resuscitation in the setting of diagnostic uncertainty combined with clot lysis (likely accelerated by active infection and exposure to the digestive ferocity of succus) leads to subsequent episodes of massive hemorrhage (less self-limited). Healthy suspicion, combined with rapid diagnosis, is vital if patients with this presentation are to be successfully treated.

Resuscitation of the patient who presents with gastrointestinal bleeding from an aortoenteric fistula is challenging. At times, massive ongoing bleeding results in severe hemodynamic instability and the patient requires full replenishment of intravascular volume to stabilize. Once the diagnosis is made and intervention is underway, a strategy of judicious hypotensive resuscitation can be employed. This decreases fluid administration and avoids the subsequent disastrous edema that results from excessive fluid administration. Additionally, passive hypotension theoretically reduces the pressure-based risk of disrupting a clot and decreases the rapidity and volume of ongoing hemorrhage. We utilize a strategy of balanced hemostatic resuscitation in our approach with low ratios of transfusion of units packed red blood cell to fresh frozen plasma and platelets. For these patients, we frequently enact our standard institutional massive transfusion protocol.

The second pattern of presentation is more insidious, and likely more common [2, 3]. Slow erosion of the bowel wall results in the continual bathing of a patch of graft with succus or stool. This continual exposure results in episodic bacteremia with poly-microbial exposure and no possibility for sterilization with antibiotic administration, unlike an uncomplicated mono-microbial graft infection (if there really is such a thing). There is often suspicion of a graft infection but not necessarily a proven etiology (imaging findings can be subtle). It is not uncommon for these patients to undergo months of several courses of escalating antibiotic therapy suffering chronic malaise and malnutrition.

Diagnosis

When the presentation is acute, expeditious diagnosis is vital. Confirmation of fistula then allows management planning (this can be a terminal event as not all patients are appropriate operative candidates). CT scanning and endoscopy are the primary modalities to confirm aortoenteric fistula [4, 5]. CT is least invasive and may be immediately diagnostic. Inflammation is generally seen at the fistula site with air, extraluminal to the GI track, as seen along the wall of the aorta or aortic graft [6] (Figs. 12.3 and 12.4). EGD or colonoscopy will often demonstrate the fistula, almost shockingly, by visualizing obvious graft material comprising a large portion of the bowel wall. This too is immediately diagnostic (Fig. 12.5).

While the CT may suggest some inflammation along the course of the aorta, it is sometimes quite difficult to confirm a fistula (Fig. 12.6). The duodenum is almost always collapsed in its third and fourth portions. Radiographically this can hide wall thickening along the posterior aspect of the duodenum. Further, there is seldom an associated pocket of purulence as the connection to the bowel effectively drains internally and in thin patients, the paucity of fat frequently precludes identification of significant inflammation.

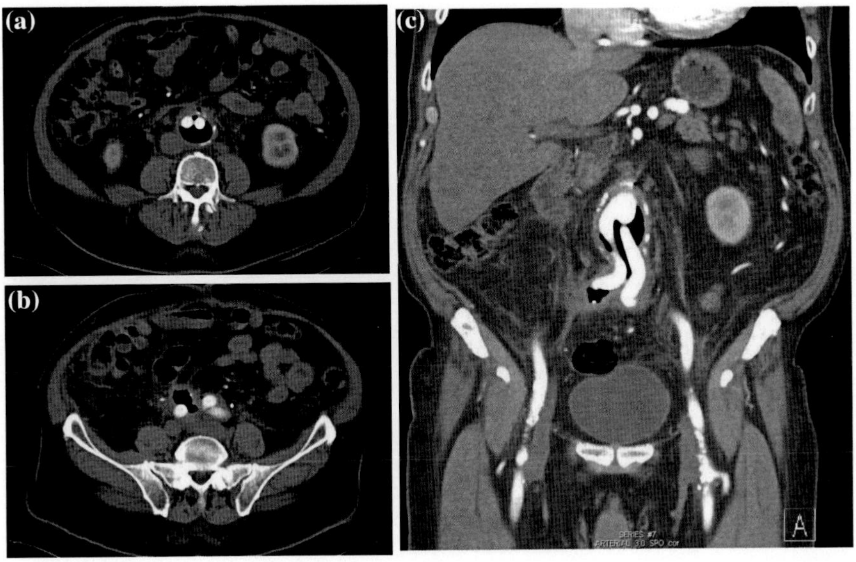

Fig. 12.3 CT of graft with massive amount of air around prosthetic graft (**a**); **b** coronal reconstruction; **c** fistulous connection with overlying sigmoid colon

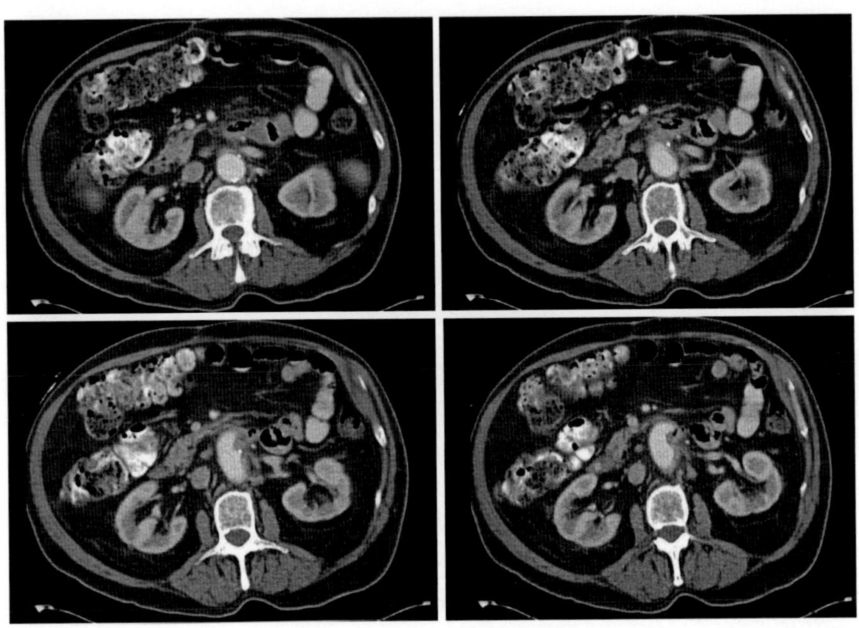

Fig. 12.4 CT of aortic graft with subtle amount of periduodenal inflammation and a spicule of air in the graft bed (*right lower frame*)

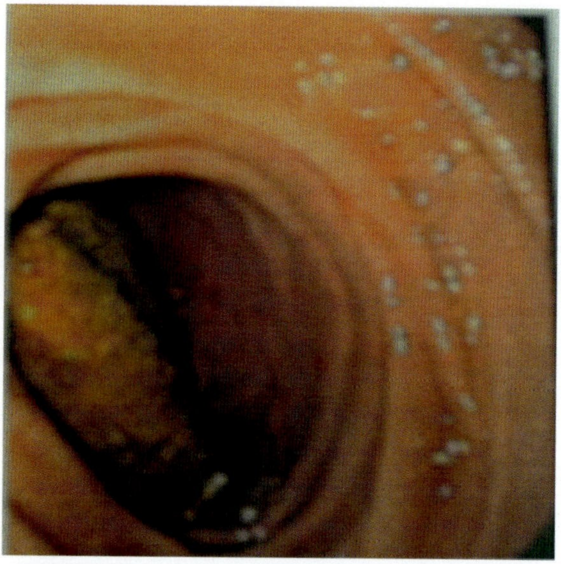

Fig. 12.5 EGD view of posterior wall of fourth portion of the duodenum with visualized prosthetic from the aortic graft

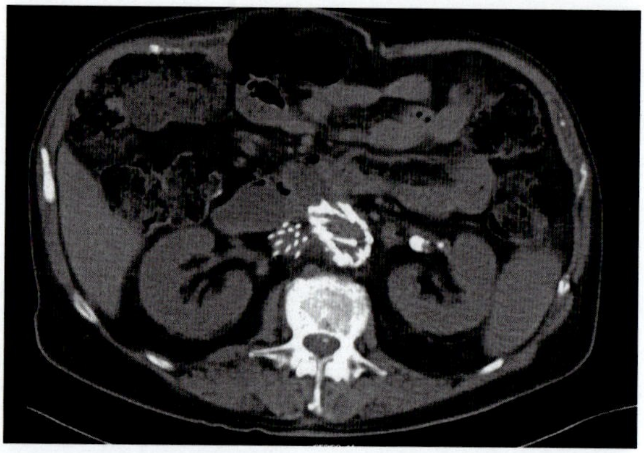

Fig. 12.6 Subtle periduodenal inflammation in a patient with an endostent; confirmed aortoenteric fistula

There is usually no pain associated with aortoenteric fistula formation (sometimes achy back discomfort) and few digestive symptoms. Chronic unwellness is nonspecific but continued elevation of inflammatory indicators, episodic illness, polymicrobial, and shifting bacteremias (especially enteric flora) should heighten suspicion and guide more aggressive diagnostic efforts.

Management

No aortoenteric fistula will heal spontaneously. Operative management is the only solution for correction of aortoenteric fistula. A decision to manage conservatively with ongoing antibiotic regimens is reasonable if the patient is unfit for operative repair, does not want to risk repair, or carries a prognosis from other comorbidities that govern life span (such as metastatic cancer). This is purely a palliative option; the natural history can be expected to be a septic or hemorrhagic death if due to the fistula.

The goals of operative therapy are to (1) assure arterial flow and adequate distal perfusion, (2) detach the connection between the GI track and the arterial system, (3) re-establish GI track integrity, (4) minimize risk of recurrence, and (5) definitively manage the systemic infection. These operations are long, technically challenging and high risk. We have chosen a multidisciplinary approach combining the efforts of both acute care and vascular surgeons with critical care anesthesia and where possible, perfusionists.

Whether the presentation is by bleeding or other, adequate access and availability of blood products are keys. Appropriate broad-spectrum antibiotics are given and redosed as per protocol. Excellent intraoperative communication is also vital as we have found that at times it is most appropriate to expect to have to truncate the repair (stage in a damage control manner) to optimize the patient's physiologic reserve. The operative plan is also of paramount importance. The patients are positioned in the supine position and the operative field that is prepared is from the neck to the mid-thighs with the axillae and femoral regions exposed. Adequate venous access for resuscitation is assured.

Arterial Flow and Distal Perfusion

With respect to arterial reconstruction, there are two overarching approaches to the management of infected aortic grafts: extra-anatomic bypass versus in situ graft placement. The advantages of extra-anatomic bypass (axillofemoral plus femoral–femoral grafts) include minimal invasive approach which can be performed prior to graft excision, removing prosthetic from an infected graft bed, assured distal perfusion to allow time to dissect and if aortic clamping is needed during fistula takedown. Disadvantages include a plan to over-sew the aortic stump in the infected field, and thus to degenerate and rupture fatally, as well as a short patency of the small diameter extra-anatomic bypass circuits. Conversely, in situ reconstruction has a longer patency and preserves native flow but leaves graft in the soiled bed, may be a longer and more complex operation, and may require a longer duration of systemic antibiotics.

In situ reconstruction of the infected aorta is gaining favor over staged reconstruction; advocates of in situ reconstruction note a durable anastomosis can be achieved and debridement of the infected graft removes the nidus of infection to reduce the risk of reinfection [7]. In situ reconstruction has better patency versus extra-anatomic bypass, and when the patient's presentation includes septic shock, limb salvage based off axillary inflow alone may be insufficient to perfuse the distal legs.

Fistula Takedown

At entry into the abdomen, it is important to preserve the omentum (the reason will be apparent later). As these cases are frequently reoperative adventures, slow and careful dissection is required. A thorough lysis of adhesions is undertaken exposing the retroperitoneum. This ultimately exposes the aortoenteric fistula. These connections are invariably characterized by dense adhesion of the bowel to the aortic structure. This is often left as the last area of dissection.

A decision must be made early in the procedure about the strategy of aortic control. For fistulas to primary aortic aneurysms, early aortic control, often supra-celiac and at the diaphragmatic hiatus, is prudent to guard against uncontrolled hemorrhage during dissection. Endovascular positioning of a Coda balloon devise is also an option. Similar consideration should be taken for patients with fistulas that present with massive bleed (indicating the connection is at a compromised aortic suture line) and in fistulas arising in the setting of endostents (Fig. 12.7). In the latter, the fixation of the proximal tines is compromised and there is a concern for disruption on the dissection of the enteric connection to the aorta. For patients with more common presentation of recurrent infection, disruption of the aortic integrity is less likely and aortic control can be deferred until the fistula is resected and the aortic dissection is performed at the stage of graft excision. With the necessary precautions, dissection of the fistulous adhesion may be undertaken

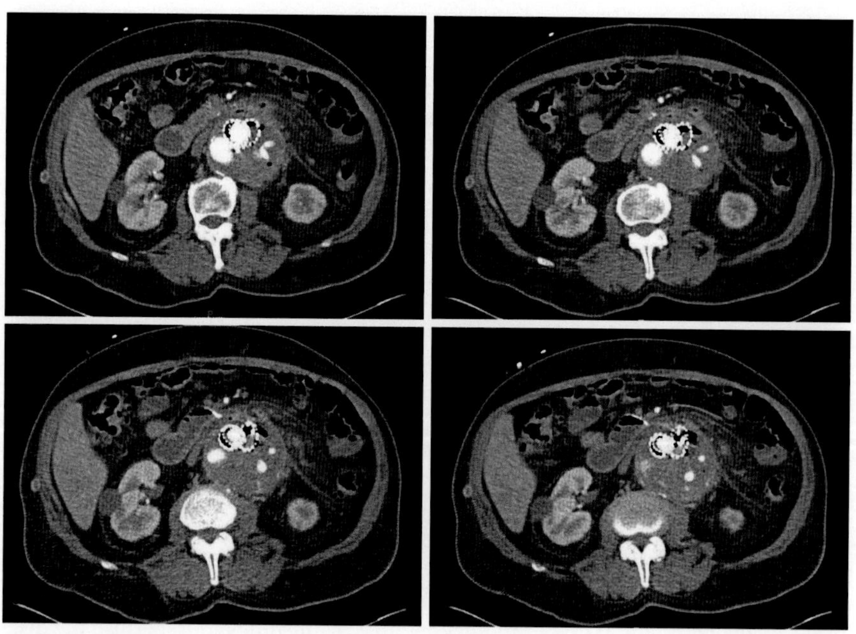

Fig. 12.7 Aortoenteric fistula with peri-graft air as well as contrast extravasation into the aneurysmal sac. This patient presented with large intermittent GI bleeding

confidently because by definition one wall of the bowel has a hole and "sealed" by the graft. This interface defines the dissection plane.

Gastrointestinal Integrity

We feel that the involved bowel segment in these cases ultimately should be managed with segmental resection rather than primary repair, no matter how small the connection that is identified. The reasons for this are multifactorial. First the bowel proximal and distal to the fistula is often inflamed and more compromised than it appears. The second principle is demonstrated in the case of the duodenal fistulas. Primary repair of the duodenal defect anatomically leaves the suture line directly anterior to the aortic replacement or an aortic stump and within the infected field. This sets this area up for the risk of recurrent adhesion and, in turn, recurrence of fistula [3].

In the case of duodenal resection, we recommend segmental resection of the fourth portion of the duodenum (and only as much of the third as is necessary), with duodeno-jejunal reconstruction to the right of the root of the SMA/SMV. We favor a hand-sewn side to side duodeno-jejunostomy. Full kocherization of the duodenum eases the technical challenge of this anastomosis and as with all anastomoses in this location; constant awareness of the location of the Ampulla of Vater is vital to avoid injury to the common bile duct. Occasionally, the reconstruction needs to be performed to the second portion of the duodenum.

The reconstruction is performed after the aortic portion of the case is completed. This avoids both needless traction on fresh anastomoses and the risk of anastomotic bleed following heparin administration given for the vascular work. The foramen posterior to the mesenteric vessels where the duodenum previously ran is closed by reapproximating the retroperitoneal tissue, further separating the beds of healing tissues.

Colonic fistulae are best managed in the acute repair with colostomy. These patients are often chronically ill and in an inflammatory state, malnourished and in the setting of acute bleed, subject to critical stress, massive transfusion, and hemodynamic lability, all potential risks for colonic anastomotic failure. The colostomy is then reversed at interval following recovery from the initial resection.

Minimize Risk of Recurrence

All patients receive broad-spectrum antibiotics and antifungals preoperatively and intraoperatively, with redosing based on blood loss of 1500 ml. At a minimum, it is vital to remove all unincorporated graft tissue; incorporated tissue can be retained. Tube grafts may be more easily excised in total than bi-limbed grafts. Similarly, tube endostents may be more readily removed as well. In addition to anatomic separation of the gastrointestinal and vascular healing tissues, it is important to cover the resection tissue. Any prior aneurysmal sac should also be debrided at this time; its blood supply is poor and it will be by definition contaminated tissue and a liability. Additionally, any pockets of purulence that are identified need to be drained, debrided, and irrigated. Adjacent psoas abscesses and infected vertebral disks are examples of such entities. The omentum that has been carefully preserved at abdominal entry is dissected from its transverse colonic attachment and an omental pedicle flap is created; the vascular supply is preserved along the greater curve of the stomach. It is brought through the transverse mesocolon to the left of the middle colic artery and the in situ replaced graft is wrapped circumferentially (not just draped). If the omentum is foreshortened, it can be split on a line radially perpendicular to the greater curve of the stomach to allow both anterior and posterior coverages of the graft. Additional length can be achieved by bringing the flap through the mesocolon as posteriorly as possible; the omental flap is then sutured in place to the retroperitoneal tissue. If the aortic stump is to be oversewn, this too should be covered with a healthy omental flap [7]. It is our practice to prepare the in situ replacement graft (Dacron) by soaking it in Rifampin for 1 h prior to placement in a solution of 1200 mg Rifmapin in 200 cc of saline. Studies have demonstrated rifampin can be detected on the graft up to 7 days postoperatively [8].

Managing Systemic Infection

Unlike infected grafts that result from hematogenous contamination, by definition, the aortoenteric fistula will be polymicrobial and enteric bacteria and fungus must be covered. Late definitive diagnosis may have resulted in episodic antibiotic exposure so perioperative broad-spectrum antibiotics are required. Culture of the excised graft and tissue is important as it may help guide and narrow appropriate antibiotic choice. We favor an aggressive antibiotic regimen with an anticipated course of at least 6–12 weeks of intravenous antibiotics, or longer until the ESR and CRP levels have normalized. At that time, oral antibiotics are started and ESR and CRP levels are checked monthly. An elevation of these proinflammatory markers should prompt a CT scan to evaluate for new retroperitoneal inflammation.

Physiologic Considerations

By definition, these are operatively complex, technically challenging, lengthy cases that potentially impose severe physiologic stress on the patient. As with all aortic operations, EBL is usually significant and intraoperative resuscitation strategies should be managed to avoid excessive crystalloid infusion. If the patient is unstable (on pressors, acidotic, and cold) following the vascular portion of the case, then a damage control approach should be employed deploying a temporary abdominal closure prior to gastrointestinal reconstruction. Once the physiologic derangements have been corrected, the patient is returned to the OR from the surgical intensive care unit.

Cell saver autotransfusion may serve to reduce non-autogenous transfusion but should not be employed until the infected graft and debridement is completed; given the substantial friability of the inflamed tissue in the periaortic region or neighboring lumbosacral discitis, substantial bleeding should be anticipated.

Clinical scenario

70-year-old woman is s/p endovascular repair of an abdominal aortic aneurysm 8 years prior to presentation. She was being followed by her primary care provider for occult GI Bleed and anemia. She is transferred from and outside hospital after a self-limited massive upper and lower gastrointestinal hemorrhage. Esophagogastroduodenoscopy demonstrated visualization of the endovascular aortic stent at the junction of D3–D4.

Author's comment:

This is the overt, dramatic presentation of aorto-duodenal fistula with a massive "heralding bleed." Though she appears to be stable at the moment, she will likely rebleed at any time and as such there is significant urgency for planning repair. Extra-anatomic vascular bypass remains an option as to the discussion or palliative care for the elderly patient with significant comorbidity. In our current practice, we would arrange a multidisciplinary procedure with both a vascular surgeon and a general surgeon (acute care). The approach for us is most frequently a midline laparotomy with the plan to excise the fistula, replace the aortic graft in situ with a rifampin-soaked Dacron graft, and re-establish GI continuity following segmental resection of the duodenum. Key operative points include: (1) *An effort to preserve omentum on entry to the abdomen.* In this case, the previous procedure was an EVAR so it is possible that there was no prior abdominal surgery. This will be used as a vascularized pedicle to wrap the new graft. (2) *Early vascular control, prior to dissection of the fistula.* As this was an EVAR the risk of dislodgement of the endostent is high, especially given that this presentation was a bleeding event suggesting possible endoleak. (3) *Confident dissection of the fistula once the vascular control is secure.* The safest approach is from the left of the fourth portion of the duodenum, following the mobilization of the ligament of Treitz. Once the adhered duodenum is off of the graft, the segmental blood supply is reliably spirals superiorly as the surgeon follows the duodenum proximally as it crosses under the superior mesenteric artery and vein. (4) *Performing a staged, "damage control" procedure as necessary.* This is well tolerated and appropriate for patients that undergo large volume resuscitation. (5) *Gastrointestinal reconstruction following vascular repair.* This too may be performed in a staged manner pursuant to the patient's physiology.

Key Questions

1. *What is the preferred operative approach to taking down an aorto-duodenal fistula?*
2. *Is there a role for a duodenal exclusion procedure?*

References

1. Saratzis N, Saratzis A, Melas N, Ktenidis K, Kiskinis D. Aortoduodenal fistulas after endovascular stent-graft repair of abdominal aortic aneurysms: single-center experience and review of the literature. J Endovasc Ther. 2008;15(4):441–8.
2. Wong JC, Taylor DC, Byrne MF. Aortoduodenal fistula: not always bleeding. Can J Gastroenterol. 2013;27(8):444.
3. Howard R, Kurz S, Sherman MA, Underhill J, Eliason JL, Coleman DM. Contemporary management of secondary aortoduodenal fistula. Ann Vasc Surg. 2015;29(8):1614–8.
4. Bussttil SJ, Goldstone J. Diagnosis and management of aorto-enteric fistulas. Semin Vasc Surg. 2001;14:302–11.
5. Tacchini S, Nicoletti R, Ghio D, Marinenghi CM, Chiesa R, Del Maschio A. CT findings of secondary aorto-enteric fistulae. Radiol Med. 2005;110:492–500.
6. Frauenfelder T, Wildermuth S, Marincek B, Boehm T. Nontraumatic emergent abdominal vascular conditions: advantages of multi-detector row CT and three-dimensional imaging. Radiographics. 2004;24(2):481–96.
7. Rodrigues dos Santos C, Casaca R, Mendes de Almeida JC, Mendes-Pedro L. Enteric repair in aortoduodenal fistulas: a forgotten but often lethal player. Ann Vasc Surg. 2014;28(3):756–62.
8. Oderich GS1, Bower TC, Hofer J, Kalra M, Duncan AA, Wilson JW, Cha S, Gloviczki P. In situ rifampin-soaked grafts with omental coverage and antibiotic suppression are durable with low reinfection rates in patients with aortic graft enteric erosion or fistula. J Vasc Surg. 2011;53 (1):99–106.

Chapter 13
Small Bowel: Pneumatosis Intestinalis

Alaina M. Lasinski, Joseph Posluszny and Fred A. Luchette

Identification of Pneumatosis and Determining Clinical Relevance

Pneumatosis intestinalis (PI) has been diagnosed more frequently in the recent years due to the increased use of computed tomography (CT) for abdominal imaging and also the improved enhancement of modern CT. In the past, PI identified on imaging was almost always considered a sign of vascularly compromised bowel and the need for emergent laparotomy. Today, it is not uncommon for PI to be an incidental finding on an abdominal CT performed for other indications, in which case it may not be clinically significant. PI is usually benign when it is secondary to the penetration of gas into the bowel wall secondary to mucosal breakdown in the setting of distension or bacterial overgrowth [1–5]. Examples of benign PI include but are not limited to COPD and other pulmonary etiologies; inflammatory bowel disease and other gastrointestinal etiologies; and autoimmune, infectious, iatrogenic,

A.M. Lasinski
Department of Surgery, Loyola University Medical Center, 2160 South First Avenue, EMS Building, Room 3210, Maywood, IL 60153, USA
e-mail: alasinski@lumc.edu

J. Posluszny
Department of Surgery, Loyola University Medical Center, 2160 South First Avenue, EMS Building, Room 3279, Maywood, IL 60153, USA
e-mail: joseph.posluszny@lumc.edu

F.A. Luchette (✉)
Department of Surgery, Loyola University Medical Center, 2160 South First Avenue, Maywood, IL 60153, USA
e-mail: fluchet@lumc.edu

J.J. Diaz and D.T. Efron (eds.), *Complications in Acute Care Surgery*,
DOI 10.1007/978-3-319-42376-0_13

drug-induced, and transplantation-related etiologies. Examples of benign PI include but are not limited to pulmonary etiologies (e.g., asthma, chronic obstructive pulmonary disorder, pulmonary fibrosis), gastrointestinal etiologies (e.g., inflammatory bowel disease, diverticulitis, infectious enteritis, adynamic ileus, peptic ulcer, carcinoma), autoimmune and systemic etiologies (e.g., connective tissue diseases, lupus, scleroderma, polyarteritis nodosa), infectious etiologies (e.g., HIV and AIDS, mycobacterium tuberculosis, and candida albicans), iatrogenic etiologies (endoscopy, enteric tube placement, mechanical ventilation, and blunt abdominal trauma), drug-induced etiologies (the use of corticosteroids or chemotherapeutic agents), and etiologies secondary to organ transplantation (e.g., graft versus host disease after bone marrow transplant or in liver, lung, or kidney transplantation) [2, 3, 5, 6] (Fig. 13.1a). Pathologic PI, in which gas within the bowel wall is consistent with ischemia, most often requires surgical intervention. Once identified on imaging, the dilemma is trying to determine the etiology of the PI, whether or not it is associated with bowel ischemia, and whether surgical intervention to assess the vascular integrity of the intestine with possible subsequent resection is necessary.

Factors Associated with Pathologic Pneumatosis Intestinalis

In the absence of obvious peritonitis, surgeons must consider the patient's clinical history, physical examination, laboratory results, and imaging findings before deciding whether operative management is appropriate in a patient with PI (Table 13.1). Patient characteristics that are associated with pathologic PI are age greater than 60 [3, 5] and comorbidities that increase the chance of a thromboembolic event, including smoking, diabetes, hypertension, hyperlipidemia, coronary artery disease, and stroke [4, 7]. Furthermore, patients who are at risk for developing a low flow state secondary to arrhythmias, heart failure, or vasopressor dependence are also more likely to have bowel ischemia. Physical examination findings include abdominal tenderness. Specifically, diffuse peritonitis with involuntary guarding and rebound tenderness is an important clinical sign that suggests the need for emergent exploration [1, 3, 4, 7]. Hypotension refractory to intravenous fluids or dependence on vasopressors is another indicator that surgery is necessary [3]. Tachycardia, tachypnea, and abdominal distension may be other less sensitive signs [3, 7]. Laboratory findings suggestive of bowel ischemia include a lactate greater than 2.0 mmol/L [1–3, 5–7], acidosis with bicarbonate less than 20 mmol/l [1, 3, 5], and leukocytosis greater than 12 c/mm [3, 5]. With regard to radiographic signs, the presence of portal venous gas [1, 2, 8–10], dilation of small bowel greater than 3 cm and large bowel greater than 6 cm, mesenteric stranding, and ascites all point toward ischemic and/or gangrenous bowel [1, 7, 11]. Regardless of which signs and symptoms are present, the decision for or against operative management must be timely as mortality rate is high in the setting of pathologic PI.

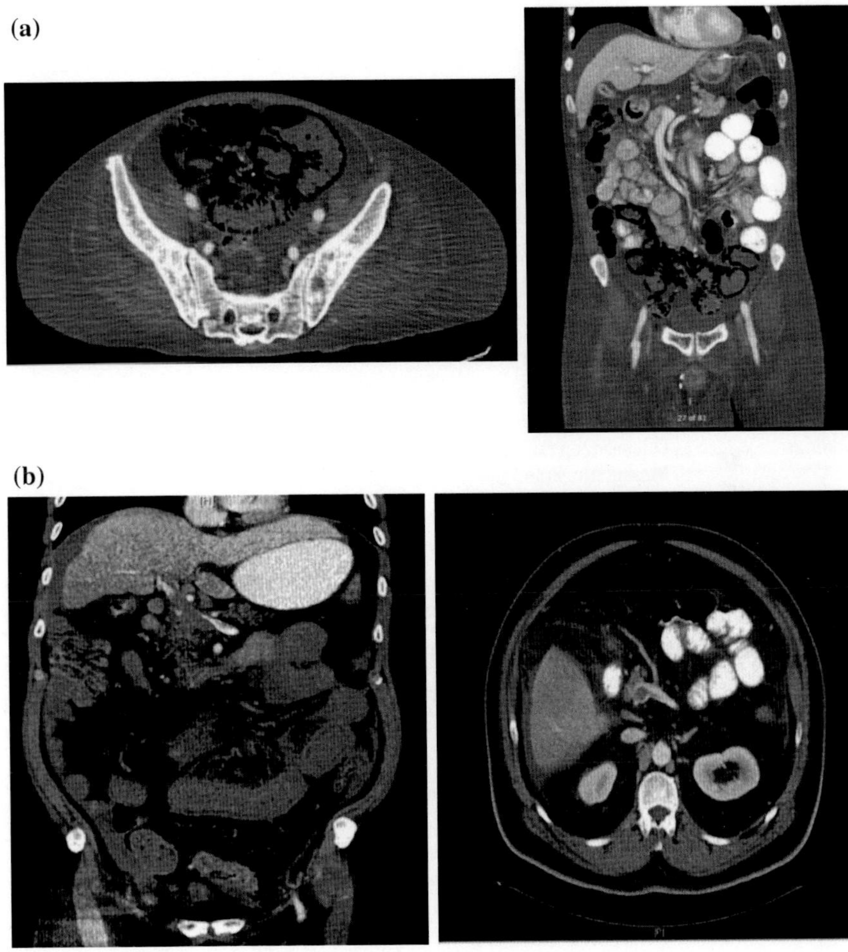

Fig. 13.1 **a** CT of patient with pneumatosis intestinalis who underwent a negative exploratory laparotomy. **b** CT of patient with ischemic bowel from venous outflow obstruction with bowel edema

Preoperative and Intraoperative Planning and Assessment

Once the decision to explore the abdomen has been made, much of the intraoperative plan can be determined preoperatively by knowing the source of ischemia. The most common causes of acute mesenteric ischemia leading to pneumatosis are arterial embolism, arterial thrombosis, nonocclusive mesenteric ischemia, and venous outflow obstruction or mesenteric venous thrombosis (Table 13.2).

An embolus in the superior mesenteric artery (SMA) in a patient recently diagnosed with atrial fibrillation or with a known hypercoagulable state with CT scan showing a clear filling defect in the SMA will often have ischemic bowel

Table 13.1 Clinical factors and radiographic findings associated with pneumatosis intestinalis that correlate with ischemic bowel

History	Age >60 Vascular risk factors (smoking history, diabetes, hypertension, hyperlipidemia) Risk factors for low flow state, including arrhythmias, vasopressor dependence, and heart failure History of cerebrovascular accident
Physical examination	Peritonitis (rebound tenderness or involuntary guarding) Hypotension not responsive to IV fluids Abdominal distention
Laboratory values	Elevated lactate (>2 mmol/L) Bicarbonate <20 WBC >12
Radiographic findings	Portal venous gas Dilated loops of small bowel (>3 cm) and large bowel (>6 cm) Mesenteric stranding Free fluid/ascites

Table 13.2 Causes of pneumatosis intestinalis, radiographic findings, and operative techniques for management

Causes of pneumatosis intestinalis	Radiographic findings	Operative techniques for management
Embolism	Discrete filling defect of SMA	Resection of ischemic bowel Embolectomy
Thrombosis	Diffuse atherosclerotic changes	Resection of ischemic bowel Vascular surgery consult Possible SMA bypass
Low flow state	Diffuse bowel wall thickening	Doppler evaluation of mesenteric vessels Warming bowel with laparotomy pads Fluorescein staining and Wood's lamp examination Temporary abdominal closure with second look after further resuscitation
Venous outflow obstruction/mesenteric venous thrombosis	Distention of mesenteric veins	Resection of ischemic bowel Second-look laparotomy Therapeutic anticoagulation

found upon exploration. Often, these emboli are small and lodge distal to the first jejunal branches. This often avoids the need for extensive bowel resection that would render the patient with short bowel syndrome (SBS). Further, this clinical scenario and radiographic finding should prompt the surgeon to prepare for SMA embolectomy in addition to bowel resection.

For patients with manifestations of atherosclerotic disease including coronary artery disease and peripheral and/or cerebral vascular disease, SMA thrombosis should be suspected. CT scan will show atherosclerotic disease throughout the aorta and within the origin of the SMA or even distally. As the ischemia may involve the entire SMA distribution, a large segment of bowel may need resection. In addition, restoration of blood flow to the bowel may require an aortomesenteric bypass, which should prompt the surgeon to involve a vascular surgeon with this expertise early in the process.

Nonocclusive mesenteric ischemia leads to a "low flow state" in which the vasculature to the small and large intestine is patent, but global flow to the bowel is compromised. High-dose vasopressors, myocardial infarction, cardiogenic shock, and the recent cardiac bypass are the more common clinical scenarios associated with a low flow state. In these instances, both the small bowel and large bowel are involved; therefore, adequate volume resuscitation, cardiac optimization, and liberation from vasopressors are keys to restoring bowel viability. When exploration is necessary and the majority of the small bowel appears ischemic, it should not be resected due to the risk of a resulting SBS. Instead, the operation should be truncated with a temporary closure of the abdomen and planned second-look laparotomy after restoration of flow.

Mesenteric venous thrombosis may involve the portal vein, the superior mesenteric vein, or both and is diagnosed preoperatively with CT scan. Therapeutic anticoagulation should start as soon as possible in hopes of resolving the clot burden and preventing propagation. CT images will show the engorgement of the mesenteric veins reflective of venous congestion secondary to stasis (Fig. 13.1b). As discussed above, if peritonitis, leukocytosis, or worsening acidosis despite fluid resuscitation occur, then exploration with bowel resection may be necessary.

Often in these scenarios, it is difficult to determine whether intestinal perfusion is compromised and may recover or clearly needs resection. Adjuncts to assessing bowel viability are palpation of the mesentery for a pulse, using a Doppler to determine the presence of a triphasic signal at the antimesenteric border of the intestine, warming of the bowel with laparotomy pads, and fluorescein staining with Wood's lamp examination. If none of these methods of assessment clearly determine bowel viability, then a second-look laparotomy should be planned. A second-look operation should be carried out in 24–48 h with the time between operations focusing on the response to resuscitation, optimization of the metabolic status, and reducing vasopressor requirements.

Complications

If a large amount of bowel is resected, SBS may develop. Although defined as the presence of less than 200 cm of residual small bowel, SBS is functionally defined as an inadequate length of bowel that results in impaired absorptive capacity and inability to maintain adequate nutrition and hydration with the patient developing diarrhea, dehydration, and malnutrition. These patients may become dependent on total parenteral nutrition (TPN) if there is less than 100 cm of residual small intestine without a functional colon or 60 cm of small bowel in patients with an intact colon. Similarly, those who undergo resection of the ileocecal valve are at an increased risk of developing SBS with TPN dependence. Roughly fifty percent of patients who initially require TPN may achieve independence from TPN because of the adaptation that the remaining bowel undergoes over time to increase its capacity to absorb nutrients. However, dependence on TPN, for a lifetime or even for a briefer time as the remaining bowel adapts, is associated with its own risks including central line infection, vascular stenosis, venous thrombosis, kidney and liver failure, and osteoporosis which leads to reduced life expectancy. The high financial costs of TPN should not be overlooked either.

Often, given the large-volume resuscitation patients undergo with the subsequent development of bowel edema and need for second-look laparotomy, the abdominal fascia may be difficult to close. This scenario renders the patient more prone to hernia formation or temporary closure with planned hernia and reconstruction at a later date. Preferably, the abdominal wall should be closed or the exposed abdominal contents covered within 5–7 days of the index laparotomy to minimize the development of an atmospheric fistula.

Clinical Scenario

You are asked to see a 67-year-old woman who had an uncomplicated mitral valve replacement one week ago. She is complaining of vague abdominal pain. On examination, there is mild tenderness but no peritoneal signs. The only abnormal laboratory studies are a white count of 18,251 and a serum lactate of 2.5. A CT scan of the abdomen demonstrates PI and portal venous air.

This patient has a few clinical characteristics and laboratory findings that are concerning for ischemic bowel in the setting of PI. Leukocytosis and lactic acidosis point toward an ischemic etiology of the PI. Additionally, the recent surgery to replace a cardiac valve increases the risk for an embolic event to the mesenteric circulation. Another risk factor for mesenteric ischemia and PI is the use of vasopressors to support the cardiovascular system. When presented with this clinical situation, the clinician is left with the options of exploratory laparotomy immediately or fluid resuscitation with re-evaluation of WBC count and lactate. If the patient is without abdominal signs and symptoms, it would be reasonable to treat with fluid resuscitation and serial physical examination with the repeat laboratory studies. If there is no change in the clinical course, emergent laparotomy is indicated.

Key Questions

1. *In the setting of mesenteric ischemia the best approach to identify and operatively expose the SMA is?*
2. *Is there a role for the Spy elite systems in identifying tissue ischemia?*

References

1. Lee H, Cho Y, Kim K, Lee JS, Lee SS, et al. A simple score for predicting mortality in patients with pneumatosis intestinalis. Eur J Radiol. 2014;83:639–45.
2. Kahlil PN, Huber-Wagner S, Ladurner R, Kleespies A, Siebeck M, et al. Natural history, clinical pattern, and surgical considerations of pneumatosis intestinalis. Eur J Med Res. 2009;14:231–9.
3. DuBose JJ, Lissauer M, Maung AA, Piper GL, O'Callaghan TA, et al. Pneumatosis intestinalis predictive evaluation study (PIPES): a multicenter epidemiologic study of the Eastern Association for the Surgery of Trauma. J Trauma Acute Care Surg. 2013;75:15–23.
4. Wayne E, Ough M, Wu A, Liao J, Andresen KJ, Kuehn D, et al. Management algorithm for pneumatosis intestinalis and portal venous gas: treatment and outcome of 88 consecutive cases. J Gastrointest Surg. 2010;14:437–48.
5. Greenstein AJ, Nguyen SQ, Berlin A, Corona J, Lee J, et al. Pneumatosis intestinalis in adults: management, surgical indications, and risk factors for mortality. J Gastrointest Surg. 2007;11:1268–74.
6. Rha SE, Hyn KH, Lee SH, Kim JH, Kim JK, et al. CT and MR imaging findings of bowel ischemia from various primary causes. Radiographics. 2000;20:29–42.
7. Duron VP, Rutigliano S, Machan JT, Dupuy DE, Mazzaglia PJ. Computed tomographic diagnosis of pneumatosis intestinalis. Arch Surg. 2011;146(5):506–10.
8. Morris MS, Gee AC, Cho D, Limbaugh K, Underwood S, et al. Management and outcome of pneumatosis intestinalis. Am J Surg. 2008;195:679–83.
9. Kernagis LY, Levine MS, Jacobs JE. Pneumatosis intestinalis in patients with ischemia: correlation of CT findings with viability of the bowel. AJR. 2003;180:733–6.
10. Wiesner W, Mortele KJ, Glickman JN, Ji H, Ros PR. Pneumatosis intestinalis and portomesenteric venous gas in intestinal ischemia: correlation of CT findings with severity of ischemia and clinical outcome. AJR. 2001;177:1319–23.
11. Tahiri M, Levy J, Alzaid S, Anderson D. An approach to pneumatosis intestinalis: factors affecting your management. Int J Surg Case Rep. 2015;6:133–7.

Suggested Reading List

12. DuBose JJ, Lissauer M, Maung AA, Piper GL, O'Callaghan TA, et al. Pneumatosis intestinalis predictive evaluation study (PIPES): a multicenter epidemiologic study of the Eastern Association for the Surgery of Trauma. J Trauma Acute Care Surg. 2013;75:15–23.
13. Duron VP, Rutigliano S, Machan JT, Dupuy DE, Mazzaglia PJ. Computed tomographic diagnosis of pneumatosis intestinalis. Arch Surg. 2011;146(5):506–10.
14. Greenstein AJ, Nguyen SQ, Berlin A, Corona J, Lee J, et al. Pneumatosis intestinalis in adults: management, surgical indications, and risk factors for mortality. J Gastrointest Surg. 2007;11:1268–74.
15. Lee H, Cho Y, Kim K, Lee JS, Lee SS, et al. A simple score for predicting mortality in patients with pneumatosis intestinalis. Eur J Radiol. 2014;83:639–45.
16. Wayne E, Ough M, Wu A, Liao J, Andresen KJ, Kuehn D, et al. Management algorithm for pneumatosis intestinalis and portal venous gas: treatment and outcome of 88 consecutive cases. J Gastrointest Surg. 2010;14:437–48.

Chapter 14
Colon: Long Hartmann and Rectal Stump Blowout

Beth R. Hochman and Patrick M. Reilly

Background

Long Hartmann or rectal stump blowout is a dreaded complication of an often already complicated patient scenario. To backtrack for a moment, consider what prompts a Hartmann operation and consequent rectal stump creation in the first place. Indications for this initial intervention are any colonic pathology requiring resection (injury, obstruction, ischemia, perforation) in a setting where primary anastomosis is deemed unsafe (poor tissue integrity, distal location of anastomosis, patient comorbidity, hemodynamic instability, all of which may negatively impact wound healing). Traditionally, the procedure involves rectosigmoid resection with end colostomy creation, leaving a defunctionalized rectal stump beginning at or just proximal to the peritoneal reflection. This stump is thus primarily extraperitoneal. However, the technique has been applied to all types of colonic resection, generating a stump comprised of any length of colon that may begin as far proximal as the ascending colon. This so-called long Hartmann extends well into the peritoneal cavity, and, particularly when the stump is filled with retained fecal matter, it is easy to appreciate that stump dehiscence can be a catastrophic event.

B.R. Hochman (✉)
Columbia University Medical Center, New York, NY, USA
e-mail: brh2106@cumc.columbia.edu

P.M. Reilly
Perelman School of Medicine, University of Pennsylvania, Philadelphia, PA, USA
e-mail: reillyp@uphs.upenn.edu

J.J. Diaz and D.T. Efron (eds.), *Complications in Acute Care Surgery*,
DOI 10.1007/978-3-319-42376-0_14

Prevention

Given the conditions in which a Hartmann stump is created, one can intuitively recognize the presence of a risk of stump dehiscence (blowout), as the very factors that preclude the safety of anastomotic healing are the same factors that threaten a stump suture or staple line (Table 14.1). Of course, the first step to combatting a complication is prevention. At the time of stump creation, optimization of tissue integrity and blood flow is paramount, starting with including only viable, noninflamed tissue at the stump margin. This helps ensure that the bowel edges are adequately apposed and that the staples or sutures successfully capture. Also, both tissue necrosis and inflammation-induced tissue edema impair blood flow, which is necessary for nutrient delivery and debris removal as the stump margin heals [1].

Meticulous surgical technique serves to preserve tissue integrity. Bleeding along wound edges may initially be taken as encouraging evidence of good blood flow, but hemostasis should be promptly achieved, as any significant hematoma formation at a wound edge can impede perfusion as well as provide a nidus for infection that would threaten the integrity of the closure. Similarly, adequate removal of any surrounding contamination is important for limiting impending infectious and inflammatory changes along the wound edge, which predispose to wound dehiscence [1]. Another very important consideration, especially when creating a long Hartmann stump, is selecting a stump margin well within the domain of segmental blood supply and avoiding watershed regions. This is less of an issue with rectal stumps due to the rectum's redundant blood supply via the inferior mesenteric artery (superior rectal artery), internal iliac artery (middle rectal artery), and pudendal artery (inferior rectal artery).

The next issue the surgeon must address is how to close the stump. Numerous studies have compared anastomotic leak rates with stapled versus handsewn and single- versus double-layer closures. The bulk of these demonstrate no clinically significant difference, though stapled and single-layer closures afford shorter operative times [2–7], which in the arena of emergency surgery can be critical. This can all presumably be extrapolated to stump closures, and a few recent studies in high-risk patient cohorts have indeed shown no difference in stump leak rates by closure method [8, 9].

Alternatively, maturation of a mucus fistula may be considered. Given the additional wound management requirements necessary with mucus fistula, stump closure is generally preferred unless a fistula can be brought up alongside the ostomy in a pseudo-loop fashion to facilitate future local restoration of continuity. Additional indications for fistula include presence of a distal obstruction, anticipated chemotherapy that may be initiated more quickly in the absence of a healing staple or suture line, and patient comorbidities that elevate concern for stump leak and/or catastrophic delay in recognition of a leak.

The heightened concern for stump leak among those patients undergoing subtotal colectomy for refractory inflammatory bowel disease—a particularly high-risk group given that they are often malnourished with recent exposure to

Table 14.1 Risk factors for intestinal wound healing

	Pathophysiology
Perioperative risk factors	
Antibiotics	Appropriate perioperative antibiosis minimizes microbial burden, which limits inflammatory response and infection risk
Blood supply	Adequate blood flow is required for delivery of nutrients and oxygen and removal of waste products
Contamination	Ongoing contamination is nidus for infection and inflammatory response, which impairs blood flow and increases collagen breakdown due to surge in MMP
Distal obstruction	Mechanical stress on bowel wall ultimately impairs perfusion
Foreign body (including suture material)	Induces persistent inflammatory response (particularly with silk suture) and serves as nidus for infection
Hemostasis	Hematoma-induced deformation of tissue impairs tissue perfusion, and hematoma is nidus for infection
Location of resection	Low dissection increases difficulty of closure, blood flow impaired if wound margins in watershed region, presence of serosa aids in bringing wound edges together when handsewn
Normothermia	Hypothermia leads to redistribution of blood flow and inhibits cell function
Operative time	Prolonged time is indicator of difficult dissection with increased tissue trauma and potentially increased bacterial exposure, especially if antibiotics not redosed appropriately
Oxygenation	Oxygen is necessary for aerobic metabolism, fibroblast proliferation, collagen synthesis, and antimicrobial oxidative burst of inflammatory cells during wound healing
Tissue integrity	Necrotic wound edges and inflammation-induced tissue edema impair perfusion
Patient risk factors/comorbidities	
Advanced age	Impairs collagen synthetic capacity and deposition
Alcohol use	Marker for malnutrition
Connective tissue disorder	Impairs collagen deposition
Diabetes	Causes microvascular disease, and impairs cell migration and proliferation
Hematologic disease	Increased viscosity and clot can impair blood flow
Hemodynamic instability/vasopressors	Impairs blood flow
Immunosuppression and chemotherapy	Impairs cell recruitment, turnover, and proliferation, and bevacizumab impairs blood flow
Inflammatory disease	Impairs perfusion and increases collagen breakdown
Jaundice	Impairs synthetic capacity and causes immunosuppression
Male gender	Increases difficulty of distal pelvic dissection
Malnutrition	Impairs collagen deposition and cell proliferation
Obesity	Increases difficulty of dissection
Radiation	Obliterates microvasculature, and alters collagen structure and fibroblast function
Tobacco use	Causes microvascular disease and impairs collagen deposition
Uremia	Impairs synthetic capacity and causes immunosuppression
Vascular disease	Impairs blood flow

high-dose steroids and/or anti-TNF agents and inherently inflamed tissue edges—has prompted a handful of studies of stump management options in this high-risk cohort. Historically, mucus fistula maturation was standard for this patient population, but a series of investigations in the 1990s demonstrated that the incidence of pelvic sepsis with stump closure was not significantly different from that with mucus fistula. Thus, incurring the added morbidity of a mucus fistula has become less popular. Instead, multiple authors have proposed leaving the stump long enough to facilitate subcutaneous placement, either at the inferior aspect of the midline incision or at a separate site in the left lower quadrant. Proponents argue that although this leaves additional potentially diseased tissue in situ, the subcutaneous location allows for safer control in the instance of a leak, which would generate a wound infection amenable to superficial management rather than pelvic sepsis requiring more invasive measures. Also, at the time of completion of proctectomy and ostomy reversal, the stump may be more readily identified than if it were left intraperitoneal. Interestingly, one recent comparison of intraperitoneal versus subcutaneous stumps found no significant difference in stump-related morbidity, including stump leak, pelvic sepsis, or wound infection, although patients with intraperitoneal stumps did experience significantly shorter time to return of bowel function, along with shorter operative times and fewer conversions from laparoscopic to open [8].

The decision to leave a drain often incites a great deal of discussion. Proponents of intraperitoneal drain placement suggest that drains offer an opportunity to remove any lingering contamination and provide a means to control any infectious complication or leak that may arise. Opponents suggest that the drains themselves generate irritation and means for pathogen exposure that potentially increase the likelihood of wound breakdown [1]. In our opinion, if any concern exists about lingering contamination, inclusion of less-than-ideal bowel in the stump margin, or presence of significant patient factors that would contribute to wound dehiscence, then drain placement is a prudent measure. Significant patient risk factors can be categorized broadly into those that compromise blood supply (hemodynamic instability, vasopressor requirement, diabetes, significant underlying vascular disease or tobacco history, pelvic irradiation, chemotherapy with anti-angiogenesis agents such as bevacizumab), and those that compromise collagen deposition and cell turnover for wound healing (advanced age, diabetes, connective tissue disorders, significant tobacco history, malnutrition or significant alcohol history, jaundice, uremia, immunosuppression, or chemotherapy). Similarly, placement of a transanal drainage catheter to encourage decompression of remnant stool is a low-risk intervention that reduces the likelihood of distal stump obstruction and may reduce the incidence of pelvic sepsis [10].

Additional perioperative considerations that have received a great deal of attention due to the Centers for Medicare and Medicaid Services Surgical Care Improvement Project (SCIP) and American College of Surgeons National Surgical Quality Improvement Program (NSQIP) initiatives include antibiotic use (specifically, appropriate selection, timing of administration, dosing, and redosing), oxygenation to optimize metabolism and collagen synthesis, and normothermia to facilitate blood flow and cell function. Also, close attention to maintaining adequate perioperative resuscitation and meeting nutritional needs is paramount [11].

Diagnosis

Unfortunately, successful prevention of complications is a luxury not always achieved. Patients suffering from stump blowout will manifest symptoms based on the location of the stump margin, extent of dehiscence, and the patient's capacity to contain the ensuing contamination. As with any infection, the initial symptoms may be nonspecific (fever, tachycardia, anorexia, ileus, leukocytosis), or the patient may suddenly develop unexplained sepsis. Vague abdominal pain may progress to frank peritonitis or focalize in the setting of a walled-off abscess. Lower pelvic stumps may precipitate urinary symptoms and/or tenesmus. While frankly peritoneal patients call for immediate operative exploration, those who are stable with unclear diagnoses are best worked up with computed tomography (CT) enhanced with oral, intravenous, and water-soluble rectal contrast [11].

Management

The overarching goals in managing a patient with stump blowout are as follows: (1) removal of infected material, (2) source control, and (3) prevention of recurrence. Specific management strategies for each of these goals vary based on the patient's clinical status and the nature of the dehiscence [12]. One advantage of these scenarios is that in all instances, diversion of the fecal stream has already been achieved.

Contained abscesses are generally treated with percutaneous drainage and/or antibiotics. Abscesses larger than 4–6 cm are unlikely to resolve with antibiotics alone. Percutaneous drainage may be achieved with image guidance and the assistance of interventional radiology colleagues. Depending on the precise location of the abscess, this results in a transabdominal, transgluteal, or transrectal drain that is generally left in place until the output is benign-appearing serous fluid.

Nonresolving or inaccessible abscesses prompt operative management. In the case of extraperitoneal collections, this involves an examination under anesthesia and potentially transanal or presacral drain placement. Intraperitoneal collections require laparoscopy or laparotomy, but in otherwise stable patients, it is important to consider the timing of such an intervention, as the extensive desmoplastic reaction induced by major surgery in the first 2–4 weeks postoperatively can make reoperations during this time extremely challenging and incur greater risk of bleeding, iatrogenic injury, and subsequent fistula formation [11].

Once the decision has been made to take the patient to the operating room, either for emergent control of peritonitis or sepsis or for delayed management of nonresolving abscess, the approach is the same. Whether the patient undergoes laparoscopic or open exploration is up to the discretion and comfort level of the operating surgeon, although typically patient instability and extent of contamination in emergent cases demand laparotomy. Upon entry, the area is debrided of frank contamination and any loosely adherent fibrinous exudates, and then liberally irrigated with warm saline. If necessary and feasible, the open end of a long Hartmann may be whip-stitched or stapled closed for temporary control before embarking on further dissection, although often the tissue is so friable in these circumstances that attempts to do so only enlarge the defect [11]. Because of this latter risk, it is advisable to avoid any unnecessary stitch placement in short rectal stumps. Before focusing on stump management, the proximal bowel should be run and inspected thoroughly to ensure that no additional area has been compromised or is in need of repair.

The ideal approach to a blown out long Hartmann or rectal stump is to resect the damaged portion down to a margin of clearly viable tissue. This is obviously more easily accomplished with a long Hartmann, where one can be more liberal with dissection and resection. As discussed in the prevention section above, the most important technical components of wound healing are tissue integrity and blood flow, so it should be no surprise that major anastomotic or stump margin disruptions are often associated with ischemia. Thus, it is crucial to reinspect the new margin not only to confirm the presence of healthy viable tissue with minimal inflammatory changes, but also to ensure robust blood flow as confirmed by tissue edge bleeding, palpable or dopplerable pulses, and no venous engorgement. The new resection margin should be far from any watershed area. Additionally, it is important to rule out a distal obstruction both by inspecting the remaining intraperitoneal stump as well by performing a digital rectal examination and/or proctoscopy. Left alone, a distal obstruction in this setting is tantamount to a closed-loop obstruction, which is ample explanation for stump blowout.

If revised stump length permits, the surgeon may next be faced with the option to leave a closed intraperitoneal stump, bury a closed stump in subcutaneous tissue, or mature a mucus fistula. This decision is best informed by considering the likely cause for initial stump breakdown. If technical concerns or prior hemodynamic instability was the likely culprit and has now been effectively addressed, then leaving the stump closed and intraperitoneal is preferable and most straightforward to perform. However, stump dehiscence due to distal obstruction mandates maturation of a mucus fistula for decompression unless the distal obstruction can be rectified. Similarly, if significant risk factors persist, a mucus fistula or subcutaneous stump might be preferable. In particular, for those patients who are expected to start chemotherapy with anti-angiogenesis agents such as bevacizumab, maturation of a mucus fistula completely removes the risk of a staple or suture line dehiscence and allows for earlier initiation of therapy. Also, in instances where both the ostomy and the stump require revision and the stump length permits, a mucus fistula can be matured alongside the new ostomy to facilitate future local reanastomosis. If one chooses to bury the stump in subcutaneous tissue, as might be the case for a patient with refractory ulcerative colitis, this can be done by either tacking the stump to left lower quadrant peritoneum, or bringing the stump through the inferior aspect of the midline incision and fixing it to the fascia at four points, leaving a 1-cm cuff above the level of the fascia. Absorbable sutures should be used for tacking, although a nonabsorbable suture might be advisable for a midline inferior tacking suture as a tag for future ostomy reversal.

When the rectal stump is already short at the index operation, further dissection and resection on reoperation may not be an option. In this instance, ensuring adequate drainage is the primary goal. This may require both transperitoneal and transanal drain placement. One might also consider pelvic exclusion with vicryl mesh draped over the pelvic inlet and secured with absorbable sutures to the periosteum of the superior pubic rami anteriorly and to the sacrum posteriorly.

Given the high potential for lingering contamination after reoperation for stump blowout, transperitoneal drain placement regardless of stump management choice is recommended, as well as coverage of any staple or suture lines with omentum. Similarly, placement of a transanal drain to encourage decompression of remnant stool is a low-risk intervention that reduces the chances of distal stump obstruction and may reduce the incidence of recurrent pelvic sepsis.

Abdominal closure options include standard closure, temporary closure with a vacuum dressing and planned reoperation, or a so-called capillary drainage closure that employs features of both. Standard closure is ideal for wound management and recovery if possible. However, temporary closure is an appropriate choice if significant contamination persists, the patient remains hemodynamically unstable, or the viability of the stump (or other portions of bowel) remains in question. One must keep in mind that this closure option is accompanied by the risk of iatrogenic injury with each operation and an increased chance of fistula formation. The capillary drainage (Mikulicz) technique is essentially a form of pelvic exclusion, whereby the upper abdomen is closed in standard fashion after bowel is wrapped inferiorly with vicryl mesh, and the pelvis is separately completely covered with a gauze bag and packed with gauze and a 16F silicone catheter. This dressing is then placed to drainage or suction and can be irrigated via the silicone drain until and after the gauze packing is slowly removed [12].

A proposed stump leak management algorithm is represented in Fig. 14.1.

Additional Considerations

Selection and duration of antibiotics is beyond the scope of this chapter, but it is worth noting that antibiotics should be initiated as soon as a leak is suspected and continued at least until source control is achieved.

Prolonged or recurrent pelvic sepsis delays eventual ostomy reversal and can ultimately impair future neorectum function. For this reason, use of the endo-sponge, an endoluminal vacuum device, has been proposed to help expedite healing of pelvic abscess cavities. This has been investigated in patients who develop anastomotic leaks after low anterior resection for malignancy or restorative

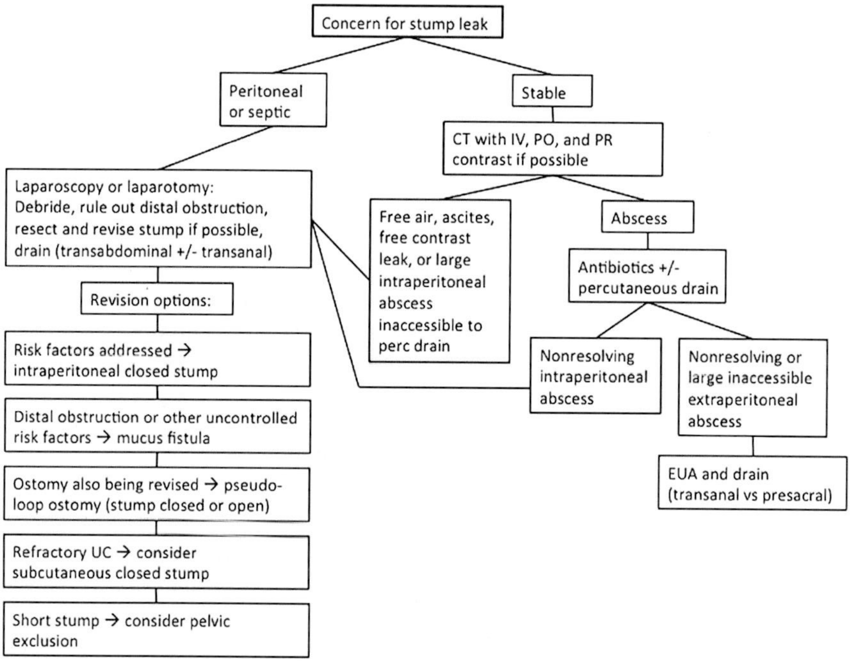

Fig. 14.1 Stump leak management algorithm. *UC*, ulcerative colitis. *CT*, computed tomography. *IV*, intravenous. *PO*, per orem. *PR*, per rectum. *EUA*, exam under anesthesia

proctocolectomy for ulcerative colitis with some positive results [13, 14]. This arguably may also have applications in patients with extraperitoneal rectal stump leaks or low pelvic stump leaks not amenable to intraoperative closure.

Long Hartmann or rectal stump dehiscence after surgery for malignancy carries an additional risk of increased locoregional recurrence and decreased survival, presumably due to spread of micrometastatic disease [11, 15]. Though this does not necessarily affect immediate management approaches to stump blowout, it may compel the surgeon to mature a mucus fistula when possible to facilitate earlier initiation of chemotherapy, and of course the patient should be counseled accordingly.

Clinical Scenario

"Patient is a 60 yo female on whom you have done a R colectomy, ileostomy, and long Hartmann for cecal perforation 1 week ago. She had cecal pneumatosis for Ogilvie's after R hip replacement secondary to R femoral head necrosis due to prolonged steroid use. She develops fever and increased abdominal pain 5 days postcolectomy. CT scan of her abdomen is obtained as part of her workup, which demonstrated free air and ascites. At laparotomy, she has a blowout of her Hartmann stump. No distal obstruction is identified."

This patient brings multiple risk factors for stump blowout to the table: (1) potentially ongoing colonic pseudo-obstruction (Ogilvie's) which would put undue mechanical strain on the stump staple line, (2) prolonged steroid use, which impairs wound healing and potentially delays recognition of a leak by hindering the initial inflammatory response, and (3) the unstated reason for her steroid use, which may be a contributor to her poor wound healing capacity. Her nutritional status is also unclear. Given that she has a long Hartmann stump, we have the luxury of resecting the unhealthy portion and presumably still having a substantial length of colon preserved. The main question is whether to mature a mucus fistula or leave her stump intraperitoneal, and this may be determined by whether the stump appears to have blown out due to mechanical forces (Ogilvie's) or poor wound healing. Given that Ogilvie's is not a true obstruction, stump closure and decompression via transanal drainage catheter would be preferable to mucus fistula, as the mucus fistula creates an additional wound to manage. However, if the blowout appears to be due to poor wound healing rather than excessive distention, then a mucus fistula would be the safest option, as none of her wound healing risk factors will be altered. In either case, transabdominal drain placement would be prudent.

Key Questions

1. *When might one consider on table distal washout of a long Hartman?*
2. *What is your preferred transanal drain and how do you manage it practically?*

References

1. Mortensen NJ, Ashraf S. Intestinal anastomosis. In: Ashley SW, editor. ACS surgery: principles and practice. Decker Intellectual Properties; 2008.
2. Burch JM, Franciose RJ, Moore EE, Biffl WL, Offner PJ. Single-layer continuous versus two-layer interrupted intestinal anastomosis: a prospective randomized trial. Ann Surg. 2000;231(6):832–7.
3. Shikata S, Yamagishi H, Taji Y, Shimada T, Noguchi Y. Single- versus two-layer intestinal anastomosis: a meta-analysis of randomized controlled trials. BMC Surg. 2006;27(6):2.
4. Sajid MS, Siddiqui MR, Baig MK. Single layer versus double layer suture anastomosis of the gastrointestinal tract. Cohrane Database Syst Rev. 2012;1:CD005477.
5. Puleo S, Sofia M, Trovato MA, Pesce A, Portale TR, Russello.
6. Choy PY, Bissett IP, Docherty JG, Parry BR, Merrie A, Figtzgerald A. Stapled versus handsewn methods for ileocolic anastomoses. Cochrane Database Syst Rev. 2011;(9): CD004320.
7. Neutzling CB, Lustosa SA, Proenca IM, da Silva EM, Matos D. Stapled versus handsewn methods for colorectal anastomosis surgery. Cochrane Database Syst Rev. 2012;2:CD003144.

8. Gu J, Stocchi L, Remzi F, Kiran RP. Intraperitoneal or subcutaneous: does location of the (colo)rectal stump influence outcomes after laparoscopic total abdominal colectomy for ulcerative colitis? Dis Colon Rectum. 2013;56(5):615–21.
9. Trickett JP, Tilney HS, Gudgeon AM, Mellor SG, Edwards DP. Management of the rectal stump after emergency sub-total colectomy: which surgical option is associated with the lowest morbidity? Colorectal Dis. 2005;7(5):519–22.
10. Alberts JCJ, Parvaiz A, Moran BJ. Predicting risk and diminishing the consequences of anastomotic dehiscence following rectal resection. Colorectal Dis. 2003;5(5):478–82.
11. Landmann RG. Surgical management of anastomotic leak following colorectal surgery. Semin Colon Rectal Surg. 2014;25(2):58–66.
12. Parc Y, Frileux P, Schmitt G, Dehni N, Ollivier JM, Parc R. Management of postoperative peritonitis after anterior resection: experience from a referral intensive care unit. Dis Colon Rectum. 2000;43(5):579–87.
13. Riss S, Stift A, Kienbacher C, Dauser B, Haunold I, Kriwanek S, Radlsboek W, Bergmann M. Recurrent abscess after primary successful endo-sponge treatment of anastomotic leakage following rectal surgery. World J Gasroenterol. 2010;16(36):4570–4.
14. van Koperen PJ, van Berge Henegouwen MI, Rosman C, Bakker CM, Heres P, Slors JFM, Bemelman WA. The Dutch multicenter experience of the Endo-Sponge treatment for anastomotic leakage after colorectal surgery. Surg Endosc. 2009;23(6):1379–83.
15. Bell SW, Walker KG, Rickard MJFX, Sinclar G, Dent OF, Chapuis PH, Bokey EL. Anastomotic leakage after curative anterior resection results in a higher prevalence of local recurrence. Br J Surg. 2003;90(10):1261–6.

Chapter 15
Rectum: Management of the Urgent APR and Dissecting the "Frozen" Pelvis

Rao R. Ivatury

Problem Analysis

Continued bleeding PR, presumably of a significant degree, requiring multiple transfusions of blood and blood products and invasive interventions in a clinical scenario of recurrent, advanced cancer with very limited palliation.

Therapeutic Interventions

These must be planned with a consideration of

1. Recurrent, fixed (inoperable for cure) cancer that makes total resection extremely difficult and dangerous.
2. Postoperative, postradiation frozen pelvis with dense adhesions that make iatrogenic injury to vital structures very likely and massive intra-operative blood loss and intra-operative mortality a distinct possibility.

Even though the editors give me the suggestion of an emergent abdomino-perineal resection, I consider it a last resort. My steps for a therapeutic solution will involve the following:

R.R. Ivatury (✉)
Department of Surgery, Virginia Commonwealth University, Richmond, VA, USA
e-mail: raoivatury@gmail.com

J.J. Diaz and D.T. Efron (eds.), *Complications in Acute Care Surgery*,
DOI 10.1007/978-3-319-42376-0_15

Preoperative [1]

1. Since this is a palliative and not a curative approach with a very limited scope for meaningful palliation, what are the patient's and family's approach to end-of-life decision?
2. If their decision is to do whatever is necessary, after a thorough discussion with them I will consider any of these following ancillary measures to control or diminish the bleeding:

   (a) Correction of all bleeding diatheses and correction of coagulopathy;
   (b) Preoperative angiography and embolization of bleeding vessels;
   (c) Preoperative angiography and occlusion of internal iliac arteries (may not succeed if the bleeding is from the anal verge and the branches of external iliac artery);
   (d) Endoscopy in the lithotomy position, debridement of the tumor with or without fulguration, and application of pressure packs with or without hemostatic substances (e.g., quick clot);
   (e) Cryoablation to stop bleeding; and
   (f) Irradiation of the tumor to stop bleeding.

3. If none of these is successful, it is mandatory to (again) have a detailed, frank discussion with the patient's family or health proxy. Encourage them to consider comfort measures and hospice treatment, since the prognosis for short-term and long-term palliation is dismal and prolonged morbidity and/or death with a need for colostomy is a distinct possibility with operation.
4. Pelvic exenteration is an option for recurrent rectal cancers, but I do not consider this fixed tumor at the anal verge as a candidate.
5. Urgent exploration for resection of the tumor to control bleeding by APR is a horrendous approach for this particular scenario. If unavoidable and the surgeon is forced into it, the following points should be kept in mind (if time and patient's hemodynamic status permit):

   (a) Preoperative ureteric stents by the urologists;
   (b) Preoperative bowel preparation and antibiotics;
   (c) Bladder catheterization;
   (d) Insertion of a rectal tube of a large size to enable easy identification of the rectosigmoid in the "frozen" pelvis;
   (e) Try to schedule the operation electively, early in the morning (first case) and have additional senior help available, if possible;
   (f) Solid grounding in pelvic anatomy, with live experience involving varying degrees of pelvic distortion;
   (g) A realistic expectation that the operation will be difficult and fraught with hazards;
   (h) Flexibility to change course when a particular pathway proves too risky, or even abandon the procedure, if necessary;

Operative [2]

Laparotomy: Use a midline low incision to attempt to get into the pelvis. Proceed from the right paracolic gutter, rather than from the left side because of previous surgery. Dissect in the retrovesical space, feel for the stented ureter, and identify the iliac vessels. Holding the colon in the left hand of the surgeon standing on the left of the patient, stay close to the rectosigmoid and try to dissect it free from the surrounding important structures.

Remembering that this is a palliative operation, if one can get around the rectosigmoid at the upper edge of the fixed, recurrent tumor, divide the colon with a stapler, and bring it up to thc left lower quadrant. Concentrate on identifying both ureters and carefully mobilize all small bowel loops out of the pelvis.

(Useful trick: There are bound to be inadvertent iatrogenic enterotomy because of radiation and past surgery in the pelvis. Use these unavoidable enterotomies to advantage by inserting your index fingers inside and judge the direction of the matted loops proximally and distally. With the finger inside guiding a "road map," mobilize the bowel loops. Accept multiple enterotomies but do your best to keep them in all the same or adjacent loops, so that we can minimize the amount of small bowel that needs to be sacrificed. It is helpful to dissect more on the anti-mesenteric walls). Once reasonably free from the rectosigmoid (the large rectal tube in the rectosigmoid will help identify the large bowel), pack the small bowel out of the pelvis. Remember, this operation is for anal recurrent tumor, so concentrate on getting into the rectosigmoid and not carry out extensive adhesiolysis of the small bowel.

Proceed to the pelvic part of the operation and complete, to the best of your ability the freeing of the lateral pelvic ligaments (even through the tumor), as long as the small bowel and the ureters are free of danger. If the major bleeder could be identified at this point, transfix it with large 0-silk sutures. Otherwise, transfix the lateral ligaments with large 0-silk sutures, sometimes multiple. Cut through the anterior portion of the recurrent tumor if adherent to the bladder and excise the anal canal, recurrent tumor surrounding skin, etc. with electrocautery turned high.

Secure the major bleeders with transfixing sutures, pack the entire pelvic wound with sheets of hemostatic substances like Quick clot, consider introducing a three-way foley catheter into the pelvic wound and inflating the balloon with a large amount of saline to compress the soft tissues of the pelvis for hemostasis. The packs can be used to supplement this pressure.

This patient is most likely not very stable at this time with the inevitable extensive blood loss and multiple transfusions. He will clearly benefit from a "damage control" approach and an abbreviated, truncated procedure, after rapid resection and stapling off of traumatized small bowel with iatrogenic perforations, temporary abdominal and pelvic closures with prosthetic mesh. He may be returned to the O.R., after physiologic improvement by SICU resuscitation within 24 h, for colostomy construction and closure of abdomen (to be very optimistic).

Potential, Anticipated Complications [3]

Continued bleeding from residual tumor
Massive blood loss, massive transfusion, and coagulopathy
Intra-operative hypotension, cardiac arrest
Iatrogenic injury to small bowel, ureter, and iliac vessels
Inability to mobilize and resect the entire recurrent tumor
Inability to close the abdomen
Pelvic wound infection, disruption, and pelvic sepsis
Multiple-organ failure and death

Much of this morbidity may be avoided by accepting the inevitability of a terminal outcome from advanced, recurrent, fixed cancer.

Summary

In summary, this is a desperate case scenario of uncontrolled bleeding from an advanced, recurrent, high-grade and fixed tumor in a male pelvis that is beyond cure and unlikely to be amenable even for meaningful palliative resection. If non-surgical approaches did not stop the bleeding, I would try very hard to convince the family to pursue only hospice care and allow the patient end of life with dignity and compassion.

Clinical Scenario
56-year-old man who presents with ongoing bright red blood per rectum. He is 2 years s/p low anterior resection for a mid-rectal cancer with accompanying chemotherapy and pelvic radiation. Rectal exam reveals a large firm fixed mass at the anal verge with ongoing bleeding.

Key Question

1. *Is there role for formalin enema to palliate rectal bleeding? Multiple studies have showed efficacy of 2 percent formalin enema to palliate rectal bleeding from* ***radiation proctitis. In one series 78.2 percent responded positively. More than one application was required in 34.7 percent of the patients. The procedure was well tolerated and most of the side effects were mild. (Raman RR : Dis Colon Rectum. 2007 Jul;50(7):1032-9.)***

References

1. Pereira J, Phan T. Management of bleeding in patients with advanced cancer. Oncologist. 2004;9:561–70.
2. Goldstein DP, Callahan MJ. Surgical strategies to untangle a frozen pelvis. OBG Manage. 2007;19(03).
3. Bonello VA, Bhangu A, Fitzgerald JE, Rasheed S, Tekkis P. Intraoperative bleeding and haemostasis during pelvic surgery for locally advanced or recurrent rectal cancer: a prospective evaluation. Tech Coloproctol. 2014;18(10):887–93.

Chapter 16
Complex Liver Abscess

Brandon R. Bruns and Thomas M. Scalea

Introduction

Liver abscesses are typically classified into one of the three categories based on the inciting organism (Table 16.1): pyogenic, amoebic, or fungal. In the United States and other developed countries, pyogenic hepatic abscess is by far the most common in the immunocompetent host. Amoebic liver abscess, caused by *Entamoeba histolytica*, is typically found in certain parts of Mexico, Indonesia, tropical Africa, and India. Fungal abscesses remain more commonly associated with the immunocompromised host and typically present in a multifocal manner; however, they remain uncommon overall.

Incidence and Demographics

Pyogenic hepatic abscesses typically originate from enteric infectious sources (appendicitis and diverticulitis), biliary sources, or via hematogenous spread from endocarditis or poor dentition. Evaluating pyogenic liver abscess from the years 1994–2005, investigators in the United States found the incidence to be 3.6 per 100,000 admissions. Additionally, they found an in-hospital mortality of 5.6 % with mortality being associated with older age, those who did not have private

B.R. Bruns (✉) · T.M. Scalea
R Adams Cowley Shock Trauma Center, University of Maryland,
22 S Greene Street S4D07, Baltimore, MD 21201, USA
e-mail: bbruns@umm.edu

T.M. Scalea
e-mail: tscalea@umm.edu

J.J. Diaz and D.T. Efron (eds.), *Complications in Acute Care Surgery*,
DOI 10.1007/978-3-319-42376-0_16

Table 16.1 Liver Abscess Etiology

Abscess type	Causative organism	Patient population	Treatment
Pyogenic	Polymicrobial (biliary and enteric organisms most likely); Klebsiella spp. increasing in incidence	Recent biliary intervention; Multiple medical comorbid conditions; Immunocompromised	Broad-spectrum antibiotics; Culture-directed antibiotics; Percutaneous drainage; Possible surgical therapy
Amoebic	*Entamoeba histolytica*	Recent travel to endemic region	Metronidazole; Surgical therapy rarely required
Fungal	Often mixed fungus and bacterial	Immunocompromised (chemotherapy likely); Indwelling biliary stents	Antifungal therapy and antibacterial; Possible surgical therapy, though rarely required

health care insurance, and medical comorbidities (cirrhosis, chronic kidney disease, and cancer) [1]. A similar investigation in China, over the years 1995–2008, showed the mean age of patients was 57 years, 59 % were male, and the case fatality rate was 10 %. The most common etiology of hepatic abscess was cholecystitis and/or cholangitis (34 %) and the following factors were associated with increased mortality: Acute Physiology and Chronic Health Evaluation (APACHE II) scores ≥15, Simplified Acute Physiology Score (SAPS 2) scores ≥28, gas within the liver abscess, and infection with anaerobes [2].

Compared to pyogenic liver abscess, amoebic liver abscess tends to be less common and appears to be decreasing in incidence. Amebiasis is derived from infection with the anaerobic protozoan *E. histolytica* after infection of the colon and subsequent invasion of the portal venous system. Patients with amebiasis typically present with fever, malaise, and right upper quadrant pain. Utilizing the United States Nationwide Inpatient Sample from 1993 to 2007, Congly et al. showed an overall incidence of hospitalization of 1.38 per million admissions, with a decreasing incidence over time during the study period. Eighty-one percent of patients were male, approximately half were of Hispanic origin, and one-third had private health insurance. The mortality in the study was 0.8 % with predictors of mortality being age greater than 60 years, female gender, and those without private health insurance [3].

Fungal abscesses are also relatively uncommon and typically present in the immunocompromised host. Over a 20-year period at The Johns Hopkins Hospital, only 8 solitary fungal and 34 mixed fungal/bacterial abscesses were identified. Biliary tract disease was much more likely in patients with combined fungal/bacterial abscesses, with 74 % of those having prior biliary surgery or indwelling biliary stents. All of the patients in the pure fungal abscess category were immunocompromised, all having received chemotherapy. Purely fungal abscesses were smaller than the mixed type [4].

Microbiology

The majority of pyogenic liver abscesses is derived from enteric or biliary sources, thus the microbiology is frequently polymicrobial in nature [5]. However, given advances in antimicrobial therapy and imaging techniques, abscess formation from pylephlebitis is decreasing in incidence in the current era. In a 2010 population-based study from the United States, streptococcal species and Escherichia coli were the most common bacterial species isolated [1]. Increasingly, *Klebsiella pneumonia* is being a reported isolate from hepatic abscess growth, with initial reports from Taiwan [6]. A 2014 study from Texas showed Klebsiella species to be the most common isolate from a series of 49 patients with hepatic abscess. Additionally, in these Klebsiella-infected patients, they found a significant number of associated malignancies [7]. Unilocular *K. pneumonia* liver abscesses are at increased risk of having associated septic pulmonary emboli and other extra-pulmonary metastatic infections [8].

Treatment

The vast majority of liver abscesses can be treated with antimicrobial therapy directed at the appropriate pathogen and percutaneous drainage with either ultrasound or CT guidance [9]. Initial therapy begins with broad-spectrum antibiotics directed at common pathogens. Culture data should be obtained from the abscess itself by aspiration with possible placement of a drainage catheter. Antibiotic therapy can then be tailored depending on culture data that return. Factors shown to be associated with failed medical treatment include the presence of a gas-forming abscess and shock present on admission [10].

Surgical therapy remains an important consideration in selected patients. Investigators in Rhode Island devised a treatment algorithm for hepatic abscesses <3 cm, unilocular hepatic abscesses >3 cm, and multilocular hepatic abscesses >3 cm. They were able to show 100 % treatment success with antibiotics alone for those with the small abscesses <3 cm. Similarly, they had 100 % treatment success with surgical therapy of the multilocular abscesses >3 cm. Percutaneous therapy combined with antibiotic therapy provided mixed results for patients with unilocular abscesses >3 cm and multilocular abscesses >3 cm [11].

Tan et al. examined two populations of patients with hepatic abscesses greater than 5 cm, one group treated with surgical and one with percutaneous drainage. They found that patients managed with surgical therapy had fewer treatment failures, required fewer procedures, and had shorter hospital lengths of stay. Additionally, they found no difference in morbidity or mortality between the two groups [12].

In another series, investigators in China studied 31 patients undergoing simultaneous treatment of biliary disease and hepatic abscess. Patients were managed with either laparoscopic or open surgical techniques. They found no difference in operating time, blood loss and transfusion rates, postoperative morbidity, or abscess recurrence between the two groups. Patients managed with the laparoscopic approach had a faster return of bowel function and had shorter hospital lengths of stay [13].

However, when compared to surgical therapies, percutaneous drainage of liver abscess appears to be associated with lower morbidity and less cost when compared to surgical therapies [5]. In a study of 264 patients with 354 liver abscesses, investigators performed ultrasound-guided aspiration in those with abscesses less than 5 cm and performed ultrasound-guided catheter drainage in those greater than 5 cm. In their series, percutaneous therapy was successful 87 % of the time, with only 8 % converted to operative therapy [14].

Patients with advanced malignancy are at higher risk for hepatic abscess and pose unique challenges as many are malnourished and may be undergoing cytotoxic therapies. At the Memorial Sloan Kettering Cancer Center, investigators examined 58 patients with hepatopancreaticobiliary malignancy and hepatic abscess. Fifty-two percent of patients had a history of bilioenteric anastomosis. Polymicrobial culture data returned in 55 % of patients. In the study, 66 % of patients were successfully treated with percutaneous drainage and only 9 % progressed to surgery [15].

As many pyogenic liver abscesses are the result of hematogenous spread from an intra-abdominal source, surgical therapy directed at control of the abdominal source may be warranted. Concomitant surgical treatment of biliary pathology contributing to hepatic abscess can also be undertaken simultaneously. Similarly, consideration for endocarditis as a potential source of ongoing showering of bacteria should be considered, as the liver's reticuloendothelial system makes it relatively resistant to infection. In addition to broad-spectrum antibiotics, tailored therapy can be provided after culture data from the abscess becomes available.

Specific Situations

Hepatic Complications After Trauma

Increasingly, the management of blunt hepatic injury in the hemodynamically normal patient is non-operative in nature. Hepatic complications after non-operative management of liver injury are common and increase as the grade of hepatic injury increases [16]. In a multicenter study, only 24-h transfusion requirement and grade of injury were accurate predictors of liver-related complications [17]. Thus, though non-operative therapy may help avoid initial laparotomy, it does mandate close follow-up and anticipation of complications.

Angioembolization of bleeding hepatic injury is commonly employed as an adjunct in non-operatively managed patients (Fig. 16.1). Major hepatic necrosis is a

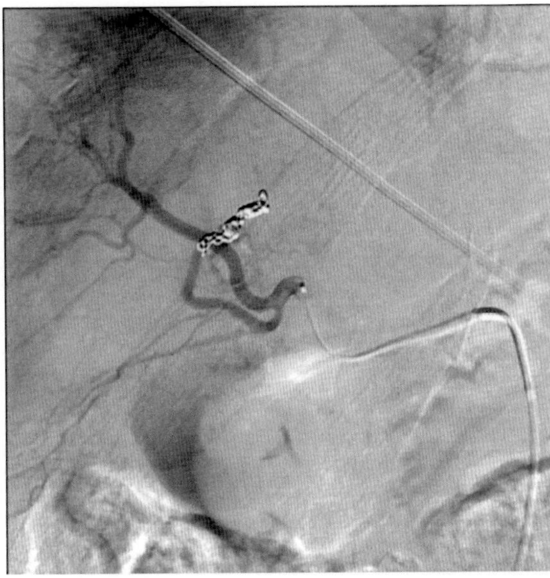

Fig. 16.1 Embolization coils in branch of right hepatic artery after stab wound to the liver

dreaded complication of this therapy and occurs in up to 40 % of embolized patients in some series. Major hepatic necrosis (Fig. 16.2) after embolotherapy is more prevalent in those with high-grade injuries and when it does develop, it is associated with increasing complications, longer length of stay, and the need for greater number of transfusions [18].

The diagnosis of hepatic necrosis is often suspected on the basis of persistent fevers, leukocytosis, and right upper quadrant pain. CT imaging is often used to secure the diagnosis. Treatment is varied, depending on the clinical scenario, but can involve watchful waiting, interventional radiologic guided drainage, debridement, and formal lobectomy. In a series of 30 patients with hepatic necrosis treated at the Shock Trauma Center, Dabbs et al. [19] showed that formal hepatic lobectomy was associated with fewer total procedures and less complications when compared to those undergoing radiologic drainage or debridement.

In our experience at the Shock Trauma Center, perihepatic fluid collections, bilomas, and abscesses are not uncommon after resectional therapy (Fig. 16.3). These are often successfully treated with a combination of percutaneous drainage and endoscopic retrograde cholangiography with stenting in an effort to decrease pressure in the biliary radicals and facilitate drainage of bile through the ampulla.

Operative Therapy

When operation is required, preparation is paramount as blood loss can be profound. The utilization of low central venous pressure techniques typically utilized in

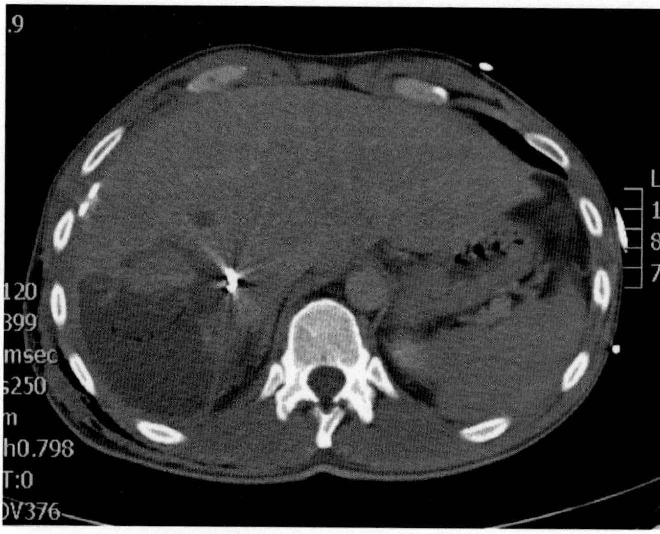

Fig. 16.2 The patient developed fever and leukocytosis. CT imaging shows embolization coils and air within an area of major hepatic necrosis

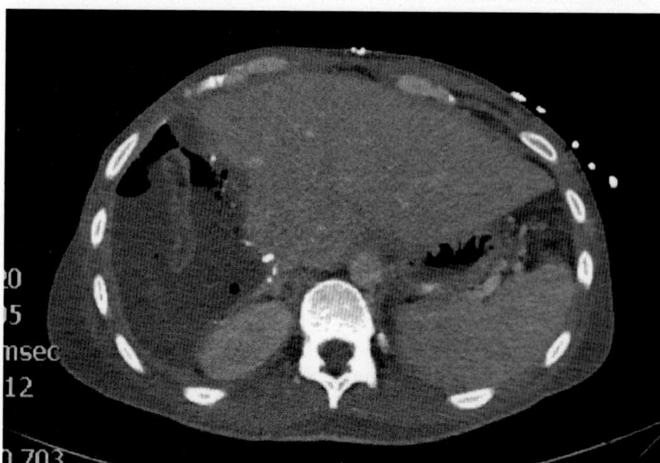

Fig. 16.3 Post-resection biliary collection noted on CT imaging was successfully treated with percutaneous drainage

elective hepatic surgery is not typically possible in the hospitalized patient with hepatic abscess as peripheral venous resistance is low and fluids are required to maintain adequate perfusion. Therefore, utilization of autotransfusion devices and rapid availability of blood products must be considered.

Another option we have employed is venovenous bypass, with a drainage cannula in the femoral vein and return via the right internal jugular vein. Though not routinely employed, its use does offer theoretical benefits, including less blood loss. Another adjunct we liberally utilize when operating on the liver is the argon beam coagulator to assist with hemostasis on cut hepatic surfaces.

A midline incision or a right subcostal incision can be utilized. The midline incision may provide more versatility and allows access to the entire abdominal cavity. However, the right subcostal allows easy access to the liver and can be extended into a thoracoabdominal incision with radial takedown of the diaphragm for better visualization if necessary. No matter the incision chosen, complete mobilization of the liver is necessary. Incision the triangular and coronary ligament allows mobilization of the liver out of the wound for proper exposure. In unique circumstances, lateral positioning and resection of the twelfth rib can allow easy access to the right upper quadrant.

Identification of the abscess cavity can be facilitated with the use of intra-operative ultrasound. This technique is particularly useful when the abscess lies within the parenchyma of the liver. After identification, the abscess cavity is widely opened and septations are incised to allow for full evacuation of the abscess contents. Lavage of the cavity to ensure evacuation of all purulent material then proceeds. Closed suction drains can be left in the abscess cavity and peri-hepatic region if deemed necessary.

Clinical Scenario

Forty-two-year-old Asian man presents with right upper quadrant pain and fever. He reports several weeks of general fatigue. He has an extensive travel history to both East Asia and Africa. WBC is 15 K. CT demonstrates a large 10 cm central liver abscess adjacent to the gallbladder with severe thickening of the GB wall, irregularity hyperemia.

The presentation of right upper quadrant pain and fever along with multiple weeks of generalized fatigue is consistent with amebiasis. Amebiasis is caused by *E. histolytica* and is endemic to certain parts of Asia and Africa. CT was performed in this case, but given the classic history, ultrasound would likely lead to a conclusive diagnosis. Treatment is with metronidazole and close clinical follow-up to ensure resolution of symptoms. Surgery is rarely indicated, but given the large size of this abscess (10 cm), percutaneous drainage or open surgical therapy may be required if symptoms fail to resolve with antibiotic therapy.

Another potential diagnosis is a pyogenic liver abscess. The etiology of pyogenic liver abscesses is typically from enteric infectious sources (classically diverticulitis and appendicitis), biliary sources, or hematogenous spread from endocarditis or poor dentition. Pyogenic liver abscesses of this size will likely require percutaneous drainage and catheter placement along with directed antimicrobial therapy directed by culture results. If surgical therapy is required, laparoscopic or open approaches can be entertained. Given the central location, drainage of the abscess would be the most appealing option as resection would likely be technically challenging.

Key Questions

1. *What are the considerations for hydatid cysts?*
2. *What is the best approach for hepatic infection: anatomic versus non-anatomic liver resection?*

References

1. Meddings L, Myers RP, Hubbard J, Shaheen AA, Laupland KB, Dixon E, et al. A population-based study of pyogenic liver abscesses in the United States: incidence, mortality, and temporal trends. Am J Gastroenterol. 2010;105(1):117–24.
2. Chen SC, Huang CC, Tsai SJ, Yen CH, Lin DB, Wang PH, et al. Severity of disease as main predictor for mortality in patients with pyogenic liver abscess. Am J Surg. 2009;198(2): 164–72.
3. Congly SE, Shaheen AA, Meddings L, Kaplan GG, Myers RP. Amoebic liver abscess in USA: a population-based study of incidence, temporal trends and mortality. Liver Int. 2011;31 (8):1191–8.
4. Lipsett PA, Huang CJ, Lillemoe KD, Cameron JL, Pitt HA. Fungal hepatic abscesses: characterization and management. J Gastrointest Surg. 1997;1(1):78–84.
5. Ferraioli G, Garlaschelli A, Zanaboni D, Gulizia R, Brunetti E, Tinozzi FP, et al. Percutaneous and surgical treatment of pyogenic liver abscesses: observation over a 21-year period in 148 patients. Dig Liver Dis. 2008;40(8):690–6.
6. Tsai FC, Huang YT, Chang LY, Wang JT. Pyogenic liver abscess as endemic disease, Taiwan. Emerg Infect Dis. 2008;14(10):1592–600.
7. Ali AH, Smalligan RD, Ahmed M, Khasawneh FA. Pyogenic liver abscess and the emergence of Klebsiella as an etiology: a retrospective study. Int J Gen Med. 2013;23(7):37–42.
8. Chang Z, Zheng J, Ma Y, Liu Z. Analysis of clinical and CT characteristics of patients with *Klebsiella pneumoniae* liver abscesses: an insight into risk factors of metastatic infection. Int J Infect Dis. 2015;33:50–4.
9. O'Farrell N, Collins CG, McEntee GP. Pyogenic liver abscesses: diminished role for operative treatment. Surgeon. 2010;8(4):192–6.
10. Alkofer B, Dufay C, Parienti JJ, Lepennec V, Dargere S, Chiche L. Are pyogenic liver abscesses still a surgical concern? A western experience. HPB Surg. 2012;2012:316013.
11. Hope WW, Vrochides DV, Newcomb WL, Mayo-Smith WW, Iannitti DA. Optimal treatment of hepatic abscess. Am Surg. 2008;74(2):178–82.
12. Tan YM, Chung AY, Chow PK, Cheow PC, Wong WK, Ooi LL, et al. An appraisal of surgical and percutaneous drainage for pyogenic liver abscesses larger than 5 cm. Ann Surg. 2005;241(3):485–90.
13. Tu JF, Huang XF, Hu RY, You HY, Zheng XF, Jiang FZ. Comparison of laparoscopic and open surgery for pyogenic liver abscess with biliary pathology. World J Gastroenterol. 2011;17(38):4339–43.
14. Zerem E, Omerovic S, Kunosic S. Sonographically guided percutaneous treatment of liver abscesses in critically Ill patients. J Clin Ultrasound. 2014;42(9):527–33.

15. Mezhir JJ, Fong Y, Jacks LM, Getrajdman GI, Brody LA, Covey AM, et al. Current management of pyogenic liver abscess: surgery is now second-line treatment. J Am Coll Surg. 2010;210(6):975–83.
16. Kozar RA, Moore JB, Niles SE, Holcomb JB, Moore EE, Cothren CC, et al. Complications of nonoperative management of high-grade blunt hepatic injuries. J Trauma. 2005;59(5): 1066–71.
17. Kozar RA, Moore FA, Cothren CC, Moore EE, Sena M, Bulger EM, et al. Risk factors for hepatic morbidity following nonoperative management: multicenter study. Arch Surg. 2006;141(5):451–8; Discussion 458–9.
18. Dabbs DN, Stein DM, Scalea TM. Major hepatic necrosis: a common complication after angioembolization for treatment of high-grade liver injuries. J Trauma. 2009;66(3):621–7; Discussion 627–9.
19. Dabbs DN, Stein DM, Philosophe B, Scalea TM. Treatment of major hepatic necrosis: lobectomy versus serial debridement. J Trauma. 2010;69(3):562–7.

Chapter 17
The Complex Splenectomy

Syed Nabeel Zafar and Edward E. Cornwell, III

The management of iatrogenic splenic injuries following abdominal procedures is a complicated undertaking. Not only because of altered anatomy produced by the original operation, but also because of deranged physiology that may be present in the convalescing patient.

The specter of an iatrogenic splenic injury produced by an attempted pleural drain placement represents a clinical embarrassment, even by the mere mention of it. However, there are mitigating circumstances that make the scenario plausible. Poor inspiratory effort following upper abdominal and thoracic operations is a common precursor to lower lung atelectasis. This is particularly likely with (a) combined procedures, (b) left upper quadrant/rib cage retraction required for esophageal and/or gastric mobilization, and (c) compromise of abdominal accessory muscles of respiration produced by upper abdominal drain placement. To the resultant loss of lung volume and hemidiaphragm elevation, we can add the possibility of left phrenic nerve dysfunction as a result of mediastinal manipulation. Lung volume loss, diaphragm elevation, and the presence of a pleural effusion can present a deceptive picture of where the chest cavity ends and the abdominal cavity begins. Standard anatomic landmarks for left chest tube placement may in fact be treacherously too low (Fig. 17.1). All told, there are series in the literature citing abdominal placement of chest tubes with incidence rates ranging from 0.8 % to as high as 22 % [1, 2].

S.N. Zafar · E.E. Cornwell, III (✉)
Department of Surgery, Howard University Hospital, Washington, DC, USA
e-mail: ecornwell@howard.edu

S.N. Zafar
e-mail: syed.zafar@howard.edu

E.E. Cornwell, III
The LaSalle D. Leffall, Jr., Professor & Chairman of Surgery, Howard University College of Medicine, Department of Surgery, Howard University Hospital, 2041 Georgia Avenue NW, Washington, DC 20060, USA

J.J. Diaz and D.T. Efron (eds.), *Complications in Acute Care Surgery*,
DOI 10.1007/978-3-319-42376-0_17

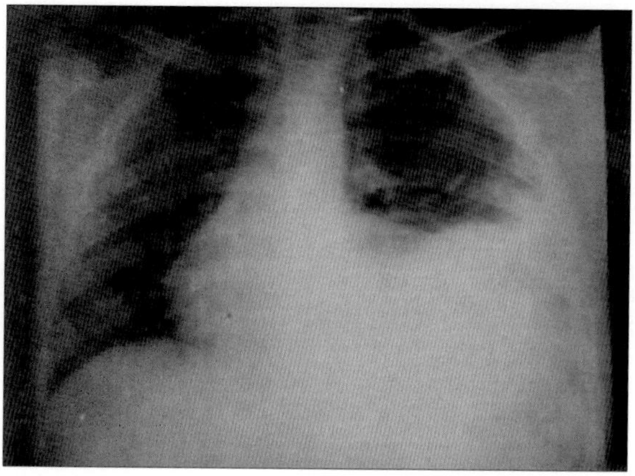

Fig. 17.1 CXR showing elevated left hemidiaphragm with permission from Kadian et al. [9, Fig. 2]

The clinical management of a bleeding splenic injury in a complicated surgical patient should, as in any patient with splenic injury, be directed by the severity of the injury, the hemodynamic status of the patient, and the response to initial therapy. The first consideration is the decision to perform a laparotomy versus a trial of non-operative management (NOM).

Non-operative Management of Splenic Injury

Enhancements in helical computed tomography (CT) and angioembolization techniques have expanded the use and success of NOM of splenic injury over the past few decades. Approximately 85 % of adult patients with blunt splenic injury now undergo NOM with success rates varying between 70 and 90 % [3]. NOM consists of observation, intensive monitoring, serial abdominal examinations, serial hemoglobin/hematocrit measurements, and occasionally repeat CT imaging. Angioembolization, in select patients, remains a useful adjunct and has increased the success of NOM significantly.

To forgo laparotomy in favor of NOM a number of criteria must be met; the patient must be hemodynamically stable, must exhibit no peritoneal signs, and the setting in which NOM is being considered must be suitable. The appropriate setting entails a dedicated area for observation and intensive monitoring (e.g., an ICU), the capability of serial and frequent abdominal examinations by the same surgical team, and easy and rapid access to an operating room if necessary (Table 17.1). If any of these criteria are not met, then attempting NOM is potentially hazardous. On the other hand, if all of these criteria are met, then the practice management guideline committee for the Eastern Association for the Surgery of Trauma (EAST) developed a level 2 guideline suggesting that NOM may be attempted regardless of age, neurologic status, injury severity or the presence of associated extra-abdominal injuries [3].

Table 17.1 Criteria for non-operative management of splenic injury

Criteria
Hemodynamic stability
Absence of peritoneal signs
Documented computed tomography injury gradation
Transfusion of fewer than 2 units of PRBCs
Appropriate environment to perform non-operative management

Adapted from Eastern Association for the Surgery of Trauma, practice management guidelines for blunt splenic injury [3]

Table 17.2 American Association for the Surgery of Trauma Organ Injury Scale for the Spleen [4]

Grades	Injury type	Description of injury
I	Hematoma	Subcapsular, <10 % surface area
	Laceration	Capsular tear, <1 cm parenchymal depth
II	Hematoma	Subcapsular, 10–50 % surface area intraparenchymal, <5 cm in diameter
	Laceration	Capsular tear, 1–3 cm parenchymal depth that does not involve a trabecular vessel
III	Hematoma	Subcapsular, >50 % surface area or expanding; ruptured subcapsular or parenchymal hematoma; intraparenchymal hematoma ≥5 cm or expanding
	Laceration	>3 cm parenchymal depth or involving trabecular vessels
IV	Laceration	Laceration involving segmental or hilar vessels producing major devascularization (>25 % of spleen)
V	Laceration	Completely shattered spleen
	Vascular	Hilar vascular injury with devascularized spleen

With permission from Wolters Kluwer Health, Inc., Moore et al. [4, Table 1]

Injury Severity

Another useful tool in the decision-making armamentarium is the severity of the splenic injury as visualized upon CT imaging. The American Association for the Surgery of Trauma Organ Injury Scale provides the clinician with an injury grading scale from which management decisions can be made [4]. This scale is detailed in Table 17.2 and Fig. 17.2. Success rates of NOM, however, do vary according to the AAST injury severity. Patients with grade III injuries with large hemoperitoneum, or with grade 4 and 5 injuries are at higher risk of failure. A multi-institutional study demonstrated failure rates of 34.5 % for grade IV injuries, and 60 % for grade V injuries [5].

Intravenous contrast enhanced CT scanning is the gold standard for diagnosing and grading splenic injury (Fig. 17.3). Multi-slice multi-phase helical CT scanning is not only rapid but also very sensitive at picking up vascular injury [6]. Large amounts of contrast extravasation indicate active splenic hemorrhage and require

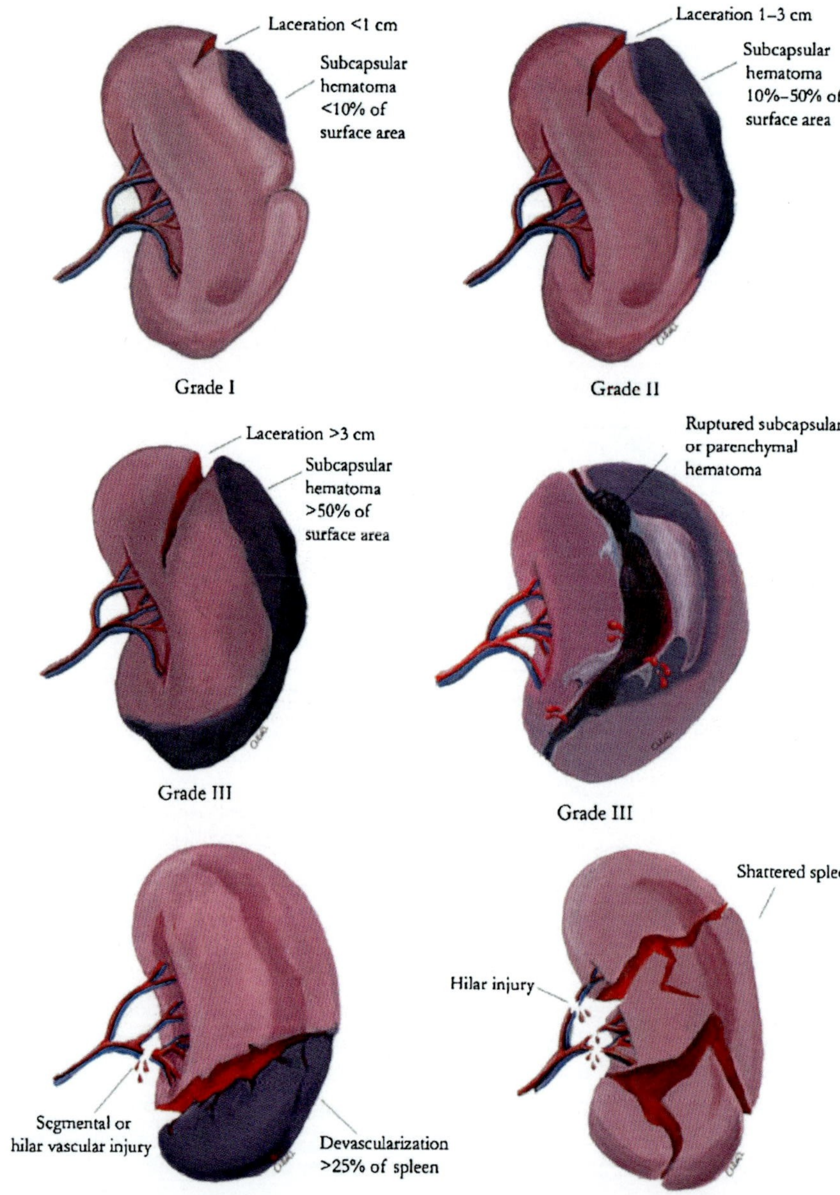

Fig. 17.2 Diagrammatic representation of the American Association for the Surgery of Trauma Organ Injury Scale for the Spleen with permission from Fischer and Jones [10, Chap. 175, Fig. 5]

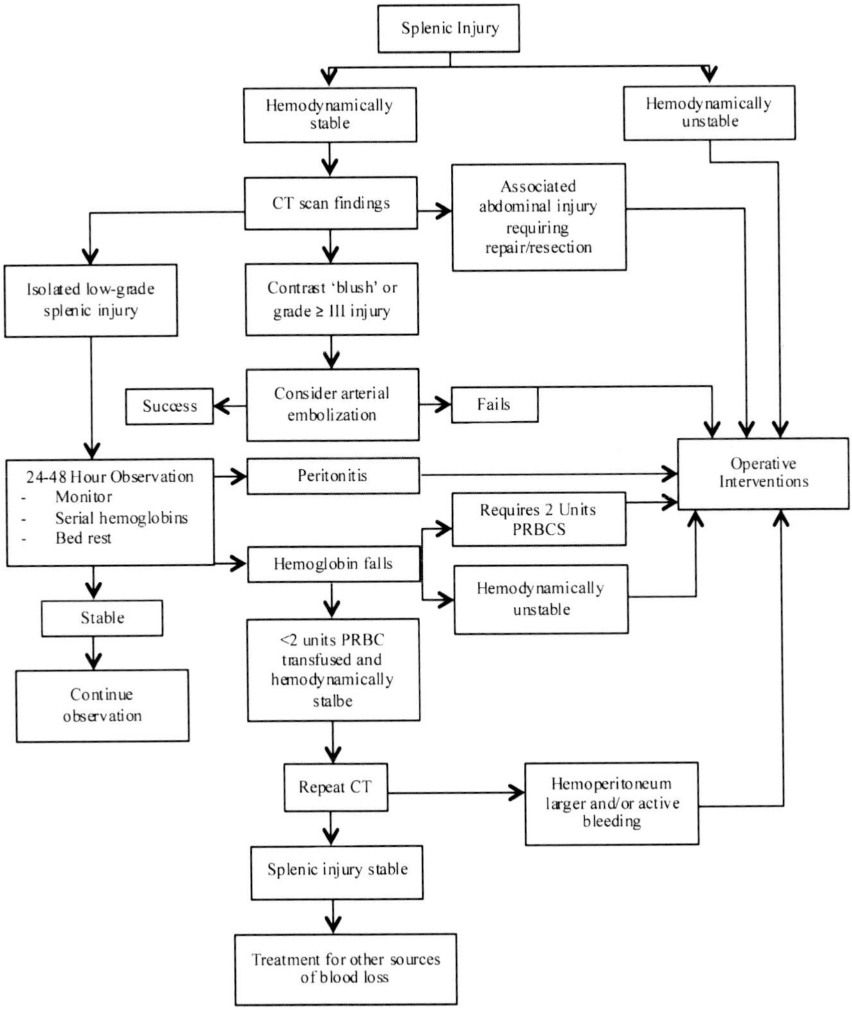

Fig. 17.3 Algorithm for non-operative management of splenic injury. Modified with permission from Haider and Cornwell [11]

urgent intervention. A focal area of hyperintensity within the splenic parenchyma signifies a contained injury. This is commonly referred to as a 'contrast blush.' The management of a blush on CT scanning is, however, controversial; many surgeons opt for angioembolization when a blush is detected on the initial CT scan while some may prefer initial NOM followed by repeat imaging to determine the need to angioembolization as many small 'blushes' may resolve spontaneously. Laparotomy on the basis of contrast blush alone is not recommended.

Failure of Non-operative Management

It is important to adhere to a preconceived definition of failure when one embarks on a trial of NOM. If the patient becomes hemodynamically unstable, or the hematocrit value drops enough to require 2 or more units of packed red blood cells (PRBCs), or the patient develops signs of peritonitis, then immediate laparotomy is mandated. Of those that fail NOM, two-thirds fail within the first two days, 88 % within five days, and 93 % within the first week of injury [7, 8].

Figure 17.4 depicts a clinical pathway for the management of a patient with splenic injury. Patients who meet criteria for NOM, in an environment where NOM is possible should be initially managed non-operatively. If the CT scan shows an active blush or grade III or higher splenic injury, then angioembolization should be considered. At any point in time if the patient becomes hemodynamically unstable, develops peritoneal signs, or requires ≥2 units of PRBCs, then immediate laparotomy is indicated. Laparotomy is also indicated if a repeat CT scan demonstrates an increase in hemoperitoneum or active bleeding.

The patient presented in the above clinical scenario is a complex surgical patient with severe physiological derangement who has suffered an unfortunate iatrogenic splenic injury. She is currently hemodynamically labile with a grade 3 injury. She would be managed in an ICU setting with an initial trial of intravenous fluid boluses, intensive monitoring, and serial abdominal exams as well as serial hematocrit measurements. If she responds well to the fluid boluses and remains hemodynamically stable, then NOM can continue according to the aforementioned algorithm. Since her CT shows a grade III injury with a blush and large hemoperitoneum, she should undergo angioembolization. However, if she does not respond to a fluid challenge and becomes unstable, or angioembolization fails, then a laparotomy is mandated.

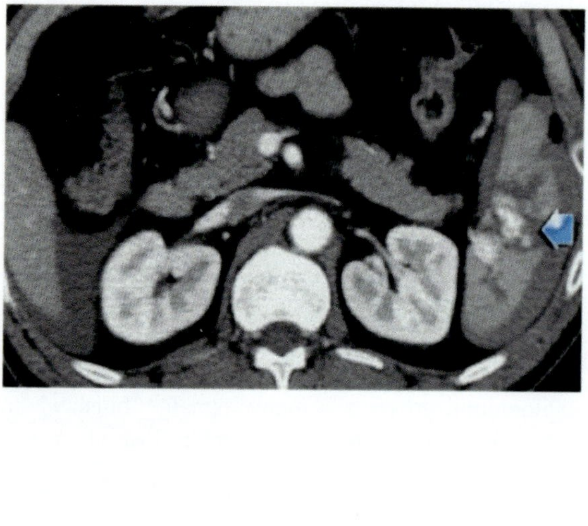

Fig. 17.4 CT of grade III splenic injury. Computed tomography image showing splenic injury with contrast blush with permission from http://www.radiologyassistant.nl/en/p466181ff61073/acute-abdomen-role-of-ct-in-trauma.html

Operative Management—the Complex Splenectomy

Even though several splenic salvage operations exist, in a surgically complex patient where a second physiological insult may prove fatal, a splenectomy is the safest and in fact the only reasonable operative option. Splenorrhaphy and other MESH maneuvers to salvage the spleen may be considered in relatively stable, healthier, younger patients.

The most important principles governing a splenectomy are exposure, mobilization, and control of hilar vessels. A midline incision and self-retaining retractors assure exposure. The surgeon may evacuate the blood in the left upper quadrant and pack laparotomy pads around the spleen. If needed, the remainder of the abdomen can be quickly and systematically explored at this point in order to rule out any other injuries. In the current scenario, it will be important to rule out other hollow viscous injuries as the spleen is in close proximity to the stomach and large and small bowels. To aide with exposure packs can be placed behind the spleen/under the diaphragm—this will elevate the spleen to bring it into view. All four ligaments attaching the spleen to stomach (splenogastric), diaphragm (splenophrenic), kidney (splenorenal), and colon (splenocolic) need to be taken down. Care should be taken while dissecting the splenogastric ligament and the short gastric vessels should be appropriately controlled. In the above-mentioned patient, a prior gastric pull up operation would have already divided the short gastric vessels. Adhesions from the prior operation need to be carefully dissected, traction on the spleen should be gentle to avoid capsular avulsion. If the previously placed jejunostomy feeding tube is hindering the operation, then this tube should be removed and replaced at the end of the procedure. Once the spleen is mobilized and elevated to the central aspect of the surgical field (Fig. 17.5), the hilum is exposed and the artery and the vein

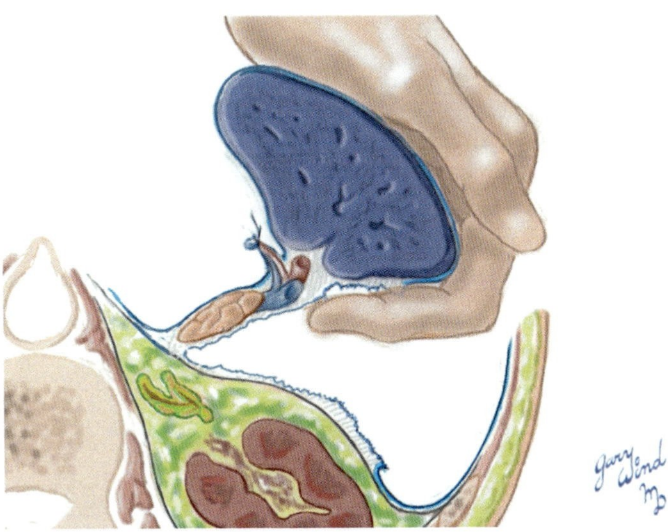

Fig. 17.5 Splenectomy, the mobilized spleen is elevated to the center of the operative field

should be individually ligated close to the hilum. The surgeon should be aware that the splenic artery may begin to branch up to 5 cm before entering the hilum and these branches should be ligated as well. Drains are placed only if there is suspected injury to the tail of the pancreas during mobilization and dissection. The splenic bed is often vascular and can be a source of extravasation, and this can be prevented with the use of argon beam to the splenic bed. Once the spleen is removed, the abdomen is closed in the standard fashion and standard postoperative care must ensue, including 24-h perioperative antibiotics, venousthromboembolism prophylaxis, incentive spirometry, pain control, fluid, and acid base management. Appropriate vaccinations should be administered after 2 weeks or prior to discharge as is typical for an unplanned splenectomy.

Clinical Scenario

A 66-year-old woman 4 weeks s/p Ivor Lewis esophagectomy (with pre-op feeding jejunostomy in the left upper quadrant) for adeno-CA complicated by intrathoracic leak. A total of 48 h following placement of a pleural drain, her hemoglobin drops 3 points with some hemodynamic lability. CT scan demonstrates large subcapsular hematoma with blush and large perisplenic blood.

Key Questions

1. *When would one consider a flank incision or subcostal incision?*
2. *What is your optimal timing for post-splenectomy vaccines?*

References

1. Kong VY, Clarke DL. The spectrum of visceral injuries secondary to misplaced intercostal chest drains: experience from a high volume trauma service in South Africa. Injury. 2014;45 (9):1435–9.
2. Seneff MG, Corwin RW, Gold LH, Irwin RS. Complications associated with thoracocentesis. Chest. 1986;90(1):97–100.
3. Stassen NA, Bhullar I, Cheng JD, Crandall ML, Friese RS, Guillamondegui OD, et al. Selective nonoperative management of blunt splenic injury: an Eastern Association for the Surgery of Trauma practice management guideline. The journal of trauma and acute care surgery. [Practice Guideline]. 2012;73(5 Suppl 4): S294–300.
4. Moore EE, Cogbill TH, Jurkovich GJ, Shackford SR, Malangoni MA, Champion HR. Organ injury scaling: spleen and liver (1994 revision). J Trauma. 1995;38(3):323–4.
5. Velmahos GC, Zacharias N, Emhoff TA, Feeney JM, Hurst JM, Crookes BA, et al. Management of the most severely injured spleen: a multicenter study of the Research Consortium of New England Centers for Trauma (ReCONECT). Arch Surg. [Multicenter Study]. 2010;145(5):456–60.

6. Shanmuganathan K, Mirvis SE, Boyd-Kranis R, Takada T, Scalea TM. Nonsurgical management of blunt splenic injury: use of CT criteria to select patients for splenic arteriography and potential endovascular therapy. Radiology. 2000;217(1):75–82.
7. McIntyre LK, Schiff M, Jurkovich GJ. Failure of nonoperative management of splenic injuries: causes and consequences. Arch Surg. [Comparative Study]. 2005;140(6):563–8; discussion 8–9.
8. Peitzman AB, Harbrecht BG, Rivera L, Heil B. Failure of observation of blunt splenic injury in adults: variability in practice and adverse consequences. J Am Coll Surg. 2005;201(2): 179–87.
9. Kadian YS, Rattan KN, Verma M, Kajal P. Congenital diaphragmatic hernia: Misdiagnosis in adolescence. J Ind Assoc Pediatr Surg. 2009;14(1):31–3.
10. Fischer JF, Jones DB. Fischer's mastery of surgery. 6th ed. Philadelphia: WK Health Book, Wolters Kluwer Health; 2011.
11. Haider AH, Cornwell EE. Splenic salvage procedure: therapeutic options. In: Cameron JL, editor. Current surgical therapy. 9th ed. Amsterdam: Elsevier.

Chapter 18
Soft Tissue Necrotizing Infection Due to Perforated Colon

Sharon M. Henry

Overview

Necrotizing Soft tissue infections (NSTI) are uncommon in a daily community practice and most surgeons encounter only a few of these cases throughout their careers. In a referral or tertiary center practice, however, they are seen more commonly. In both settings prompt identification and treatment are essential to optimal outcome. Lack of familiarity with the presentation can make this challenging. Unfortunately, these infections may be life-threatening and frequently occur in patients with limited physiologic reserve. A tentative approach or failure to recognize this problem as a surgical emergency can lead to inadequate treatment with increased morbidity and mortality.

Epidemiology

Multiple intraabdominal conditions may lead to NSTI. Perforated appendicitis, colon cancer, diverticulitis, inflammatory bowel disease and complex, neglected or inadequately treated perianal abscesses are the leading etiologies related to colon and rectal pathology. Additionally, gastroduodenal or small bowel perforations and gangrenous cholecystitis are other potential intraabdominal causes of NSTI. NSTI can also follow elective or emergency gynecologic, genitourinary, abdominal, or rectal surgical procedures. The abdominal wall is the site of NSTI in approximately 5–10 % [1] infections.

S.M. Henry (✉)
Department of Trauma, University of Maryland Medical center,
22 South Greene Street, Baltimore, MD 21201, USA
e-mail: shenry@umm.edu

J.J. Diaz and D.T. Efron (eds.), *Complications in Acute Care Surgery*,
DOI 10.1007/978-3-319-42376-0_18

Table 18.1 Organism producing necrotizing soft tissue infection [3]

Gram + aerobic	Gram − aerobic	Anaerobic	Marine vibrio	Fungi
Group A streptococcus	*Escherichia coli* (cirrhosis)	*Bacteroides* sp. (DM)	*Vibrio vulnificus* (cirrhosis)	*Candida* (immunosuppression)
Group B Streptococcus (DM)	*Pseudomonas aeruginosa* sp. (immunosuppression and burns)	*Clostridium* sp. (Intravenous drug use, colonic neoplasms, contaminated wounds)	*Vibrio parahaemolyticus* (cirrhosis)	*Aspergillus* (immunosuppression)
Staphylococcus aureus (DM)	*Enterobacter cloacae*	*Peptostreptococcus* sp	Vibrio damsela	Zygmocetes (immunosuppression)
Coagulase negative staphylococci	*Klebsiella* sp. (cirrhosis and DM)	*Peptococcus* sp.	*Vibrio alginolyticus* (cirrhosis)	
Enterococci (DM)	*Proteus* sp.			
Bacilli	*Seratia* sp. (chronic renal failure and DM)			
	Acinetobacter			
	Citrobacter freundii			
	Pasteurella multocida (intravenous drug use)			

Sources Morgan [2], Vinh and Embil [26], Brook [27], Paramythiotis et al. [28]

Pathophysiology

In general, necrotizing infections result from bacterial invasion into the subcutaneous fat or superficial fascia. Enzymes and toxins produced by the bacteria facilitate the spread along the fascial planes deep below the skin surface [2]. Bacterial invasion produces tissue necrosis by causing vascular thrombosis leading to tissue death. This environment favors the growth of anaerobic or facultative anaerobic bacteria. The hallmark of NSTI is the accumulation of gas formed by these bacteria. A variety of gases are produced in the low-oxidative reduction potential environment including hydrogen, nitrogen, hydrogen sulfide, and methane which then accumulate in the soft tissue spaces [3]. Perforation of the retroperitoneal colon or pelvic portion of the rectum may introduce air and bacteria into the retroperitoneum or peritoneum. Abscesses may subsequently develop in these spaces and extend along fascial pains or necessitate to the skin surface.

Anatomy

The site of perforation in the bowel will govern the route of spread to the subcutaneous position. Intraperitoneal perforations dissect through defects in the peritoneum or mesenteric attachments. A violation of the peritoneum or fascia neighboring the injury leads to the intramuscular and subcutaneous surfaces. The infection can spread contiguously to extend from the retroperitoneum to the deep abdominal fascia and ultimately through the abdominal skin or exit through the obturator foramen to spread to the gluteal region or the thigh (see Fig. 18.1). This can lead to involvement of the limb by following the iliacus or psoas muscle to their insertions on the greater and lesser trochanters, respectively (see Figs. 18.1 and 18.2).

Solid organs or intact fibrous membranes offer good resistance to extension while areolar and loose fascial tissues offer significantly lower resistance. Muscular insertions and vascular investing fascia may conduct the spread of intrapelvic and retroperitoneal infection to the buttocks, hip, thighs, and perineum (see Figs. 18.1 and 18.3). Studies using cadavers show that air injected into the posterior peritoneum produced air in the anterior peritoneal area while air injected into the presacral space produced air in the lower abdominal wall, thighs, scrotum, and buttocks [4]. The routes of spread include passage along neurovascular bundles that penetrate muscle and abdominal wall fascia, through natural defects such as the inguinal ring, along the femoral vessels and over the inguinal ligaments and through the pelvic floor to the tissues of the buttocks and thighs and over the abdomen [5]. Air present in the soft tissues may represent dissected air from the aerodigestive tract or air produced by infecting organisms. Perforation of the bowel should be excluded when subcutaneous emphysema of the abdominal wall is identified.

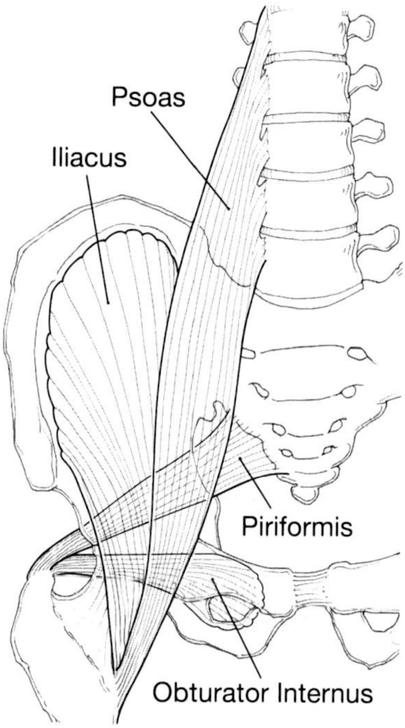

Fig. 18.1 Four major pelvic muscles and their extremity attachements, Psoas major origin transverse processes of lumbar spine inserts on lesser trochanter, Iliacus origin upper portion of the iliac fossa and sacrum and inserts on lesser trocanter, Pyriformis origin sacrum and sciatic foramen and inserts on greater trochanter, Obturator internus origin obturator foramen margins and inserts on lesser trochanter

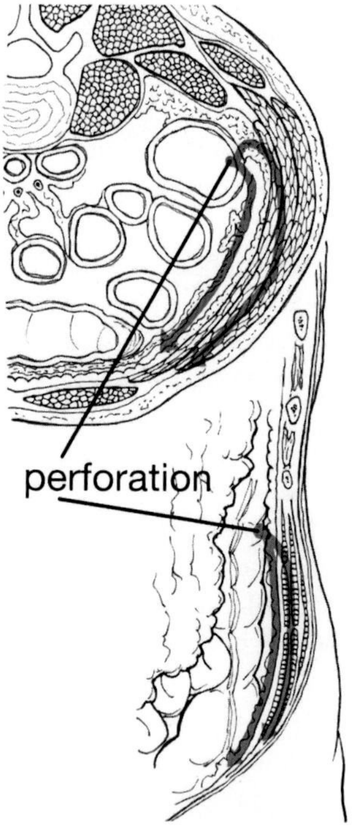

Fig. 18.2 Demonstrates path of bacterial spread from colon perforation with relationship to abdominal wall

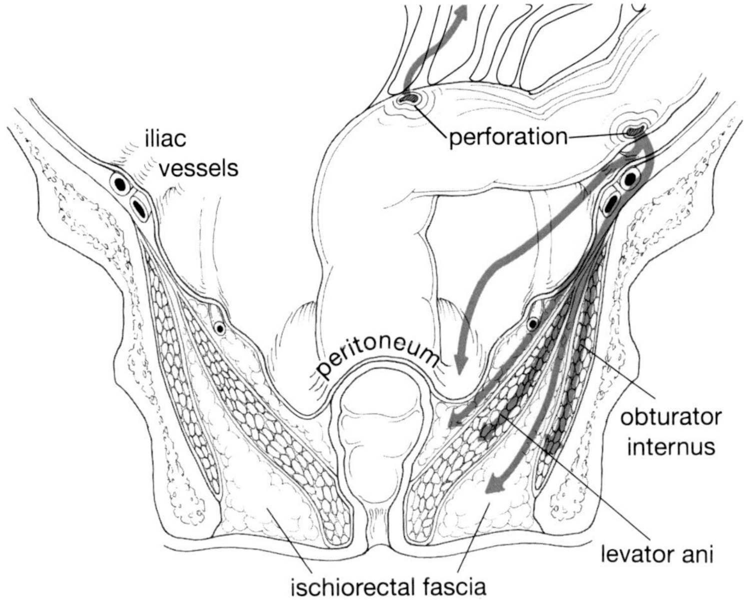

Fig. 18.3 Note endopelvic fascia covers major pelvic muscles, *Arrows* demonstrate path of potential bacterial spread from colonic perforations

Bacteriology

NSTI related to perforations are overwhelmingly polymicrobial reflecting the microbiota of the colon. However, patient factors may alter host defenses favoring the growth of particular organisms. See Table 18.1. Antibiotics should be directed against likely pathogens including anaerobic organisms. Fungal infection is possible with perforated bowel especially with nosocomial infections or an immunocompromised host. See Table 18.2 for microbes and effective anti-infective therapy.

Presentation

Hard signs of necrotizing fasciitis are classically tense edema, violaceous bullae, and crepitance. When necrotizing fasciitis results from bowel perforation, it is usually because of a delay in the recognition of the problem or presentation of the patient. Intraperitoneal colonic perforation usually presents overtly with signs of peritonitis, fever, and tachycardia. Abdominal-wall skin changes and crepitus are not a part of the usual presentation. A retroperitoneal perforation may be at least partially walled off and sequestered from the peritoneum. This would limit the peritoneal irritation and subsequent discomfort that would be anticipated. Further

Table 18.2 Microorganisms associated with necrotizing fasciitis and antibiotic therapy

Microbe	First line therapy	Penicillin allergy
Mixed infections	Piperacillin-tazobactam and vancomycin Imipenem-cilastatin Meropenem Ertapenem Cefotaxime and Metronidazole or clindamycin	Clindamycin or metronidazole with an aminoglycoside or fluroquinolone
Streptococcus	Penicillin plus clindamycin	Vancomycin, linezolid, quinupristin/dalfopristin, daptomycin
Staphylococcus aureus (SA)	Nafcillin Oxacillin Cefazolin Vancomycin (for resistance) Clindamycin	Vancomycin, linezolid, quinupristin/dalfopristin, daptomycin Bacteriostatic; inducible resistance in methicillin resistant SA
Clostridial species	Clindamycin plus penicillin	
Aeromonas hydrophila	Doxycycline plus ciprofloxacin or ceftriaxone	
Vibrio Vulnificus	Doxycycline plus ciprofloxacin or ceftriaxone	
Candida albicans	Caspafungin, micafungin or fluconazole	
Aspergillus	Voriconazole, lipid formulation amphotericin B	

With permission from Oxford University Press, Stevens [29]

extension into the flank musculature and fascia may produce pain that can be confused with an extra abdominal source confounding the diagnosis. As the infection spreads and tissue destruction progresses, skin changes may become evident. The most common signs include tenderness (often out of proportion to physical findings), erythema, and induration. Unfortunately, these findings are rather nonspecific and are seen with non-necrotizing soft tissue infections and trauma. Alternatively, depending on the cause of the perforation, gastrointestinal symptoms may be more prominent and influence the diagnostic evaluation or lead to urgent laparotomy. Nausea, vomiting, diarrhea, constipation or obstipation, melena, hematochezia, and weight loss are evidence of a likely intraabdominal problem. When these symptoms coincide with the presence of abdominal wall, flank or even limb skin changes or crepitus, abdominal imaging to identify the source of pathology will be useful. Patients with NSTI related to bowel perforation present with signs related to the bowel perforation or to the soft tissue infection or with some combination of the two (see Table 18.3).

There are a variety of patient factors that effect the clinical presentation. Patients with altered pain perception are a group at high risk for delayed presentation or

Table 18.3 Signs and symptoms associated with necrotizing fasciitis

General	Frequency (%)	Systemic	Frequency (%)	GI related
Erythema	70	Fever	40	Nausea Vomiting Constipation Diarrhea Abdominal pain Hematochezia Melena Bloating Anorexia Draining (fecalent) sinus
Warmth	44	Hypotension	21	
		Tachypnea (>20)	26	
Tenderness	79	+ Blood culture	35	
Induration	66	Mental status changes	5	
Bullae/blisters	25	Tachycardia	59	
Creptius	20	Tachypnea	26	
Skin necrosis	24			
Swelling	80			
Drainage	19			

Sources Shimizu and Tokunda [30], Wang and Lim [31], Goh et al. [32]

diagnosis. Both patients and providers easily ignore early subtle findings. This group includes patients who abuse narcotics and alcohol. They may self-medicate thereby masking their symptoms or their symptoms may be overlooked when they do seek medical care. As a result, some of these patients have obvious skin necrosis and/or are in septic shock when they present.

The host's ability to contain the bacteria can impact the development of NSTI. Immunosuppressed patients are at high risk for a delay in diagnosis of perforation [6]. Without the normal inflammatory response to injury, these patients lack a classical presentation. Fever, erythema, and pain may be mild or absent.

Diabetes Mellitus and morbid obesity can interfere with the presentation of signs and symptoms. Many diabetic patients have neuropathy that may alter their pain perception, and poor glycemic control certainly alters immune function. Abdominal evaluation in the morbidly obese patient is notoriously difficult. Elderly patients may also present with atypical symptoms or blunted responses making prompt diagnosis difficult (see Table 18.4 for a list of associated medical conditions).

Investigation

In addition to a comprehensive physical examination, laboratory tests may help to confirm or raise the level of concern for NSTI. As is true of the physical examination, many routine laboratory tests results are nonspecific, but in combination with physical findings, laboratory abnormalities can improve diagnostic precision [7–9] (see Table 18.5). Serum carcinoembryonic antigen (CEA) should be measured when perforated colon carcinoma is suspected. The patient that presents in septic shock with "hard signs" of NSTI does not usually require further diagnostic

Table 18.4 Associated medical conditions

Associated medical condition
Diabetes
Advanced age
Cirrhosis
Renal failure
Immunosupression
Peripheral vascular disease
Intravenous drug use
Alcohol abuse
Obesity

Sources Childers et al. [33], Lamagni et al. [34], Sharkawy et al. [35], Geusens et al. [36], Cox [37]

Table 18.5 Useful laboratory studies

Blood test	Value	Laboratory risk nccrotizing fasciitis indicator score (LRINEC) >6	
WBC per mm^3	>15	<15	0
		15–25	+1
		>25	+2
Na meq/dL	<135	≥135	0
		<135	+2
Glucose mg/dL	>180	≤180	0
		>180	+1
Creatinine mg/dL	>1.6	≤1.6	0
		>1.6	+2
C reactive protein mg/dL	>15	<15	0
		≥15	+4
Hemoglobin g/dL	<11	>13.5	0
		11–13.5	+1
		<11	+2
Myoglobin mcg/L	Elevated		
Lactate mmol/L	>2		
$HC0_3$ mmol/L	<15		
pH	<7.3		
Platelet × 10^9/L	<100		
PT seconds	>15		
CPK IU/L	>600		

Sources Wong et al. [38], Murphy et al. [39], Erol et al. [40], Kinasewitz et al. [41]

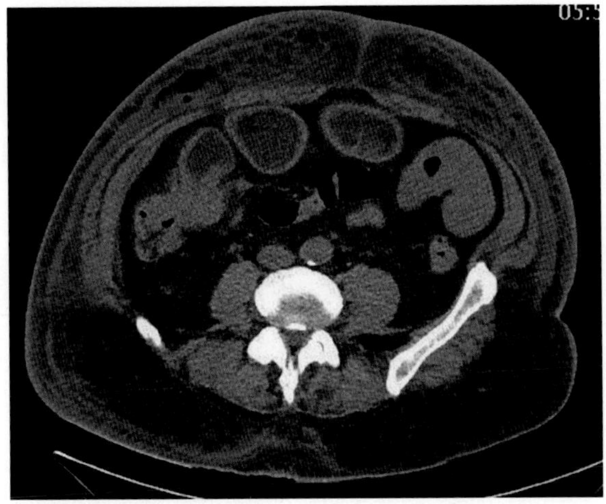

Fig. 18.4 CT image demonstrating air in the subcutaneous tissue with bowel thickening and dilated small bowel

investigation. Laboratory studies are used to gauge the degree of shock and organ dysfunction and to monitor resuscitation.

For those patients without significant physiologic derangement and in whom the diagnosis remains in question, radiologic imaging may be vitally important. Plain abdominal X-rays are more sensitive than physical examination to the presence of air in the soft tissues. They may also reveal free intraabdominal air or bowel dilation associated with obstruction. Ultrasound can detect soft tissue air and fluid collections.

By far, the most useful study is the contrast enhanced computed tomography scan (CT scan). It is very sensitive to the detection of air and fluid in the soft tissues and gives very specific information regarding the intraperitoneal and retroperitoneal structures (see Fig. 18.4). Magnetic resonance imaging (MRI) provides excellent images of the soft tissue and intraabdominal regions but is not more useful than CT scan in this clinical setting.

Treatment

Resuscitation

For the reasons outlined above, the patient with perforation of the colon and NSTI is likely to have been ill for several days. In addition, the inflammatory response to the soft tissue injury and infection may be intense. Significant physiologic and laboratory abnormalities need to be addressed rapidly prior to operative intervention [10]. Excessive delay to prepare the patient for surgery can increase mortality. Metabolic and lactic acidosis should be addressed with volume resuscitation. Electrolytes abnormalities should be addressed with supplements or rarely dialysis.

Coagulation abnormalities may not be fully correctable. Intravenous access for fluids, blood products, medication, and resuscitation are mandatory. The stomach should be decompressed with insertion of a nasogastric tube. A Foley catheter is necessary to monitor urinary output and response to resuscitation. Arterial catheters are particularly helpful to continuously monitor blood pressure and facilitate blood draws to monitor ongoing resuscitation.

Antibiotics should be administered quickly and redosed in the operating room if indicated.

Operation

Preoperative discussion with nursing and anesthesia providers is important. Potential blood loss is significant and all staff should be prepared for this in the operating room. Blood products should be on hand immediately and replenished as needed. Topical hemostatic products may be useful to control surface oozing especially when coagulopathy is present at the outset.

Positioning is usually supine with the upper extremities extended laterally. In circumstances, when there is involvement of the thigh, groin, or perineum, lithotomy positioning may be necessary to access these areas and the abdomen. When the NSTI extends to the flanks, a gel or blanket roll may increase the exposure of this area and allow simultaneous access to the abdomen. Do not hesitate to reposition the patient when needed to visualize all the affected areas. Self-retaining abdominal wall retractors are very helpful particularly in the obese patient. Extra long instrument sets may be necessary as well.

The initial procedure is potentially lengthy given that it is essentially two procedures. One is the laparotomy to treat the intraabdominal pathology and the other is the debridement of the NSTI. It may be necessary to truncate one or both of the procedures depending on patient stability. In any case, planned reoperation within 24–48 h is mandatory. The laparotomy is usually carried out first. The source of contamination is controlled rapidly. This is usually accomplished with a segmental or hemicolectomy depending on the problem encountered and the patient's stability. At times, proximal diversion and/or defunctionalization may be required. I favor deferring the creation of a stoma in cases with significant skin, fascia, and muscle involvement. Evolution of the infection may alter the placement. Furthermore, reanastomosis may be an option at a subsequent procedure. Stoma creation is particularly challenging in morbidly obese patients.

Then, the NSTI is debrided. Many times, there is an area of obvious skin involvement. This area is characterized by intensive erythema, warmth, tense induration or bogginess, bullae, or necrosis and represents the primary site of involvement or "ground zero". Adjacent to this area is an area of less severe erythema and induration. More distantly, there is a third region where erythema without induration is found. The debridement begins at site of maximal skin abnormality but should encompass all three regions. The incision should be

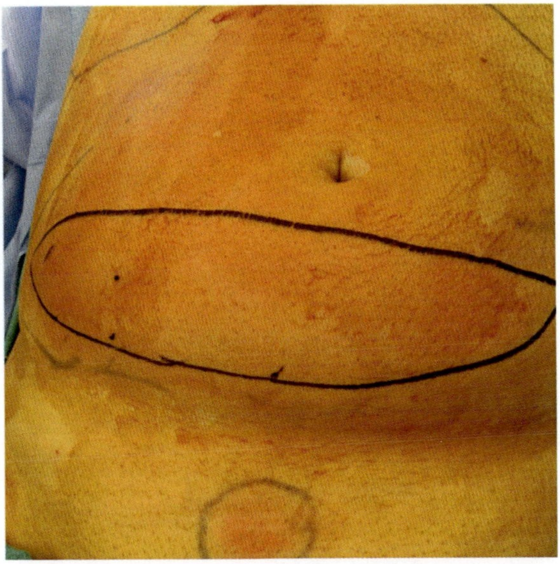

Fig. 18.5 Area of maximal erythema marked with *dark marker* area also indurated. *Lighter marked* areas with less pronounced erythema without induration

extended to the deep fascia to allow evaluation of all tissue layers (see Fig. 18.5). At this point take tissue cultures or samples of pus that is encountered. Both aerobic and anaerobic cultures should be taken. Next, manually probe the tissues to ascertain the limits of extension. Bacterial enzymes and toxin elaboration release tissue bonds allowing the surgeon's finger to easily pass through the tissue above the deep fascia. The incision is extended until healthy deep fascia with adherent subcutaneous tissue is encountered. Undermining the skin may produce dermal ischemia and skin loss. This is unavoidable in many circumstances as removal of the subcutaneous tissue is required when there is evidence of necrosis, abscess, or vascular thrombosis. The quantity of skin debridement requires clinical judgment (see Fig. 18.6a). The primary objective is to control the infection. In severely septic patients, failure to remove all involved tissue may allow the infection to progress [11]. This may result in further tissue loss and delay in control of the infection. All unhealthy tissue is removed. The deep fascia is incised to inspect the muscle. The muscle is inspected and assessed for viability and contractility. A separate incision might be needed depending on the location. Avoid multiple parallel incisions as this may compromise skin blood flow. Debride all abnormal subcutaneous fat and fascia. Remove all nonviable muscle. Large defects are the rule, and reconstructions will be complicated. Do not focus on the future task but on controlling the current infection.

After completing the debridement, the wound is irrigated with copious amounts of fluid. I use normal saline 6–9 L. Irrigation is commonly performed but the best solutions, volumes, and temperature is not well defined. A metaanalysis evaluating the practice of intraabdominal irrigation to decrease surgical site infection concluded that using any solution compared with no irrigation resulted in reduction of

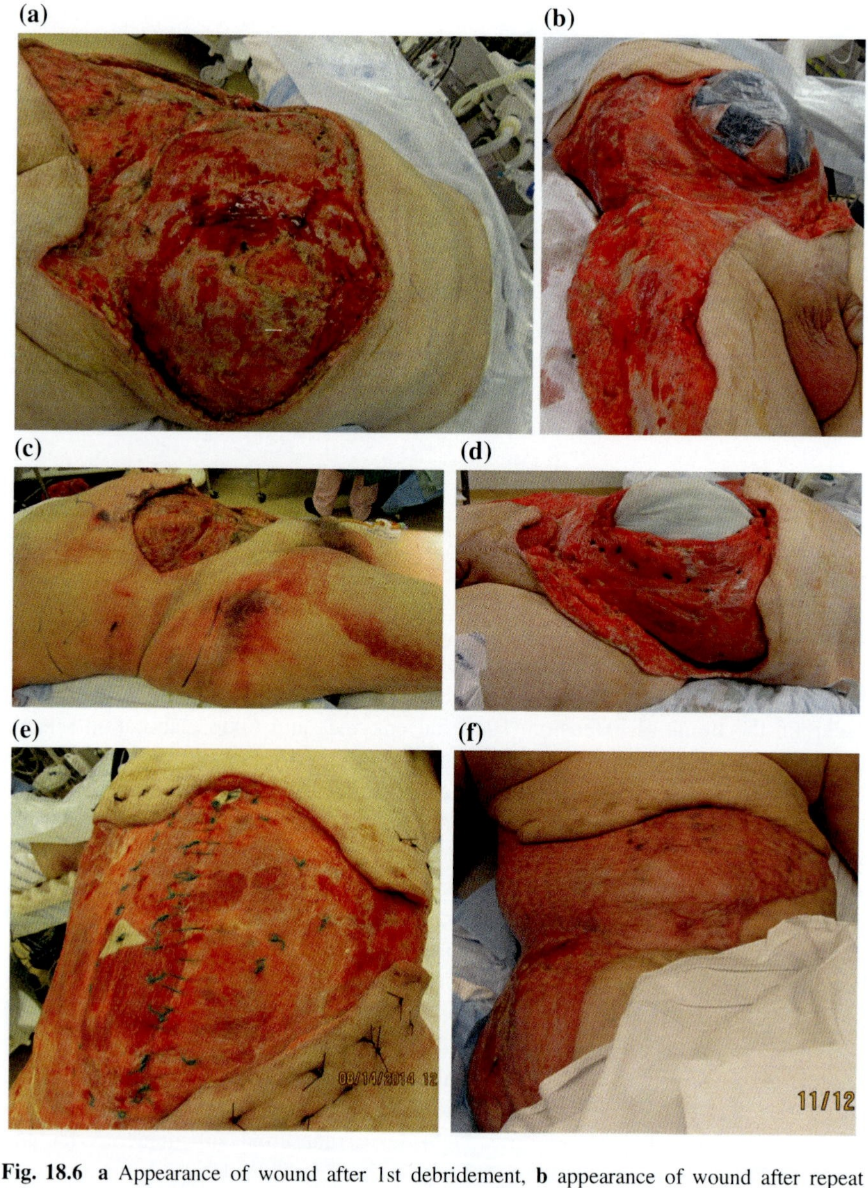

Fig. 18.6 **a** Appearance of wound after 1st debridement, **b** appearance of wound after repeat debridement and laparotomy left open with Abthera™, **c** progression of infection after 1st debridement, **d** abdominal wall closure using biologic mesh, **e** abdominal wall closure over biologic mesh, and **f** skin grafted wound

surgical site infection. The effect was the strongest in colorectal surgery subgroup of the analysis [12]. Some commonly used solutions and additives for irrigation are listed in Table 18.6.

Table 18.6 Irrigation solutions and additives

Irrigant	Advantages	Disadvantages
Normal Saline	Does not interfere with wound healing	Does not reduce SSI
	Removes clot and debris	
Povidone iondine 1 %	Broad spectrum antimicrobial solution	Potential iodine toxicity cytotoxicity
	Decreased SSI compared to no irrigation	Dries and may discolor skin
Hydrogen peroxide 3 %	Effervescence acts as chemical debriding agent to lift debris	Cytotoxicity
		Should not be used in wounds with sinuses
		Over use can actually reduce the speed and effectiveness of healing and protection from infection
Bacitracin 50,000 U		Report of anaphylaxis
Cefazolin	Combined with systemic antibiotics reduced mortality in animal studies	Animal studies show increased adhesions
Kanamycin	Decreased infectious complications compared to saline in obese patients	Potential for development of resistance
Chloramphenicol 2 g	Stimulating effect on peritoneal macrophages in vitro	Potential for development of resistance
	Effective when used after irrigation	
Sodium hypoclorite 0.25 %	Bacteriocidal to most organisms found in wounds	Cytotoxicity
		Should not be used in wounds with sinuses
		Should not be used for longer than 7–10 days
0.05 % Chlorhexidine gluconate solution	Non-cytotoxic	Bacteriostatic
	No irritating	
	Only FDA approved antiseptic for surgical irrigation	
Hypochlorous acid 0.01 %(HOCl)	Rapid bactericidal activity	
	Safe for human cells	

Sources Fry [42], Chundamal and Wright [43], Rodeheaver [44], Damm [45], Rappaport et al. [46], Yelon et al. [47], Nomikos et al. [48], Barnes et al. [49], Sakarya et al. [50]

Closure of the abdomen is frequently impossible given the quantity of tissue debrided. A fabricated or manufactured negative pressure wound therapy (NPWT) device is a popular management strategy. This device has the advantage of controlling exudate and decreasing the likelihood of abdominal compartment syndrome (ACS) developing. NPWT is also an option for management of the NSTI wound as well whether contiguous or separate from the laparotomy incision. Irrigating systems can be added that allow for intermittent irrigation with saline or antimicrobial solutions. Contours and extension to the genitalia and perineum can make placement challenging particularly in obese patients. It is unwise to use NPWT in circumstances when coagulopathy or thrombocytopenia is significant. NPWT should never be used in cases where the debridement is incomplete. Topical hemostatics can be useful when oozing persists. Tissues are highly exudative, so absorptive dressings are necessary. A nonadhering contact layer is applied to the wound surface to diminish adherence to structures in the wound bed. A variety of gauze, cellulose, or foam dressings can be chosen to dress the wound. Securing the dressing using an abdominal binder, stretch netting, roll gauze, or ace bandages avoids the use of tape on weepy fragile skin.

Most patients will require reoperation at least once to complete the abdominal procedure. Further abdominal procedures may include performing bowel resection, anastomosis, placement of drains, placement of feeding access, and abdominal wall closure or reconstruction (see Fig. 18.6b). The soft tissue wound is reinspected to assure the adequacy of the debridement (see Fig. 18.6c). Areas of new or persistent erythema or induration require exploration and possibly debridement. Large tissue defects will require wound care, which in some cases requires repeated operative trips. NPWT with serial dressing changes in the operating room or at the bedside is an excellent method to prepare the wound bed [13, 14]. Secondary bacterial or fungal infections are possible and the wound must be monitored to detect this. Biologic and synthetic tissue substitutes may be needed to complete wound reconstruction (see Fig. 18.6d). Final wound closure may require skin grafts (see Fig. 18.6f) or fascio or myocutaneous flaps.

Comprehensive Care

Tissue culture results are used to guide antimicrobial therapy. Temperature and white blood cell count (WBC) are followed to monitor recovery from the infection. Antibiotics are continued until the infection resolves. This is usually not longer than two weeks. Blood glucose control is important. Diabetes is present in 40–60 % [15] of patients with necrotizing fasciitis.

Nutritional support should begin as soon as physiologically possible and should continue until wound closure. Protein loss through tissue exudate and hypermetabolism associated with the infection make adequate nutrition vitally important. Vitamin supplementation may also be useful to correct deficiencies and assure adequate supply for healing to occur (see Table 18.7).

Organ system support with mechanical ventilation and renal replacement therapy is frequently needed. Early physical therapy and mobilization are important to minimize nosocomial infections and complications.

Pain management using multiple modalities is required to aid in the management of these large wounds.

Table 18.7 Vitamins and minerals associated with wound healing

Nutrient	Affect	Dosage
Vitamin A	• Reverses decrease tensile strength effect of cortisone • Anti-oxidant activity • Increased fibroblast proliferation modulation of cellular differentiation and proliferation • Hyaluronate synthesis, and decreased MMP mediated extracellular matrix degradation	25,000 IU daily
Vitamin E	• Anti-oxidant, maintains and stabilizes cellular membrane integrity by providing protection against destruction by oxidation • Decreasing excess scar formation in chronic wounds • Increase breaking strength and normalize healing of wounds exposed to irradiation	800 IU daily
Vitamin C	• Important to the synthesis of collagen and the growth of new blood vessels • Enhances neutrophil function	1–2 g daily
Zinc	• Essential for DNA synthesis, cell division and protein synthesis • Processes for tissue regeneration and repair	220 mg daily

Source Guo and Dipietro [51]

Outcome

Many patients with NSTI resulting from bowel perforation are elderly and have multiple comorbidities. These patients are a challenge to manage. Their care needs to be thoughtful and meticulous. They are prone to complications related to nosocomial infection and thromboembolic phenomenon. Acalculous cholecystitis, ischemic bowel, ulcer perforation, clostridium difficile colitis, ventilator associated pneumonia, myocardial infarctions, arrhythmias, urinary tract, and catheter associated infections are among the serious complication that can also occur in this critically ill patient group. This is a particularly risk when prolonged vasopressors or steroids have been used. Family meetings to discuss potential outcome and to define goals of care should begin early and occur regularly. It is important to understand acceptable outcomes to the patient and their family.

The mortality for NSTI in modern times is less than 30 %. The addition of organ failure increases the mortality to up to 70 % [16]

A study using NSQIP (National Surgical Quality Improvement Program) data from 2005 to 2010 identified several variables through logistic regression modelling to predict 30 day mortality (see Table 18.8).

Hospital stays are lengthy, averaging 24.5 days. Intensive care unit stays are necessary in 50 % of patients and average 8.6 days [17, 18]. Annual patient charges for patients with NSTI was over $18 million in a 2007 study of patients hospitalized

Table 18.8 Multivariable logistic regression model for 30 day postoperative mortality from NSTI

Variable	Odds ratio	95 % CI	P Value
Older than 60 years	2.47	1.72–3.55	<0.001
Dependence level			
Partially dependent	1.61	0.95–2.69	0.072
Completely dependent	2.33	1.43–3.80	0.001
Dialysis before operation	1.89	1.15–3.10	0.012
ASA class >4	3.55	2.25–5.59	<0.001
Emergent operation	1.56	1.03–2.34	0.035
Preoperative septic shock	2.35	1.55–3.56	<0.001
Platelet count			
<150,000	1.67	1.21–2.87	0.005
>50,000/mm^3	3.48	1.65–7.37	0.001
<50,000/mm^3			

With permission from Elsevier, Faraklas et al. [52]

in Florida. In general, involvement of the trunk is associated with higher likelihood of death [19–22]. Recovery is lengthy, and post discharge care at an acute or subacute rehabilitation facility is frequently needed. One single institution study noted 1/3 of patients were discharged to skilled nursing or rehabilitation facilities [23]. Despite this, truncal involvement was surprisingly independently associated with better functional outcome [24]. Patients well enough to be discharged home will usually need home nursing and outpatient or home rehabilitation [25]. Readmissions are common. Patients with associated comorbidities often fail to return to their preadmission health status.

Case Continued

Summary

Colon perforation is an uncommon cause of NSTI. Failure to identify it as a cause of NSTI can lead to delay in source control and thereby increase morbidity and mortality. Managing both the colon pathology and the soft tissue infection can lead to technical challenges. Judgement is required to choose the patient who requires diversion and in choosing the site for diversion on the abdominal wall. Successful management requires attention to wound care, nutrition, pain management, and rehabilitation.

Clinical Scenario

A 50-year-old man presents to his local emergency department with complaints of abdominal pain. The pain is localized to the right lower abdomen. On examination, there is erythema and tenderness of the lower abdomen without diffuse peritoneal signs (Fig. 18.5). He has no past medical or surgical history but admits to weight loss and fatigue over the last month.

His WBC was 7.8, Hematocrit 30, lactate 4.1, sodium 131, BUN 96, and creatinine 2.42. A non-contrast enhanced computed tomography (CT) scan was performed (Fig. 18.4). Extensive soft tissue gas and fat stranding are noted over the right side of the abdomen. Dilation and thickening of the distal ileum suspicious for inflammation, Crohn's disease, ischemia, or neoplasm were reported by the radiologists.

He was transferred to a tertiary referral center where after the initial evaluation and stabilization his abdominal wall was debrided (Fig. 18.6a, c). His operative cultures grew alpha hemolytic strep, group C strep, E. coli, clostridium, and bacteroides. There were clear intraabdominal abnormalities with concern for neoplasm or inflammation on his CT scan. However, since he did not appear to be completely obstructed or to have on going fecal contamination, abdominal exploration was deferred. Carcinoembryonic antigen was measured and was elevated at 34-ng/mL. An urgent colonoscopy and biopsy of a cecal mass was performed. He underwent exploratory laparotomy and right hemicolectomy with anastomosis. His abdomen was left open (Fig. 18.6b) He was ultimately closed over biologic mesh (see Fig. 18.6d, e). He was then skin grafted (Fig. 18.6f). He had eleven operative procedures. This hospital course was complicated by the development of pulmonary embolus and clostridium difficille colitis. He was able to receive his chemotherapy 4 months after presentation.

Key Question

1. *Where do you bring the ostomy out when a significant part of the abdominal wall has been resected? How is this fashioned and how much normal skin do you need to place a stoma?*

References

1. Howell GM, Rosengart MR. Necrotizing soft tissue infections. Surg Infect (Larchmt). 2011;12 (3):185–90.
2. Morgan MS. Diagnosis and management of necrotizing faucitis: a multi parametric approach. J Hosp Infect. 2010;2010(75):249–57. doi:10.1016/j.jhin.01.028.
3. Roje Z, Matic D. Necrotizing fasciitis: literature review of contemporary strategies for diagnosing and management with three case reports: torso, abdominal wall, upper and lower limbs. World J Em Surg. 2011;6:46.
4. Meyers M, Goodman K. Pathways of extrapelvic spread of disease: anatoic-radiologic correlation. AJR. 1975;125(4):900–9.
5. Fiss T, Cigtay O, Miele A, Twigg H. Perforated viscus presenting with gas in the soft tissues (subcutaneous emphysema). AJR. 1975;125(1):226–33.
6. Tsitsilonis S, Druschel C, Wichlas F, Haas NP, et al. Necrotizing fasciitis: is the bacteria spectrum changing? Langenbecks Arch Surg. 2013;398:153–9.

7. Wong CH, Chang HC, Pasupathy S, Khin LW, Tan JL, Low CO, et al. Necrotizing fasciitis: clinical presentation, microbiology, and determinants of mortality. J Bone Joint Surg Am. 2003;85(A):1454–60.
8. Wall DB, Klein SR, Black S, de Virgilio C. A simple model to help distinguish necrotizing fasciitis from non-necrotizing soft tissue infection. J Am Coll Surg. 2000;191:227–31.
9. Stevens D, Bisno AL, Chamber HF, Everett ED, Dellinger P, et al. Management of skin and soft-tissue infections. Clin Infect Dis. 2005;41:1373–406.
10. Ecker KW, Baars A, Topfer J, Frank J. Necrotizing fasciitis of the perineum and the abdominal wall surgical approach. Eur J Trauma Emerg Surg. 2008;34:219–28.
11. Wong CH, Yam AK, Tan AG, Song C. Approach to debridement in necrotizing facitis. Am J Surg. 2008;196:19–24.
12. Mueller TC, Loos M, Haller B, Mihaljevic AL, Nitsche U, Wilhelm D, et al. Intraoperative wound irrigation to reduce surgical site infection after abdominal surgery: a systematic review and meta-analysis. Langenbecks Arch Surg. 2015;400:167–81.
13. Silberstein J, Grabowski J, Parsons JK. Use of a vacuum-assisted device for fournier's gangrene: a new paradigm. Rev Urol. 2008;10:76–80.
14. Moues CM, vandenBemd GJ, Heule F, Hovius SE. Comparing conventional gauze therapy to vacuum-assisted closure wound therapy: a prospective randomized trail. J Plast Reconstr Aesthet Surg. 2007;60672–81. doi:10.1016/j.bjps.2006.01.041.
15. Misiakos EP, Bagias G, Patapis P, Sotiropoulos D, Kanavidis P, Machairas A. Current concepts in the management of necrotizing fasciitis. Front Surg. 2014;1:36. doi:10.3389/fsurg.2014.00036.
16. Piedra T, Martin-Cuesta L, Arnaiz J, Marco de Lucas E, Pellon R, Garcia-Bolado A, et al. Necrotizing fasciitis secondary to diverticulitis. Emerg Radiol. 2007;13:345–8.
17. Ecker KW, Baars A, Topfer J, Frank J. Necrotizing fasciitis of the perineum and the abdominal wall surgical approach. Eur J Trauma Emerg Surg. 2008;34:214–28.
18. Nisbet M, et al. Necrotizing fasciitis: review of 82 cases in South Auckland. Int Med J. doi:10.1111/j.1445-5994.2009.02137.
19. Mulla ZD, Gibbs SG, Aronoff DM. Correlates of length of stay, cost of care and mortality among patients hospitalized for necrotizing fasciitis. Epidemiol Infect. 2007;135:868–76.
20. Tsitsilonis S, Durschel C, Wichlas F, Haas N, Schwabe P, Hermann J, et al. Necrotizing fasciitis: is the bacterial spectrum changing? Langenbecks Arch. 2013;398:153–9.
21. Pessa ME, Howard RJ. Necrotizing fasciitis. Surg Gynecol Obstet. 1985;161:357–61.
22. Bosshardt TL, Henderson VJ, Organ CH Jr. Necrotizing soft tissue infections. Arch Surg. 1996;131:846–55.
23. Eggerstedt M, Gamelli R, Mosier MJ. The care of necrotizing soft tissue infections: patterns of definitive intervention at a large referral center. J Burn Care Res. 2015;36(1):105–10.
24. Hakkarainen TW, et al. Curr Probl Surg. 2014;51:344–62.
25. Martinschek A, Evers B, Lampl L, Gerngrob H, Schmidt R, Sparwasser C. Prognostic aspects, survival rate, and predisposing risk factors in patients with fournier's gangrene and necrotizing soft tissue infections: evaluation of clinical outcome of 55 patients. Urol Int. 2012;89(2): 173–9.
26. Vinh DH, Embil JM. Rapidly progressive soft tissue infections. Lancet Infect Dis. 2005;5:501–13.
27. Brook I. Mircrobiology and management of soft tissue and muscle infections. Int J Surg. 2008;6:328–38.
28. Paramythiotis D, Koukoutsis H, Harlaftis N. Necrotizing soft tissue infections. Surg Prac. 2007;11(1):17–28.
29. Stevens DL, Bisno AL, Chambers HF, Patchen Dellinger E, Goldstein EJC, Gorbach SL, Hirschmann JV, Kaplan SL, Montoya JG, Wade JC. Practice guidelines for the diagnosis and management of skin and soft tissue infections: 2014 Update by the Infectious Diseases Society of America. Clin Infect. Dis. 2014;59(2).
30. Shimizu T, Tokunda Y. Necrotizing fasciitis. Int. Med. 2010;49:1051–57.

31. Wang JM, Lim KH. Necrotizing fasciitis: eight-year experience and literature review. Braz J Infect Dis. 2014;18(2):137–43.
32. Goh T, Goh LG, Ang CH, Wong CH. Early diagnosis of necrotizing fasciitis. BJS. 2014;101: e119–25.
33. Childers BJ, Potyondy LD, Nachreiner R, Rogers FR, Childers ER, Oberg KC, Hendricks DL, Hardesty RA. Necrotizing fasciitis: a fourteen-year retrospective study of 163 consecutive, patients. Am Surg. 2002;68:109–16.
34. Lamagni TL, Neal S, Keshishian C, Alhaddad N, George R, Duckworth G, Vuopio-Varkila J, Efstratiou A. Severe *Streptococcus pyogenes* infections, United Kingdom, 2003-2004. Emerg Infect Dis. 2008;14:2002–9.
35. Sharkawy A, Low D, Saginur R, Gregson D, Schwartz B, Jessamine P, Green K, McGeer A. Severe group a Streptococcal soft-tissue in Ontario: 1992-1996. Clin Infect Dis. 2002;34: 454–60.
36. Geusens E, Pans S, Van Breuseghem I, Knockaert D. Necrotizing fasciitis of the leg presenting with chest wall emphysema. Eur J Emerg Med. 2004;11:49–51.
37. Cox NH. Streptococcal necrotizing fasciitis and the dermatologist. Br J Dermatol. 1999;141:613–4.
38. Wong CH, Khin LW, Heng KS, Tan KC, Low CO. The LRINEC (Laboratory Risk Indicator for Necrotizing Faciitis) score: a tool for distinguishing necrotizing fasciitis from other soft tissue infections. Crit Care Med. 2004;32(7):1535–41.
39. Murphy G, Markeson D, Choa R, Armstrong A. Raised serum lactate: a marker of necrotizing fascitis? JPRSAS. 2013;66:1712–6.
40. Erol B, Tuncel A, Volkan H, Tokgoz H, Yildiz A, Akduman B, Kargi E, Mungan A. Fournier's gangrene: overview of prognostic factors and definition of new prognostic parameter. Urology. 2010;75:1193–8.
41. Kinasewitz G, Zein J, Lee G, Nazir S, Taylor F. Prognostic value of a simple evolving disseminated intravascular coagulation score in patients with severe sepsis. Crit Care Med. 2005;33(10):2214–21.
42. Fry DE. The prevention of surgical site infection in elective colon surgery. Scientifica. 2013; Article ID 896297:19.
43. Chundamal J, Wright JG. The efficacy and risks of using povidone iodine irrigation to prevent surgical site infection: an evidence-based review. Can J Surg. 2007;50:6.
44. Rodeheaver GT. Wound cleansing, wound irrigation, wound disinfection. In: Krasner D, Kane D, editors. Chronic wound care: a clinical source book for healthcare professionals. 2nd ed. Wayne: Health Management Publications, Inc.; 1997. p. 97–108.
45. Damm S. Intraoperative anaphylaxis associated with bactracin irrigation. Am J Health-Syst Pharm. 2011;68:323–7.
46. Rappaport WE, Holcomb M, Valente J, Chvapil M. Antibiotic irrigation and the formation of intraabdomincal adhesions. Am J Surg. 1989;158:435–7.
47. Yelon JA, Green JD, Evans JT. Efficacy of an intraperitoneal antibiotic to reduce the incidence of infection in the trauma patient: a prospective, randomized study. J Am Coll Surg. 1996;182:509–14.
48. Nomikos IN, Katsouyanni K, Papaicannou AN. Washing with or without chloramphenicol in the treatment of peritonitis: a prospective, clinical trial. Surgery. 1986;99:20–5.
49. Barnes S, Spencer M, Graham D, Johnson HB. Surgical wound irrigation: a call for evidence-based standardization of practice. Am J Infect Control. 2014;42:525–9.
50. Sakarya S, Gunay N, Karakulak M, Ozturk B, Ertugrul B. Hypochlorous acid: an ideal wound cre agent with powerful microbicidal, antibiolfilm and wound healing potency. Wounds. 2014;26(12):342–50.
51. Guo S, Dipietro LA. Factors affecting wound healing. JDR. 2010;89(3):219–29.
52. Faraklas I, Stoddard GJ, Neumayer LA, Cochran A. Development and Validation of a Necrotizing Soft-Tissue Infection Mortality Risk Calculator Using NSQIP. J Am Coll Surg. 2013;217(1):153–60.

Chapter 19
The Planning for the "Planned Ventral Hernia"

Danielle L. Barnard and Timothy C. Fabian

Introduction

Temporary abdominal closure has become an important component of the armamentarium of many surgeons. Several scenarios, including abdominal compartment syndrome, damage-control laparotomy for trauma, or repeated laparotomies with intra-abdominal catastrophe, call for surgeons to have an algorithm for the management of open abdomens. Attempts at fascial closure under tension often lead to fascial necrosis and/or abdominal compartment syndrome.

Various techniques have been utilized in the final phase of abdominal wall reconstruction. When prosthetic materials are used for reconstruction, the most severe complications are mesh infection and recurrent hernia. Many of the prosthetic infections occur when the mesh is inserted in conjunction with intestinal contamination such as stomal or fistula closure. Many of the patients that we care for with the planned ventral hernias have stomas that require concurrent reversal of these stomas at the time of abdominal wall reconstruction.

In 1990, Ramirez and associates [1] first described the component separation technique that allows closure of the abdominal wall using the native fascial layers without the use of prosthetics. We found that the standard component separation was insufficient to close the giant defects that represent a large portion of our patient population. For that reason, we developed a modification that we refer to as the Memphis modification for the component separation [2] that allows more extensive mobilization and advancement of autologous tissues. We have found that the

D.L. Barnard · T.C. Fabian (✉)
Department of Surgery, The University of Tennessee Health Science Center, 910 Madison Avenue Suite 201, Memphis, TN 38163, USA
e-mail: tfabian@uthsc.edu

D.L. Barnard
e-mail: dbarnar1@uthsc.edu

J.J. Diaz and D.T. Efron (eds.), *Complications in Acute Care Surgery*,
DOI 10.1007/978-3-319-42376-0_19

modification allows us to close a large portion of giant abdominal wall defects without the use of permanent mesh.

Factors that have been identified which are predictors of failure to achieve native fascial closure of open abdomens during initial hospitalization after trauma include greater number of subsequent explorations, intra-abdominal abscess/sepsis, blood stream infections, acute renal failure, development of enteric fistula, and higher injury severity score [3]. Others have identified that waiting greater than 48 h before the first take back after initial damage-control laparotomy is negatively associated with achieving primary fascial closure. The failure to return to the operating room within 48 h has been found to carry with it a real and increased risk of not achieving fascial closure of 1.1 % per hour of delay [4]. These predictors can help identify patients early in their hospital course that are high risk for needing future abdominal wall reconstruction and can be managed using a staged algorithm.

Staged Management Approach

We apply a 3-staged management algorithm to critically ill patients with abdominal catastrophes that may require future abdominal wall reconstruction. Figure 19.1 demonstrates this management scheme. Stage I is the damage-control laparotomy and temporary abdominal closure. The use of damage control is highly selective at our institution, and only critically ill patients with major physiologic derangements have planned re-exploration. Temporary abdominal closure materials used at our institution include plastic materials such as X-ray cassette covers, blue towels placed to suction, as well as commercially available negative-pressure devices such as the ABThera (KCI). If we are unable to achieve delayed fascial closure with these materials, we then place vicryl mesh. After the placement of vicryl mesh, we continue to attempt to tighten or cinch the mesh at bedside. The patients that are not amendable to fascial closure at this point, despite aggressive attempts, progress to the next stage. This group of patients comprises the patients that will have future abdominal wall reconstruction. Stage II occurs approximately 2 weeks after granulation tissue has developed under the temporary closure. The temporary closure is removed, and a split-thickness skin graft is placed over the viscera. Stage III is the definitive reconstruction of the abdominal wall and is usually performed 8 months later. The assessment of the readiness to remove the skin graft is determined by "pinching" the graft to see whether it can be easily lifted from the underlying viscera as seen in Fig. 19.2. Occasionally, this can occur as early as 6 months. If definitive reconstruction is attempted too early, the adhesions are very dense, and this leads to unwanted enterotomies and deserosalization of the bowel, which can lead to subsequent intra-abdominal abscesses and/or enteric fistulas. The reason to proceed with the reconstruction no later than 12 months is that further delay can lead to fascial retraction laterally and loss of domain that makes reconstruction more difficult and carries a high chance of needing to use prosthetic mesh.

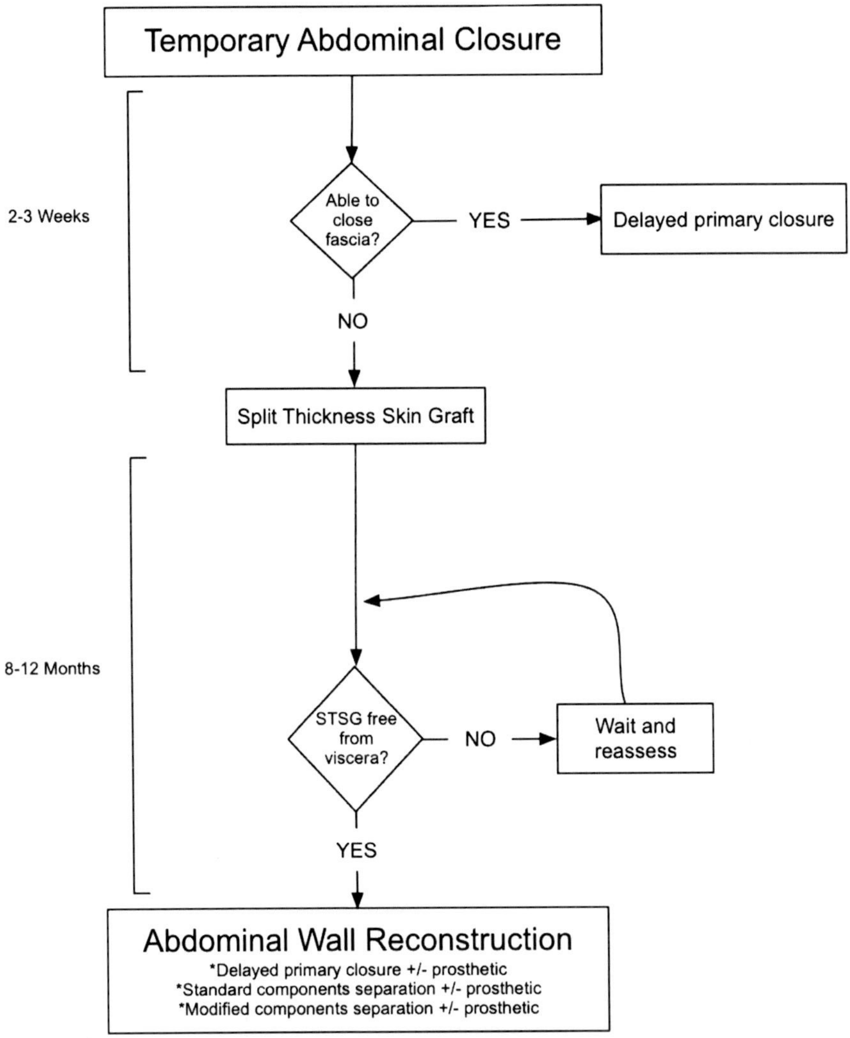

Fig. 19.1 Flow diagram representing the 3-staged approach to abdominal closure. Reproduced with permission from Dicocco et al. [7]

Lessons Learned from Previous Studies

We would like to share some practical lessons that we have learned after studying abdominal wall reconstruction for the past 25 years. In our initial years of planned ventral hernia management, the choice of temporary abdominal closure prosthetic was a decision that was left to the operating surgeon, and the prosthetics included polypropylene mesh, woven vicryl mesh, expanded PTFE soft tissue patch, and

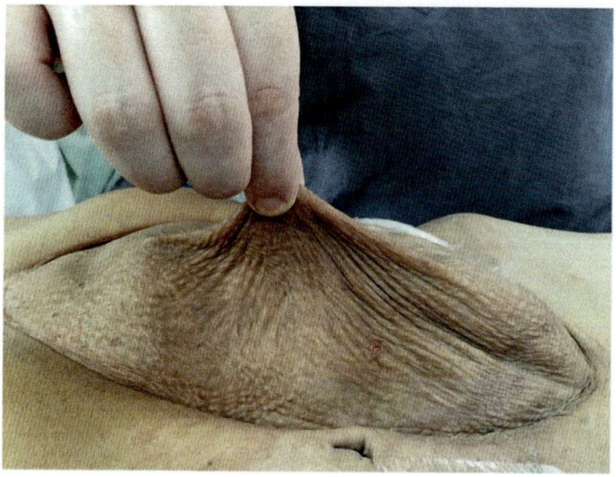

Fig. 19.2 Pinching the split-thickness skin graft from the underlying viscera, indicating the appropriate time for definitive reconstruction

plastic (intravenous fluid bag or X-ray cassette cover). The application of a variety of prosthetic materials in our institution in the past has provided a perspective on merits and drawbacks of each material. The removal of polypropylene mesh is not a simple procedure and is very time consuming and carries a higher risk of injury to bowel. The cost and difficulty of removal of expanded PTFE were made evident in the past studies, and the lack of durability of plastic material used for coverage has led to a change in our practice. These factors have been responsible for the gradual switch to absorbable mesh with woven vicryl being chosen most frequently at our institution [5].

Another lesson that we have learned over the past decade is that it is best to immediately place the skin graft at the time of vicryl mesh removal. In our early experience, we performed dressing changes for a couple of days to diminish nosocomial bacterial colonization of the granulated wounds before applying the skin graft. However, we had patients during those few days that eviscerated and had resulting derserosalization that resulted in difficult to management enteric fistula [2]. This has led to our change in practice, and now all patients receive immediate STSG at the time of mesh removal.

We have also determined that it is best to remove the mesh and place the skin graft no later than 3 weeks after mesh placement [2]. Those patients who had mesh retention beyond 3 weeks were found to have a significant increased risk of intestinal fistula. For this reason, we strive to remove the vicryl mesh and place STSG on these patients approximately 2 weeks after placement of the vicryl mesh.

There have also been many proponents of vacuum-assisted closure (VAC) to aid in the delayed primary fascial closure rates. We performed a prospective randomized trial to address the rates of delayed fasical closure and fistula rates comparing temporary closure with vicryl mesh versus VAC in patients with open abdomens [6]. Our results indicated that the VAC group trended toward increased morbidity. There was an increase in fistula rates in the VAC group, and we believe this was due to the need for repeated vacuum changes that are not required with vicryl mesh.

We also found that enteral gastrostomy and jejunostomy tubes that were placed had a higher rate of becoming dislodged with the repeated vacuum dressing changes. We also had patients with loss of domain and massive visceral edema that experienced evisceration with VAC closure. The study found that neither method was superior in regard to the rates of delayed fascial closure. For these reasons, we have adopted absorbable vicryl mesh followed by skin grafting for those patients in whom delayed fascial closure seems unlikely.

We have also found that delaying definitive abdominal wall reconstruction beyond 1 year directly contributes to the need for prosthetic mesh as well as increases the rate of hernia recurrence [2]. Delay beyond 1 year leads to loss of domain and decreased fascial compliance due to contraction and consequent retraction of the abdominal wall fascia laterally. For this reason, we carefully follow all patients discharged with planned ventral hernias at 3-month intervals to assess the readiness of removal of their skin graft and definitive reconstruction.

Review of Abdominal Wall Anatomy

Published in 1990 by Ramirez et al. [1], component separation is based on subcutaneous lateral dissection, fasciotomy lateral to the rectus abdominis muscle, and dissection on the plane between external and internal oblique muscles with the medial advancement of the block that includes the rectus muscle and fascia. This release allows 3–5 cm of the additional length on each side. Because of the giant abdominal wall defects (Fig. 19.3) that occur after open abdomens, we developed a modification that results in an additional 20 cm in the umbilical region that allows the closure of many giant planned ventral hernias with native tissue only.

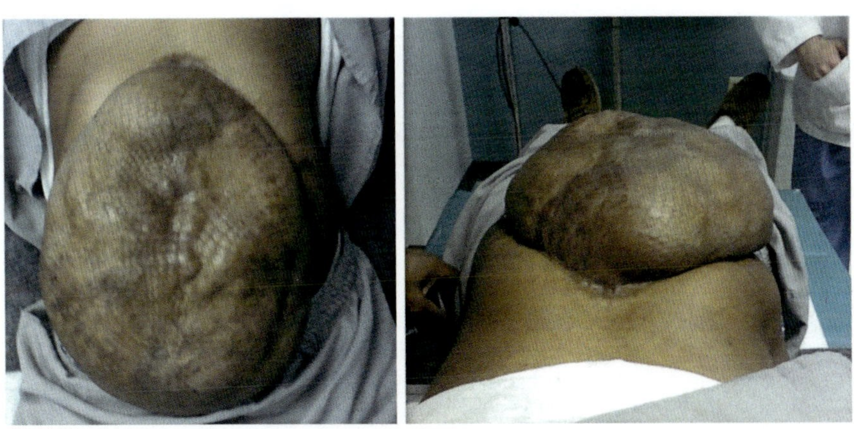

Fig. 19.3 Preoperative images of a patient with a planned ventral hernia. Giant abdominal wall defect is covered with skin graft over the abdominal viscera. Reproduced with permission from Dicocco et al. [7]

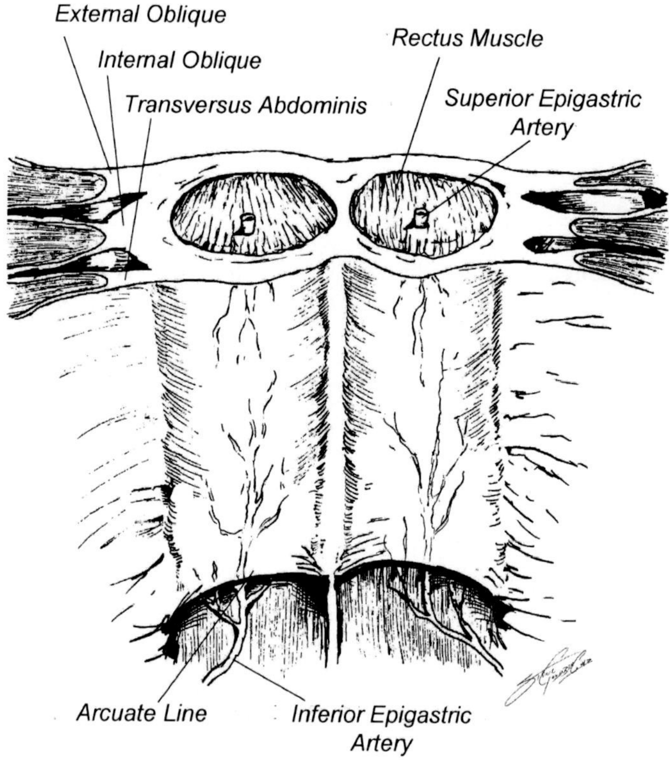

Fig. 19.4 Diagram of abdominal wall anatomy, shown from the intraperitoneal surface, with cut edge representing the cephalad portion. The arcuate line, vascular supply, and components of the rectus fascia can be seen. Reproduced with permission from Dicocco et al. [7]

Before describing the technique in depth, a brief review of the abdominal wall anatomy (Fig. 19.4) will facilitate understanding the procedure. The rectus muscle is surrounded by the anterior and posterior rectus sheaths. The external is a component of the anterior rectus sheath for the entire length of the rectus. The internal oblique splits and contributes to both the anterior sheath and posterior sheath above the arcuate line. However, below the arcuate line, the entirety of the internal oblique joins the anterior sheath. The transversus abdominis also contributes to the posterior sheath above the level of the arcuate line, but likewise joins the anterior sheath inferior to this landmark. This leaves no posterior sheath below the arcuate line and where only the peritoneum is present.

The blood supply to the rectus is supplied by the superior epigastric and the deep inferior epigastric arteries, with the inferior providing the major component. The inferior epigastric artery lies between the internal oblique and transversus abdominis muscles. It enters the rectus sheath around the arcuate line. Therefore, separation of the anterior rectus sheath laterally does not compromise blood supply. Blood supply to the anterior sheath is also from epigastric vessels. For this reason, separation of the anterior sheath from the rectus is not ideal. The posterior sheath obtains its vasculature from the vessels supplying the peritoneum and can be separated from the rectus without becoming devascularized.

Preoperative Evaluation in Preparation for Planned Ventral Hernia Repair

Patients that are managed with an open abdomen and a staged management algorithm often have a prolonged hospital course. Upon discharge, we closely follow these patients in clinic. Once out of the acute phase, we see these patients at 3-month intervals to assess the readiness of the skin graft for removal. The technique, as mentioned before and seen in Fig. 19.3, requires lifting and "pinching" the graft to see whether it can be lifted off the underlying viscera. The technique takes some experiences, and the decision to proceed with definitive abdominal wall reconstruction is made by the attending physician. In preparation for reconstruction, many of these patients also have diverting ostomies that require endoscopy and/or contrasted enemas to determine whether they are ready to be reversed. These studies are obtained concurrently with the preparation for their planned ventral hernia repair. Because we use the modification of the component separation at our institution frequently, if we anticipate the patient will have a planned ventral hernia, the initial ostomy location can be placed lateral to the rectus sheath so that the fascial defect from the ostomy can be closed primarily or with a small piece of biologic mesh. Again, we strive to repair all planned ventral hernias between 8 and 12 months after the placement of the skin graft to avoid the loss of domain that comes if the operation is delayed for more than 1 year.

Preoperative assessment can be deceiving, so the reconstruction technique should be decided intraoperatively. Patients who have very large defects may have mobile fascia and can be closed with a standard component separation. Conversely, some patients with small defects may require the Memphis modification and possible addition of prosthetic material.

This patient population has had significant physical and psychological stress due to their major trauma and prolonged hospital course. We have long discussions with these patients before proceeding with definitive reconstruction. They are again faced with a 7- to 10-day hospital stay, if no complications arise. We review in-depth complications that can occur and make patients aware that abdominal wall reconstruction results in a significant abdominal pressure and transient discomfort postoperatively. We often use epidural catheters perioperatively in these patients to help with pain control.

Operative Technique of Memphis Modification for Component Separation

Now we would like to provide a step-by-step description of our technique and include some intraoperative pearls and pitfalls that we have learned [7].

1. **Removal of the skin graft**. Beginning in an area that is loosely adherent, there will be areas with dense adhesions. In these areas, a plane between the dermis and epidermis is developed. Small areas of skin graft can be left on the viscera to avoid serosal injuries without any consequence. The skin graft is excised from the native abdominal wall laterally to preserve skin edges. Once the graft is removed, the bowel is examined thoroughly for serosal injuries or enterotomies, which are not uncommon. Ostomy reversal is done at this point.

Pearls/Pitfalls: It is started at the midpoint of the skin graft because this is the least adherent area. The graft is often very densely adhered to the liver so the use of sharp dissection can avoid violation of Glisson's capsule. The musculofascial junction is left for last, and the rest of the dissection is completed circumferentially dissecting the skin graft from the underlying viscera and omentum.

2. **Raise full-thickness skin flaps**. After the skin graft has been removed, skin flaps are raised on each side with the plane of dissection being just superficial to the fascia. There are perforating vessels that are encountered, and we attempt to preserve these. We raise flaps laterally to the level of the mid-axillary line (Fig. 19.5).

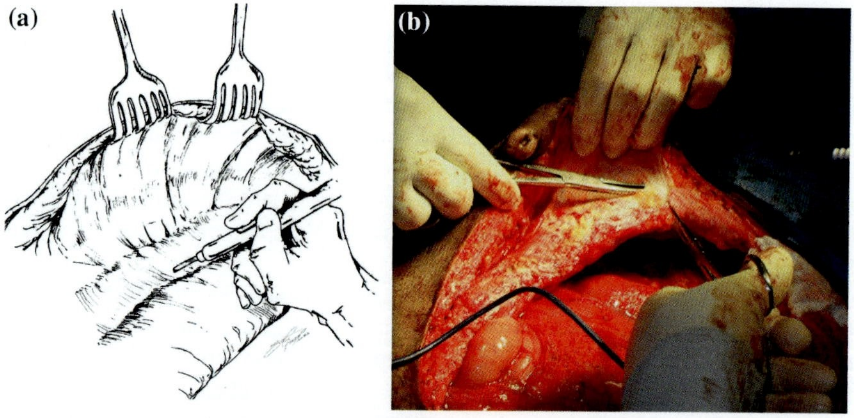

Fig. 19.5 Step 2. Skin flaps, with attached subcutaneous tissue, are raised to expose the underlying fascia. **a** The skin flap is raised several centimeters lateral to the border of the rectus sheath. **b** Skin and subcutaneous tissue flap are being raised. Reproduced with permission from Dicocco et al. [7]

(a) (b)

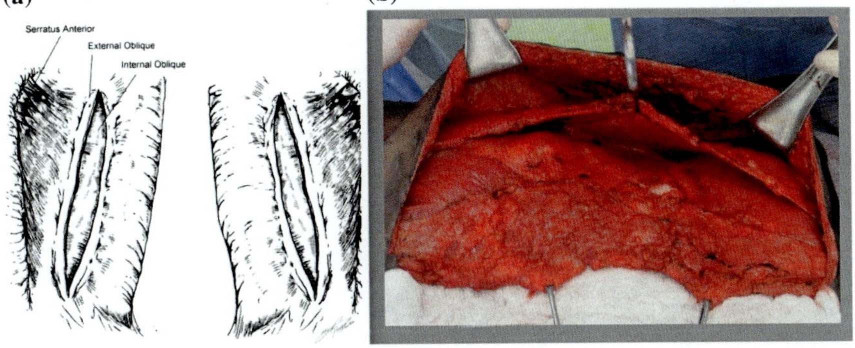

Fig. 19.6 Step 3. The external oblique release is extended cephalad toward the costal margin and caudally to the level of the pelvis. **a** Once the external oblique fascia is incised, the internal oblique can be visualized deep to this. **b** The elevated skin flap and cut external oblique fascia are shown. Reproduced with permission from Dicocco et al. [7]

Pearls/Pitfalls: The correct plane is found just superficial to the fascia. Failure to do so will result in a longer and bloodier dissection. Going too deep will result in defects in the fascia and complicate the reconstruction. Be cautious and avoid devascularization of the skin by keeping as much fat as possible with the cutaneous flap. This is very important with thin patients.

3. **Release of the external oblique**. The lateral edge of the rectus muscle is identified. The location can be confirmed by placing a hand in the abdomen with the palmar surface deep to the rectus and the thumb on top. The external oblique is nicked 1 cm lateral to the rectus border using a scalpel. A hemostat is inserted into the opening to elevate the external oblique and extend the incision with electrocautery. The extent of the release of the external oblique is from the costal margin to the level of the pubic symphysis (Fig. 19.6). There is a loose areolar tissue between the external and internal oblique laterally. Blunt dissection of this plane allows improved medial mobilization. Also, the serratus anterior may be encountered during the cephalad dissection, and release of this muscle will help with mobilization.

Pearls/Pitfalls: Care must be taken to only incise the external oblique. The internal oblique can be easily pulled up and inadvertently incised, and this will compromise the repair. It is important to make sure that you correctly identify the lateral border of the rectus and make a nick 1 cm lateral to this landmark. If the incision is too medial (over the lateral border of the anterior sheath), there will be much less ability to mobilize the rectus.

Steps 1–3 constitute a standard component separation. The Memphis modification begins with the remaining steps.

4. **Dissection of the posterior rectus sheath**. The medial portion of the rectus sheath is incised for the entire length of the muscle. This exposes the anterior

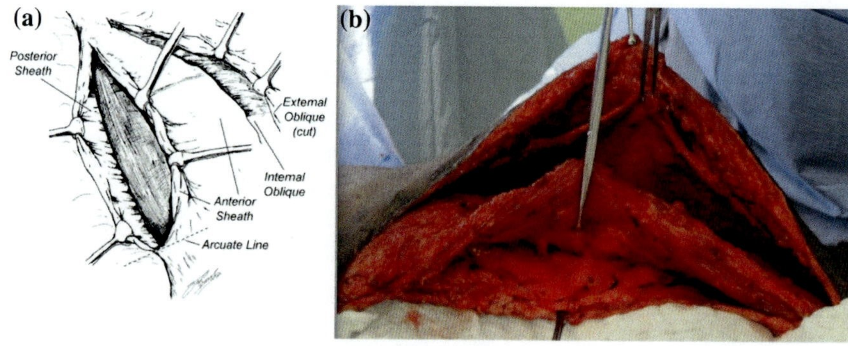

Fig. 19.7 Step 4. The medial edge of rectus sheath is divided, as seen from midline. **a** The posterior sheath is dissected off the rectus muscle to the level of the arcuate line caudally. **b** The 4 layers apparent at this stage: Skin flap, released external oblique, rectus muscle with the attached anterior sheath, and posterior sheath. Reproduced with permission from Dicocco et al. [7]

and posterior fascia and rectus muscle as 3 distinct layers (Fig. 19.7). Next the posterior sheath is freed from the rectus muscle. This dissection is carried out to the level of the arcuate line. At this level, the posterior rectus sheath is comprised only of peritoneum.

Pearls/pitfalls: The dissection plane between the rectus and the posterior sheath is relatively avascular. Usually, the epigastric vessels are intramuscular, but can run deep to the rectus muscle so be cautious so as not to avulse them.

5. **Release of internal oblique**. Once the posterior sheath is freed, a hand is placed between the rectus muscle and the posterior sheath. With this hand cupping the rectus, the index finger is used to identify the lateral border of the rectus muscle. Now the anterior fascia is sharply incised over the index finger 1 cm lateral to the rectus. This maneuver opens the anterior portion of the internal oblique fascia and protects the posterior sheath. The incision extends the length of the rectus from the costal margin down to the arcuate line (Fig. 19.8). The rectus muscle with the adherent anterior sheath is now free medially and laterally.

Pearls/Pitfalls: The technique of placing your hand between the posterior fascia and rectus muscles is the key to this step that allows your index finger to identify the correct location to incise the anterior component of the internal oblique. Cutting laterally to this (where the anterior and posterior portions of the internal oblique have combined) will result in a lateral defect. The umbilicus is generally close to the level of the arcuate line and can be used as a landmark. It is imperative that the dissection not be extended below the arcuate line because a lateral hernia will occur since there is no fascial component below this level.

6. **Translocation of the anterior fascia and muscle**. At this point, the rectus muscle and the anterior fascia are attached only at their superior and inferior portions. These remaining attachments ensure that the blood supply is

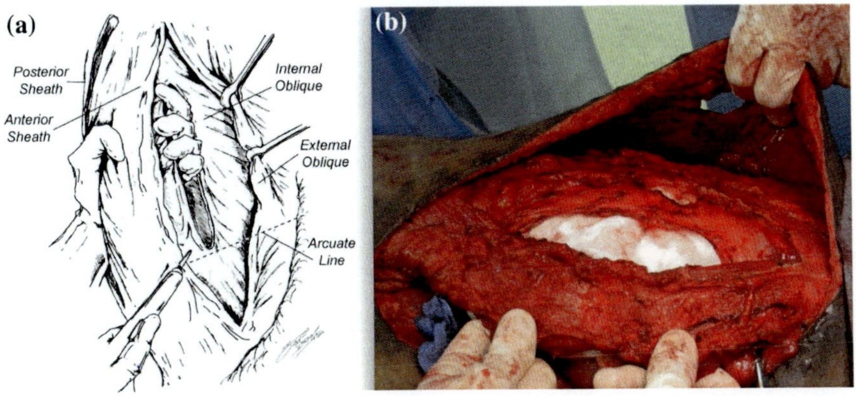

Fig. 19.8 Step 5. Release of internal oblique component. **a** Technique used to open the internal oblique component of the anterior rectus sheath. The dorsum of the hand is lying on the posterior sheath with the palmar surface cupping the rectus muscle. The incision is made directly over the surgeon's finger to ensure that only the anterior component is divided. **b** Once step 5 is completed, the anterior sheath and rectus muscle are attached at only the cephalad and caudad portions. The posterior sheath is still in continuity with the native abdominal wall. Reproduced with permission from Dicocco et al. [7]

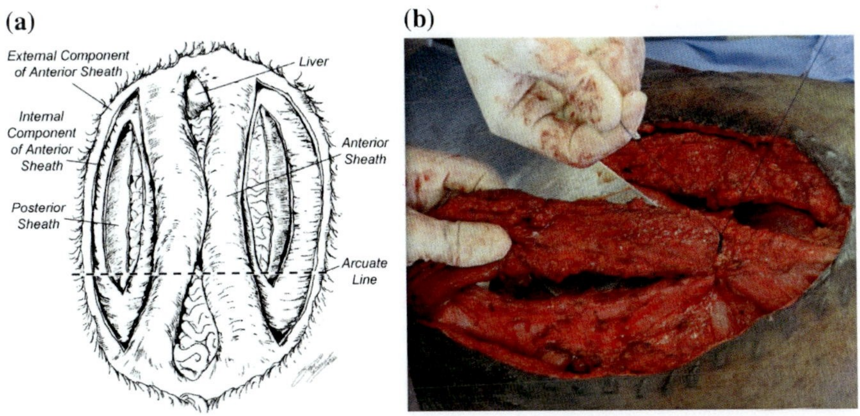

Fig. 19.9 Step 6. The rectus muscle, along with the anterior sheath, is translocated medially. The posterior rectus sheath remains in continuity with the native abdominal wall laterally. **a** The rectus fascia is being mobilized. **b** The anchoring stitch is being placed, attaching the lateral border of the anterior fascia to the medial border of the posterior sheath. Reproduced with permission from Dicocco et al. [7]

maintained. The posterior sheath remains in continuity with the native abdominal wall laterally. The rectus muscle and the anterior fascia can be pulled medially, and this provides the additional length that is obtained with the modification (Fig. 19.9). Now the medial aspect of the posterior sheath is

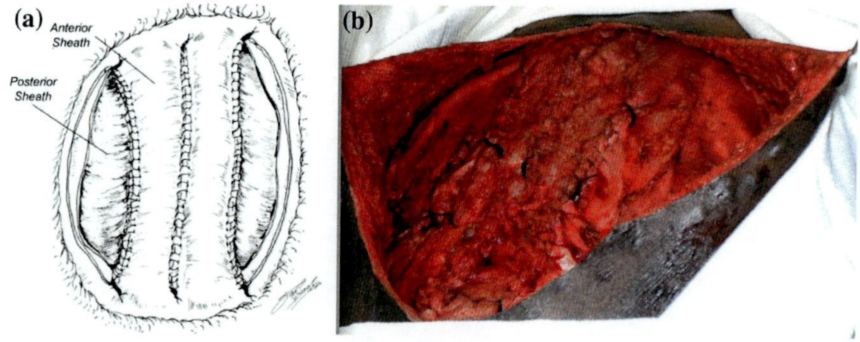

Fig. 19.10 Step 7. Final closure. **a** Final fascial closure with 3 suture lines. The mobilized anterior sheath is sutured in midline. **b** Four closed suction drains are placed, and the skin flaps are reapproximated in the midline. Reproduced with permission from Dicocco et al. [7]

sutured to the lateral aspect of the anterior sheath. This can be accomplished with running or interrupted figure-of-eight sutures.

Pearls/Pitfalls: Because fascia from 2 separate planes is being approximated, care is taken when placing the anchor stitch to close the potential space. The superior and inferior aspects of the suture lines will be puckered.

7. **Closure**. The anterior sheath is then sutured in the midline in the normal fashion. This results in 3 separate suture lines (Fig. 19.10). The most difficult area to gain adequate length is in the epigastrium. If the fascia cannot be closed in the midline without tension, a prosthetic bridge may be necessary. We always closely communicate with anesthesia during closure to ensure that peak airway pressures are monitored and that we are notified with any significant change. Because we often combine ostomy reversal with abdominal wall reconstruction and the high incidence of enterotomies with this procedure, we prefer a biologic when a mesh is needed. The skin flaps are re-inspected to ensure hemostasis has been obtained. We insert four flat, closed suction drains (2 superiorly and 2 inferiorly). After debriding skin edges, the skin is reapproximated in the midline using interrupted nylon sutures.

Pearls/Pitfalls: Hemostasis is critical because postoperative hematomas can lead to reoperation, skin necrosis, and failure of the repair. We place abdominal binders on all patients and instruct them to avoid heavy lifting for 6 weeks.

Wound Complications

Wound infection and/or skin necrosis are among the top reasons for failure of the repair. Wound seroma and hematoma prevention are imperative because both contribute to wound complications. Hematomas can be prevented intraoperatively with meticulous attention to hemostasis. All patients will have serous output from their drains due to the extent of mobilization. We only remove 1 drain at a time and generally remove the last drain between postoperative days 5–7.

Patients with high BMIs are especially at high risk for superficial skin necrosis due to the tension that their increased abdominal girth places on the skin edges and closure. If this occurs, the non-viable skin is debrided and local wound care is initiated. Thin patients are more susceptible to large areas of skin necrosis. This is thought to be due to the devascularization that can occur during the creation of skin flaps as a result of their decreased subcutaneous tissue and limited perforating vessels. After debridement of large areas, the fascia can be exposed, and we have utilized negative-pressure dressings to salvage repairs in these situations. A skin graft can be placed after granulation tissue develops. Although an infrequent complication, these patients have a high risk of recurrence.

Long-term Follow-up and Recurrence Rates

We have reviewed our experience with planned ventral hernias over a 15-year period with a mean follow-up greater than 5 years [8]. The spectrum of repairs ranged from patients that required no component separation or prosthetic to patients that required the modified component repair with the addition of a prosthetic mesh bridge. The highest rate of recurrence occurred in those patients with prosthetic-assisted closure with this group having a fourfold increase in the incidence of recurrence.

Higher BMI and female gender were also found to be risk factors for recurrence in this review. We were not surprised that increasing BMI was associated with recurrence. These patients often have larger defects and seem to have more substantial loss of domain. The reason for female gender being associated with recurrence is unclear. Theories that we have proposed include the weakening of the abdominal wall due to pregnancy and/or inherent anatomic muscular differences in men and women. We also noted that the presence of a fistula or ostomy was not associated with hernia recurrence.

For our patients who underwent a modified component separation without any prosthetic material, our recurrence rate with long-term follow-up was 5 %. This low recurrence rate with the excellent follow-up intervals provides good data which we feel shows that the Memphis modification for component separation is the procedure of choice for repair of giant planned ventral hernias.

We have also had the opportunity to review our long-term follow-up data on the quality of life after abdominal wall reconstruction [9]. These patients are essentially undergoing a "second hit" at the time of abdominal wall reconstruction after having a prolonged initial hospitalization that has left them physically and psychologically weakened. However, the results from this study show that the majority of patients can return to near normal quality of life after abdominal wall reconstruction, but this process can take several years. We follow these patients long term and provide support to assist them at achieving both physical and psychological goals.

Clinical Scenario

48-year old woman 3 years s/p Hartman's for perforated diverticulitis. She has a right-sided transverse colostomy and a known complex hernia (two defects, the length of the incision, largest with a neck diameter 12 cm and a bulge diameter 20 cm, and a sizable medial paracolostomy hernia). She presents with bowel obstruction, intermittently decompressed with NG tube and intermittent air and stool from stoma.

The patient presented here represents a very different patient population than the population that has been the focus of our chapter on planned ventral hernias. Incisional hernias and planned ventral hernia are different entities. The fascia in a patient with a planned ventral hernia is usually normal, because most trauma patients are young and healthy. Incisional hernias often occur in patients who are older, have multiple comorbidities, and have shown that their fascia is compromised. The modified component separation technique is not ideal for patients with poor fascia or problems with wound healing, because it will likely result in recurrent hernia.

For the patient in this scenario, we would plan to take the patient to the operating room for reversal of her stoma, lysis of all adhesions, and repair of her midline incisional and parastomal hernia. Given the concomitant reversal of her colostomy, we would use a biologic mesh of choice of the operating surgeon. We would choose a piece of mesh large enough to obtain good overlap in the area of the parastomal hernia. The mesh would be fixated in an underlay fashion with an attempt to close the patient's attenuated fascia over the mesh.

Key Questions

1. *What is the best way to reduce the risk of skin/flap necrosis?*
2. *Which patients are at increased risk of failure of primary fascial repair?*

References

1. Ramirez OM, Ruas E, Dellon AL. "Component Separation" method for closure of abdominal-wall defects: an anatomic and clinic study. Plast Reconstr Surg. 1990;86:519–26.
2. Jernigan TW, Fabian TC, Croce MA, Moore N, Pritchard FE, Minard G, et al. Staged management of giant abdominal wall defects: acute and long-term results. Ann Surg. 2003;238: 349–55.
3. DuBose JJ, Scalea TM, Holcomb JB, Shrestha B, Okoye O, Inaba K, et al. Open abdominal management after damage-control laparotomy for trauma: a prospective observational

American Association for the Surgery of Trauma Multicenter Study. J Trauma Acute Care Surg. 2012;74:113–22.
4. Pommerening MJ, DuBose JJ, Zielinski MD, Phelan HA, Scalea TM, Inaba K, et al. Time to first take-back operation predicts successful primary fascial closure in patients undergoing damage control laparotomy. Surgery. 2014;156:431–8.
5. Fabian TC, Croce MA, Pritchard FE, Minard G, Hickerson WL, Howell RL, et al. Planned ventral hernia. Staged management for acute abdominal wall defects. Ann Surg. 1994;219: 643–50.
6. Bee TK, Croce MA, Magnotti LJ, Zarzaur BL, Maish GO, Minard G, et al. Temporary abdominal closure techniques: a prospective randomized trial comparing polyglactin 910 mesh and vacuum-assisted closure. J Trauma. 2008;65:337–44.
7. Dicocco JM, Fabian TC, Emmett KP, Magnotti LJ, Goldberg SP, Croce MA. Components separation for abdominal wall reconstruction: the memphis modification. Surgery. 2011;151: 118–25.
8. Dicocco JM, Magnotti LJ, Emmett KP, Zarzaur BL, Croce MA, Sharpe JP, et al. Long term follow-up of abdominal wall reconstruction after planned ventral hernia: a 15-year experience. J Am Coll Surg. 2009;210:686–95.
9. Zarzaur BL, Dicocco JM, Shahan CP, Emmett KP, Magnotti LJ, Croce MA, et al. Quality of life after abdominal wall reconstruction following open abdomen. J Trauma. 2010;70:285–91.

in practice, the RYGB remains the most effective operation for treatment of the comorbid diseases associated with obesity. This operation is highly effective at treating medically complicated obesity. After RYGB, patients can expect to lose about 70 % of their excess weight. Moreover, obesity-related comorbid diseases, such as type 2 diabetes mellitus, hypertension, hyperlipidemia, obstructive sleep apnea, and gastroesophageal reflux disease, are treated quite effectively. Although in the past, these operations were performed via the open approach, today greater than 95 % of primary bariatric procedures are performed via the laparoscopic approach [2].

The overall morbidity of the RYGB is reported about 5 %. Complications from RYGB include pulmonary embolism, hemorrhage, wound infection, ventral hernia, bowel obstruction, venous thromboembolism, and gastrointestinal leak. A gastroenteric leak from one of the anastomoses or from a staple line occurs in about 2 % of operations and is perhaps the most serious of the complications, with an associated mortality estimated at 15 %. The overall mortality is less than 1 % for laparoscopic RYGB [3].

Enteric Leaks

The reported risk of leak after laparoscopic and open bariatric operations ranges from 0.5 to 5 % for primary procedures [4–17]. The reported risk of leaks after bariatric surgical revisions is as high as 35 % [18]. Leaks can be categorized temporally from the time of operation—early versus late, and according to the extent of spillage—localized versus free/non-localized. There is a substantial overlap with these classification schemes; nonetheless, these distinctions are important, because the etiology, diagnosis, and the approach to treatment of each type of leak are different. In the literature, leak has been defined as "evidence of extravasation of contrast material on an upper gastrointestinal contrast study or abdominal computed tomography (CT), or by identification of enteric spillage from a gastrointestinal anastomosis, staple line, or enteric lumen at the time of laparotomy (laparoscopy)" [4].

Enteric leaks after bariatric surgery are generally divided into early leaks and late leaks. Early leak is defined by some authors as occurring prior to dismissal from the hospital during the time period when it is easiest to re-operate, and by others as occurring within 10 days postoperatively. Late leaks may be defined as occurring after the patient is discharged from the hospital or occurring after the onset of dense adhesions, which increases markedly the risk of reoperation. The authors use the 10-day cut-off to define early leaks.

Contained leaks, also termed fistulas, are those in which a small amount of contrast material or enteric contents is spilled in a localized area. Other terms describing this scenario are Type I or subclinical leaks, which occur through a fistulous track to the pleural or abdominal cavity. Leakage with dissemination into the pleural or abdominal cavities by an irregular pathway may be termed Type II or uncontained leaks and are usually accompanied by clinical signs and symptoms; these patients are often very ill.

In our discussion of the clinical scenario of a late leak occurring after Roux-en-Y gastric bypass, we will examine the signs and symptoms that should catch the clinician's attention and prompt early workup and diagnosis of this complication, as well as the management strategies that can improve the outcome for our patient.

Diagnosis

Recognizing the specific signs and symptoms of an enteric leak after bypass is paramount in providing effective patient care after bariatric procedures. The signs of an early, uncontained leak are usually acute and severe. Several clinical predictors have been identified and published in the literature. First, the most sensitive indicators of early leak are respiratory distress and heart rate exceeding 120 beats per minute (bpm) [4]. In fact, 90 % of patients with a leak demonstrate severe tachycardia, whereas only 16 % of patients without a leak have this sign. Less severe tachycardia (100 bpm) occurs in virtually all patients with a leak and only half of patients without a leak [4]. Respiratory distress is six-times more common in patients with a leak, and marginal urine output is five-times more common. Tachycardia and respiratory distress have been shown to be independent predictors of leak [4]. Conversely, lack of fever should not decrease the level of suspicion for leak, because only one-quarter of patients with a leak will be febrile; in fact, low-grade increases in temperature are more common in patients without a leak. Likewise, hypotension has been shown to have a low sensitivity for a leak but does occur twice as commonly in patients with a leak than those without [4]. Abdominal pain is an important clue but only occurs in 30 % of patients [4]. Two additional, lesser-known clinical signs that are found by the authors to be highly sensitive for enteric leak are a left sided sympathetic effusion and/or atelectasis and pain referred to the left shoulder caused by diaphragmatic irritation. If there is a suspicion that the patient is not progressing as expected, and the patient complains of left shoulder pain, it is crucial to investigate for possible leak.

In contrast, the signs of a contained leak may be much more subtle. Often, the patients do not look as sick or as acutely ill. Left shoulder pain, left pleural effusion, low-grade fever, and mild leukocytosis are more common than severe tachycardia, respiratory distress, or decreased urinary output. Some patients will have intermittent symptoms that recur and disappear transiently with antibiotic treatment. They may also have recurrent subphrenic or left upper quadrant abscesses or recurrent pleural effusions that resolve with percutaneous drainage, but then continue to recur secondary to a persistent fistula to the region of the abscess.

Our patient presents with food intolerance, focal epigastric discomfort, leukocytosis, and fever 6 months after a RYGB. She has several nonspecific symptoms for anastomotic leak. As she is several months from her procedure, even a low-grade temperature should raise the suspicion of an infection. In addition to a

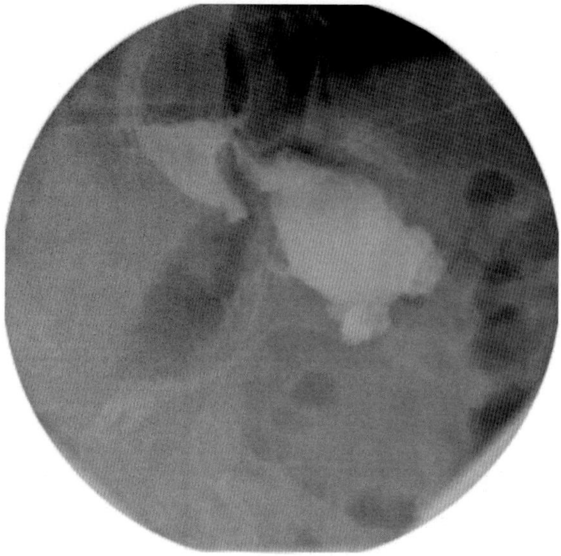

Fig. 20.1 Leak demonstrated on UGI 2 weeks after laparoscopic sleeve gastrectomy

leak, the differential diagnosis should also include marginal ulceration with or without perforation, gastroenteritis, cholecystitis, bowel obstruction, and pancreatitis.

Once a leak is suspected, whether it is from a RYGB or a sleeve gastrectomy, the first step is to obtain imaging of the anastomosis, usually either an upper gastrointestinal (UGI) swallow study with absorbable contrast or CT of the abdomen with oral contrast; endoscopy is not a part of the initial evaluation. Several studies support utilizing CT for superior sensitivity and with the ability to visualize intra-abdominal abscesses concomitantly [19]. Conversely, UGI is less expensive and more useful in identifying the precise location of the leak. UGI is the preferred imaging modality of choice at the authors' institution for suspected early leak (Fig. 20.1). If both CT and UGI are planned as investigation of potential leak, the CT should be performed prior to the UGI to avoid interference from UGI contrast. Any late leak should undergo urgent CT, because there is substantial risk of an associated intra-abdominal abscess.

Of note, many practices obtain routine UGI as part of postoperative algorithm for management, whether the patient is or is not exhibiting any specific signs of leak. Routine contrast studies, however, have low sensitivity for leaks, and prior work has shown alarmingly inconsistent detection rates for a leak, ranging from 50 to 79 % [20–22]. One important factor to consider is that the jejunojejunal anastomosis is difficult to assess by UGI, and although the risk of leak at this anastomosis is very low, it is still a possibility.

Treatment

Late leaks generally have a very different etiology and treatment strategy than early leaks, with the exception of late leaks that are associated with abscess formation, because this presentation may represent a contained early leak but with a delayed clinical presentation. In this case, immediate operation is not recommended due to prohibitive inflammation of the tissues and associated adhesions. Our patient underwent a CT of the abdomen and pelvis demonstrating a contained, 5 cm fluid collection anterior to the gastrojejunostomy.

Intraoperative Management

According to the literature, once a leak is suspected by clinical signs and symptoms, and then confirmed with CT, the rate of therapeutic laparotomy is 100 % [4]. Although in this scenario, the risk of false negative for abdominal exploration is virtually zero, other management approaches should be considered. Reoperation after bariatric procedures is associated with substantial potential morbidity and mortality. A nonoperative approach may be justified in certain patients. Patients with controlled leaks who are hemodynamically stable are candidates for nonoperative management. The nonoperative approach may include placement of a percutaneous drain, manipulation of indwelling surgical drains, percutaneous placement of a tube gastrostomy in the remnant stomach, NPO status, intravenous antibiotics, and gut rest/nutritional support via TPN. Innovative strategies with endoscopic drainage and endoscopic therapies may offer safe and efficacious alternatives to laparoscopic or open abdominal exploration (Fig. 20.2).

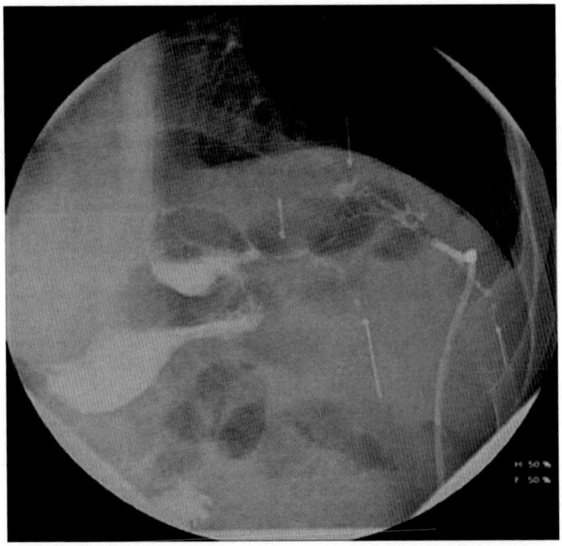

Fig. 20.2 Strictured vertical sleeve gastrectomy with leak and percutaneously placed drain

If operative management is necessary, several surgical principles are important to remember. Because of the many possible scenarios one might encounter intraoperatively, the surgeon should be prepared for diagnostic and technical challenges, and good surgical judgement is essential. A patient with a perforated marginal ulcer is managed ideally by closure of the edges of the perforated tissue and bolstered with omental tissue. If the ulcer edges are not amenable to the primary closure, an omental patch is the best option. Another option is the placement of a form of gastrostomy tube (use a Malecot) into the perforation and closure or patching of the area. For some patients with a history of marginal ulcers and stricture at the gastrojejunostomy, a complete revisional bariatric procedure of the gastrojejunal complex may be indicated in the hemodynamically stable, non-septic patient and when there is no local sepsis present. In our clinical scenario, the CT suggests a perforation at the gastrojejunostomy; however, the entire Roux-en-Y anatomy should be examined for factors that could contribute to the development of a marginal ulcer, such as a short Roux limb leading to the bile reflux or a breakdown in the gastric staple line closing the proximal pouch with a gastrogastric fistula to the remnant stomach. If the Roux limb is too short, then lengthening of the Roux limb with revision of the jejunojejunostomy is indicated. If there is a gastrogastric fistula, then closure of the fistula is imperative with placement of autogenous tissue between the staple lines.

One challenging scenario occurs when the site of perforation has sealed, so that on abdominal exploration, the exact site of perforation is not evident, although surrounding inflammation and fluid collection may be present. In this case, careful yet provocative maneuvers should be performed to identify the site of perforation, such as a leak test by insufflation under saline immersion. Uncovering of suspected areas by removal of adhered tissues and even gentle probing may be necessary to identify the site of leak. If no definitive leak can be identified at the gastrojejunostomy, other etiologies should be considered, particularly a duodenal or gastric perforation from indolent peptic ulcer disease or a leak at the staple line closure of the proximal pouch. If no other site of leak is identified, omental covering and wide drainage of the most likely site is recommended. When there is strong evidence of a healed marginal ulcer, some consideration should be entertained for revision of the size of the proximal pouch with reconstruction of the gastrojejunostomy.

After repair of the site of perforation, anastomotic revision, or downsizing of too large a proximal pouch, the authors advocate performing an intraoperative leak test by air insufflation using endoscopy or other means with submersion of the anastomosis under normal saline. If air bubbles are seen, the bubble stream is followed to the point of leak and the area is oversewn, as the condition of the tissues allow. The authors have used fibrin glue in the past but have abandoned this adjunctive measure due to concern that a heavy layer of fibrin glue may prevent adherence of omentum to the serosa; rather, a vascularized omental patch is utilized with tacking sutures.

An important adjunct to the treatment of anastomotic leak or perforation is the placement of a gastrostomy tube in the gastric remnant. This tube provides the ability to maintain a favorable nutritional status using enteric supplementation or full nutritional support to maximize healing. In obese patients, it is often impossible to use a proper Stamm technique because the stomach may not reach the abdominal wall due to immobility of the stomach and prominent visceral obesity. In these cases, a double purse-string suture is used to secure the tube at the stomach, and omentum can be wrapped around the tube in its course from the stomach to the abdominal wall; this technique will quickly provide a tissue tract and is safe and effective.

Practice is evolving in terms of a laparoscopic or open approach to abdominal exploration. For surgeons with advanced laparoscopic skills the authors suggest beginning with a laparoscopic exploration, but the operative approach should depend on the operating surgeon and their experience managing leaks with a laparoscopic intervention. The same principles of leak management apply. One consideration is that the laparoscopic exploration allows better visualization of the gastroesophageal junction, especially in the setting of morbid obesity. Additionally, laparoscopy lessens the risk of wound-related morbidity and slow healing time for larger incisions should they get infected, which can be the major problems in these patients. In contrast, the conventional benefits of laparoscopic surgery, including shorter stay, less pain, and quicker recovery, may not apply in this setting.

When the leak is identified and repaired, the authors suggest wide abdominal drainage using a drain which transverse the abdominal wall in a nondependent region to minimize drainage from around the tube. The authors prefer 19 F, channel drains placed with the tip in the left subdiaphragmatic space, coursing between the gastric remnant and the gastrojejunostomy, posterior to the Roux limb, and exiting the abdomen anteriorly in the right upper quadrant. Additional drains may be necessary along the medial aspect of the anastomosis depending on the extent of local sepsis and suppuration.

Enteric drainage via a nasogastric tube placed across the gastrojejunal anastomosis protects the repair from excessive intraluminal pressure. This drain can be guided intraoperatively under direct vision. Alternatively, an endoscopic technique is used most frequently by the authors. This technique is designed to prevent iatrogenic disruption of the repair: A flexible guidewire with a soft, flexible tip is passed from the mouth through anastomosis under direct vision with the endoscope; the endoscope is withdrawn leaving the wire in place across the anastomosis; then a soft rubber, non-sump enteric tube (such as "red Robinson" catheter) is advanced over the wire. Once the enteric tube is confirmed to be in optimal position across the anastomosis, the wire is removed, and the proximal end is passed from an oral to nasal location; this repositioning of the tube is accomplished by passing a traditional nasogastric tube from the nasal cavity out through the mouth where it is sutured to the soft rubber enteric tube and then threaded back through the nasal passage. The tube is then placed to gravity drainage.

Postoperative Management

Postoperatively, the patient is vulnerable to several potential complications, including septic shock, multi-system organ failure, prolonged ventilator dependence, pneumonia, intraabdominal abscess, central venous catheter sepsis, a persistent fistulas, deep vein thrombosis, and even pulmonary embolus. Patients should be treated with intravenous, broad spectrum antibiotics. The authors' current practice is to use piperacillin-tazobactam combined with an antifungal agent; additional anaerobic coverage is added if the patient does not respond to antibiotics within the first day. Addition of metronidazole has the additional benefit of potentially avoiding Clostridium difficile colitis. Patients should be treated with prophylactic, subcutaneous heparin or low molecular weight heparin while hospitalized. If the patient demonstrates signs of pulmonary embolism, including tachycardia and hypoxia, a chest CT angiography with a PE protocol should be performed urgently.

After operative or nonoperative intervention and convalescence, verification of a successful repair can be accomplished with a negative UGI. The patient should be kept strictly NPO until this study is conducted, usually at least 3–5 days or more after the repair depending on the security of the repair and the amount of local inflammation and suppuration. After a negative contrast UGI study, a clear liquid diet was begun and advanced slowly. The abdominal drains are left in place until the diet is advanced, and there is no sign of leakage.

Alternative Operative Approach

Natural endoscopic transluminal endoscopic surgery (NOTES) procedures are gaining acceptance as safe and effective treatments for leaks after bariatric procedures. These procedures require advanced endoscopic technique and specialized instrumentation and are proving to be exceedingly useful in treating a variety of complications [23]. In particular, the utility of an endoscopic approach in treating a late leak seems instinctive given the potentially hostile environment of the abdomen after a surgical procedure and the inflammatory insult of an enteric leak; the endoscopic approach is also unaffected by body habitus. Using this approach, the advanced endoscopist can debride and drain the space around the anastomotic defect, place endoscopic endoluminal stents across the defect effectively sealing the area of leak and/or utilize endoscopic sutures and adhesives to repair the leak [23, 24]. This approach requires off-label use of an esophageal or colonic endoluminal stent as a device specific for the esophagogastric anastomosis and the anatomy of a small gastric pouch. These stents have advantages and disadvantages. Distal migration of the stent is common (17–47 %), and multiple procedures are often required to achieve complete seal of the leak [24, 25]. In contrast, effective placement of the stent can arrest further leakage immediately. At our institution, stents are often secured to the esophageal mucosa using endoscopic suturing, which appears to decrease the risk of stent migration [23, 24]. Additionally, the anastomosis may take several months to heal. Nevertheless, the endoscopic approach to management of anastomotic leaks is becoming a useful tool for the bariatric surgeon, because serious complications of this approach are rare, and the ultimate success rate for healing of the leak is reportedly 88 % [24]. Use of these stents is

(a) (b)

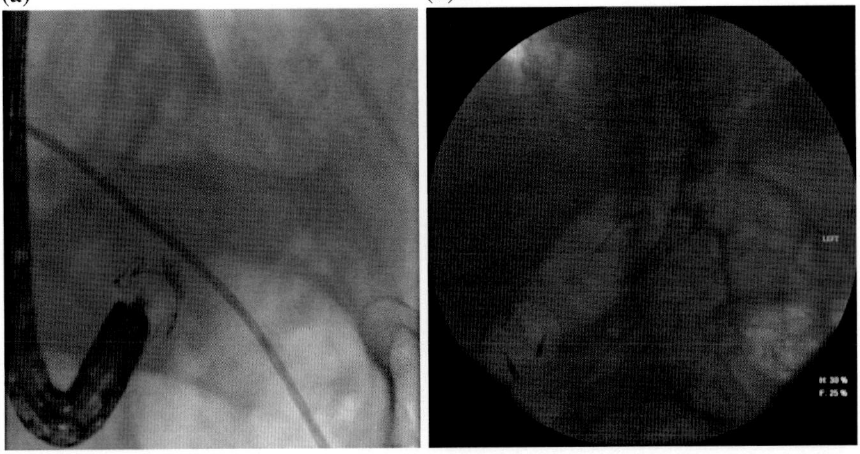

Fig. 20.3 Leak and fistula formation at the proximal staple line 6 weeks after laparoscopic sleeve gastrectomy. **a** The fistula was closed with an over the scope clip that is 12 mm in diameter (12/6T Ovesco Clip). **b** The defect was bypassed with a fully covered SEMS anchored to the distal esophagus with three endoscopic sutures to avoid migration

much more effective for early leaks than for the more established, late contained leaks, especially if the leak involves a long fistula to a more distant site of abscess.

Endoscopic clips (Endoclips) have also been used to "close" leaks in stable bariatric patients with a delayed leak. Endoscopic clips can be an option for cases not amenable to stent placement or for leaks that have failed endoscopic stenting [26]. Clip closure is usually used for small defects (less than 20 mm). Larger defects or defects with everted edges are difficult to close with clips, and in these cases, stents might be a better option [27] (Fig. 20.3). Other emerging interventions include endoscopic injection of glue at the anastomotic site and endoscopic suturing; there is not yet substantial data to recommend these novel therapies [27]. Broad spectrum antibiotics, nothing by mouth, and parenteral nutrition are important for healing after endoscopic attempts at closure.

Conclusion

Although rare after primary bariatric operations, anastomotic and staple line leaks can present a challenging clinical scenario for the surgeon. Many nuances to their management depend on the stability of the patient, time from initial procedure, surgeon's experience, and the characteristics of the leak. A tailored approach for each patient will rely on key principles of management, namely providing adequate resuscitation, achieving source control, treating infection, and provision of nutritional support. In addition to standard and reliable operative management of the

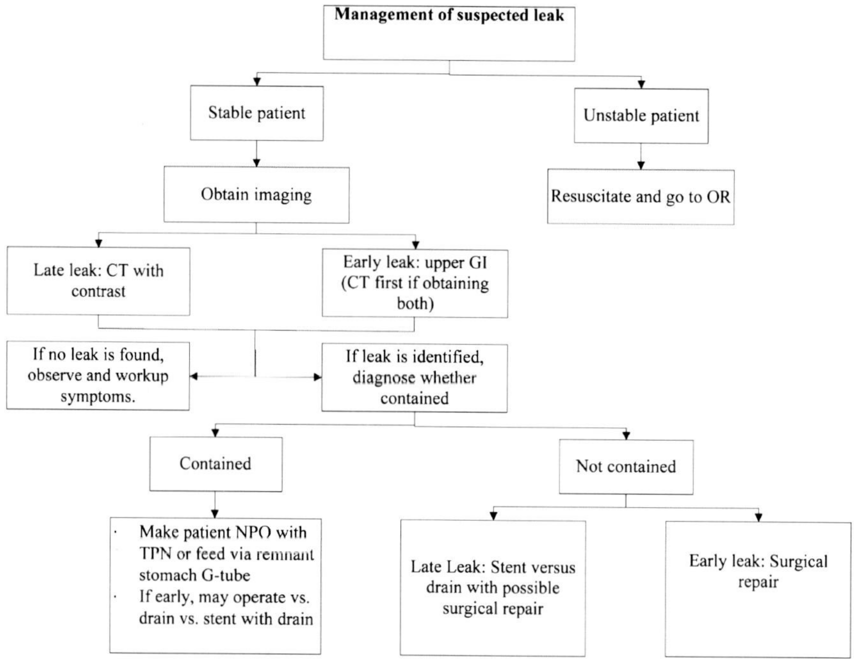

Fig. 20.4 Management of suspected leak

leak, multiple innovative treatment strategies have emerged to address these complex scenarios (see management algorithm in Fig. 20.4). Collaboration with other specialists, including interventional gastroenterologists and radiologists, provides a multidisciplinary approach that can optimize the treatment outcomes.

Clinical Scenario

A 34-year-old woman presents 6 months after a routine laparoscopic Roux-en-Y gastric bypass. She complains of progressive food intolerance and during the week prior to presentation has only been able to tolerate liquids. She presents with 24 h of focal epigastric discomfort and has an increased WBC and low-grade fever. CT of the abdomen and pelvis demonstrates a 5 cm diameter fluid collection anterior to the gastrojejunal anastomosis. A water soluble contrast study suggests a contained perforation anterior to the gastrojejunostomy as well as a gastrogastric fistula between the pouch and the excluded stomach.

References

1. Finkelstein EA, Trogdon JG, Cohen JW, Dietz W. Annual medical spending attributable to obesity: payer-and service-specific estimates. Health Aff. 2009;28(5):w822–31.
2. Buchwald H, Oien DM. Metabolic/bariatric surgery worldwide 2011. Obes Surg. 2013;23:427–36.
3. Lim RB. Bariatric operative procedures: thirty-day morbidity and mortality. UptoDate, Jones DJ, editor. Waltham, MA; 2015.
4. Hamilton EC, Sims TL, Hamilton TT. Clinical predictors of leak after laparoscopic Roux-en-Y gastric bypass for morbid obesity. Surg Endosc Interv Tech. 2003;17:679–84.
5. Podnos YD, Jimenez JC, Wilson SE, et al. Complications after laparoscopic gastric bypass: a review of 3464 cases. Arch Surg. 2003;138(9):957–61.
6. Gonzalez R, Sarr MG, Smith CD, et al. Diagnosis and contemporary management of anastomotic leaks after gastric bypass for obesity. J Am Coll Surg. 2007;204(1):47–55.
7. Biertho L, Steffen R, Ricklin T, et al. Laparoscopic gastric bypass versus laparoscopic adjustable gastric banding: a comparative study of 1,200 cases. J Am Coll Surg. 2003;197 (4):536–44; Discussion. 544–5.
8. DeMaria EJ, Sugerman HJ, Kellum JM, et al. Results of 281 consecutive total laparoscopic Roux-en-Y gastric bypasses to treat morbid obesity. Ann Surg. 2002;235(5):640–5; Discussion. 645–7.
9. Fernandez AZ Jr, DeMaria EJ, Tichansky DS, et al. Experience with over 3,000 open and laparoscopic bariatric procedures: multivariate analysis of factors related to leak and resultant mortality. Surg Endosc. 2004;18(2):193–7.
10. Higa KD, Ho T, Boone KB. Laparoscopic Roux-en-Y gastric bypass: technique and 3-year follow-up. J Laparoendosc Adv Surg Tech A. 2001;11(6):377–82.
11. Nguyen NT, Goldman C, Rosenquist CJ, et al. Laparoscopic versus open gastric bypass: a randomized study of outcomes, quality of life, and costs. Ann Surg. 2001;234(3):279–89; Discussion. 289–91.
12. Papasavas PK, Hayetian FD, Caushaj PF, et al. Outcome analysis of laparoscopic Roux-en-Y gastric bypass for morbid obesity. The first 116 cases. Surg Endosc. 2002;16(12):1653–7.
13. Schauer PR, Ikramuddin S, Gourash W, et al. Outcomes after laparoscopic Roux-en-Y gastric bypass for morbid obesity. 2000;232(4):515–29.
14. Wittgrove AC, Clark GW. Laparoscopic gastric bypass, Roux-en-Y 500 patients: technique and results, with 3-60 month follow-up. Obes Surg. 2000;10(3):233–9.
15. Nesset EM, Kendrick ML, Houghton SG, Mai JL, Thompson GB, Que FG, Thomsen KM, Larson DR, Sarr MG. A two-decade spectrum of revisional bariatric surgery at a tertiary referral center. Surg Obes Relat Dis. 2007;3:25–30.
16. Fernandez Jr AZ, DeMaria EJ, TIchansky DS, et al. Experience with over 3,000 open and laparoscopic bariatric procedures: multivariate analysis of factors related to leak and resultant mortality. Surg Endosc. 2004;(18):193–7.
17. Podnos YD, Jimenez JC, Wilson SE, et al. Complications after laparoscopic gastric bypass. Arch Surg. 2003;138:957–61.
18. Lim RB. Bariatric operations: perioperative morbidity and mortality. Uptodate, Jones DJ, editor. Waltham, MA; 2015.
19. Burgos AM, Braghetto I, Csendes A, et al. Gastric leak after laparoscopic-sleeve gastrectomy for obesity. Obes Surg. 2009;19:1672–7.
20. Bingham J, Shawhan R, Parker R. Computed tomography scan versus upper gastrointestinal fluoroscopy for diagnosis of staple line leak following bariatric surgery. Am J Surg. 2015;209:810–4.
21. Quartararo G, Facchiano E, Scaringi S, et al. Upper gastrointestinal series after Roux-en-Y gastric bypass for morbid obesity: effectiveness in leakage detection. A systemic review of the literature. Obes Surg. 2014;24:1096–101.

22. Schiesser M, Guber J, Wildi S. Utility of routine versus selective upper gastrointestinal series to detect anastomotic leaks after gastric bypass. Obes Surg. 2011;21(8):1238–42.
23. Bege T, Emungania O, Vitton V, et al. An endoscopic strategy for management of anastomotic complications from bariatric surgery: a prospective study. Gastroint Endosc. 2011;73:238–44.
24. Puli SR, Spofford IS, Thompson CC. Use of self-expandable stents in the treatment of bariatric surgery leaks: a systemic review and meta-analysis. Clin Endosc. 2012;75(2):287–93.
25. Puig CA, Waked TM, Baron Sr TH, Wong Kee Song LM, Gutierrez J. The role of endoscopic stents in the management of chronic anastomotic and staple line leaks and chronic strictures after bariatric surgery. Surg Obes Rel Dis. 2014 Jul–Aug;10(4):613–7.
26. Ritter LA, Wang AY, Sauer BG. Healing of complicated gastric leaks in bariatric patients using endoscopic clips. JSLS. 2013 Jul–Sep;17(3):481–3.
27. Goenka MK, Goenka U. Endotherapy of leaks and fistula. World J Gastrointest Endosc. 2015;7(7):702–13.

Chapter 21
The Problem Stoma

Leslie Kobayashi and Raul Coimbra

A junior colleague recently consulted me for assistance with a patient who was, at that time, postoperative day 2 from an emergent laparotomy and Hartmann's procedure for Hinchey grade 4 diverticulitis. The patient was still febrile with a leukocytosis, but was hemodynamically stable and respiring comfortably on minimal supplemental oxygen via nasal cannula. Upon examination, I found a morbidly obese patient with an end colostomy in the left lower quadrant, and the mucosa was edematous and gray–black in color (Fig. 21.1). The abdomen was obese, distended, soft, and mildly tender. The surgical incision was closed loosely with staples without surrounding cellulitis. My colleague had requested my advice as to whether or not the patient should be taken back to the operating room for stoma revision [1–3].

While edema and venous engorgement in the immediate postoperative period is common, this was a case of stoma necrosis, which is one of the more common early complications following creation of stomas which also include stoma retraction, dermatitis, leakage, and high output dehydration. Stoma necrosis is characterized by discoloration of the mucosa ranging from dusky blue/purple to gray and black as ischemia progresses and poor or absent blood flow from raw surfaces. Stoma necrosis occurs in 1–20 % of colostomies and 1–10 % of ileostomies [4] and is more frequently observed in obese patients and following emergency surgeries [3]. Necrosis is due to inadequate perfusion and usually presents within the first few postoperative days [4, 5]. Treatment includes fluid resuscitation, reversal of hypotension, and hypoxia to improve overall tissue perfusion. Adequate bowel decompression with a nasogastric tube may reduce abdominal girth and tension on

L. Kobayashi (✉) · R. Coimbra (✉)
Division of Trauma, Surgical Critical Care, Burns and Acute Care Surgery,
University of California, San Diego Health Sciences,
200 W. Arbor Dr. #8896, San Diego, CA 92103-8896, USA
e-mail: lkobayashi@ucsd.edu

R. Coimbra
e-mail: rcoimbra@ucsd.edu

J.J. Diaz and D.T. Efron (eds.), *Complications in Acute Care Surgery*,
DOI 10.1007/978-3-319-42376-0_21

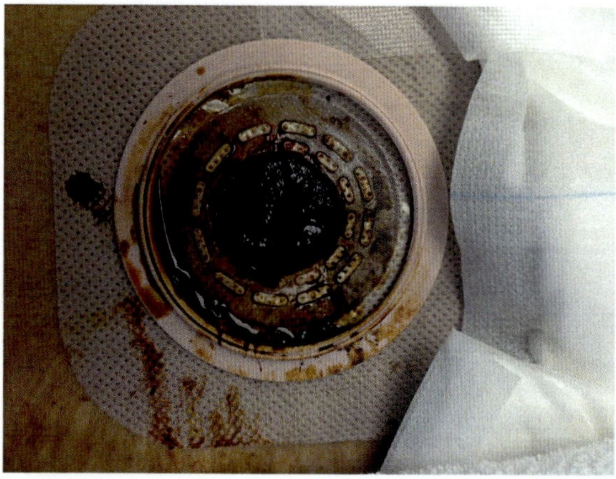

Fig. 21.1 Full-thickness ischemia of stoma

the bowel mesentery. Partial ischemia involving mucosa only and not extending below the level of the fascia (Fig. 21.2) may be managed expectantly, although risk of long-term stoma stricture and retraction is increased [1, 5]. Full-thickness necrosis and necrosis extending below the level of the fascia require immediate surgical revision to prevent perforation and peritoneal contamination [3, 5]. To determine whether tissue loss is full thickness, a dry gauze pad can be used to gently debride devitalized superficial tissue, underlying submucosa that is pink and bleeding is reassuring. To evaluate depth of ischemia, a small lubricated test tube can be inserted into the lumen of the stoma and a flashlight used to illuminate the interior to assess tissue viability below the skin and above the fascia.

Because the necrosis in this case was full thickness and complete, I advised a return to the operating room for revision. In order to maximize success of revision, the patient's physiology should be optimized with resuscitation, nasogastric decompression, and reversal of any coagulopathy, hypothermia and acidosis. Additionally, appropriate antimicrobial coverage should be anticipated and dosed to ensure therapeutic circulating levels at the time of the procedure. If not utilized previously, an enterostomal therapist should be consulted to mark the skin for optimal stoma placement in case stoma relocation is required. If no enterostomal therapist is available, or in the case of emergency surgery, the optimal site for stoma placement is generally within the rectus sheath at the apex of the subumbilical fat roll, approximately two-thirds of the way along an imaginary line from anterior superior iliac spine and the umbilicus [3, 6].

The most common causes of stoma necrosis are tension upon the stoma due to inadequate mobilization or short bowel mesentery, external compression of mesentery by an overly small abdominal wall opening, and over trimming or ligation of the mesentery. In the operating room following a general abdominal inspection for other pathology and evacuation of any bloody, purulent or feculent material attention should be turned to the bowel. For descending colostomies as was the case for this patient, complete mobilization along the left lateral white line of

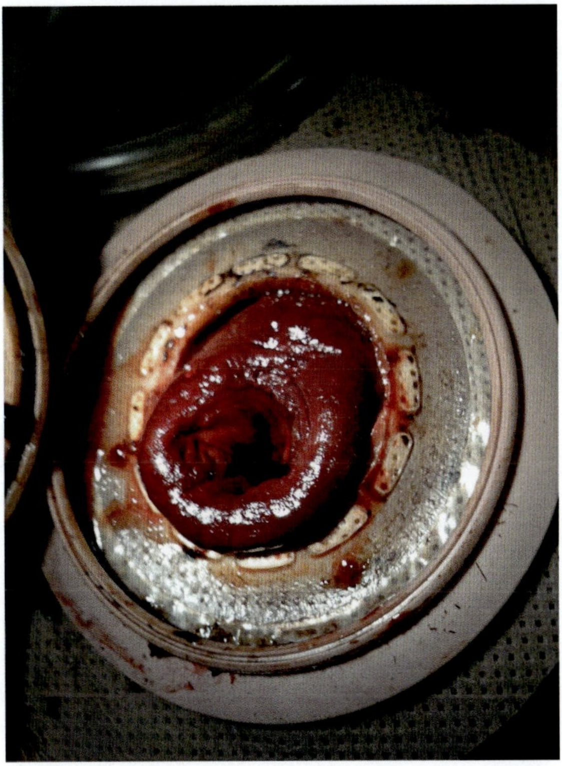

Fig. 21.2 Partial ischemia of superficial (above *skin*) stoma

Toldt and release of the splenic flexure are imperative. Particularly in obese patients who tend to have a short and fatty mesentery, the mobilization of the mesentery off of the retroperitoneum should extend to the midline medial to the ligament of Treitz. Additional length can be obtained by dissecting the distal transverse colon from its attachments to the greater curvature of the stomach and removing a portion of the greater omentum. The goal of mobilization should be easy movement of the bowel through the abdominal wall and protrusion of at least 3–4 cm of bowel above the skin without any tension. In extreme circumstances, this may require ligation of the inferior mesenteric vein at the lower border of the pancreas, and if further length is still required this can be followed with ligation of the inferior mesenteric artery (IMA) near its origin releasing the medial and most proximal tether on the colonic mesentery [1, 6]. It is essential to preserve the marginal artery and the collateral blood supply to the descending colon when required to ligate the IMA. When artificially foreshortened due to peritoneal inflammation, additional length can be obtained by pie-crusting of the mesentery creating several staggered partial thickness incisions in the thickened overlying peritoneum without disrupting the underlying vasculature.

After establishing adequate length for stoma creation, attention is then turned to the abdominal wall opening. In the case of my colleague's patient, the stoma aperture had already been created but when creating a de novo aperture it is important to localize the opening within the rectus sheath and limit the aperture size. Location within the rectus muscle, as opposed to lateral to the rectus sheath, has been associated with reduced risk of parastomal hernia and stoma prolapse [6]. Several studies have also found that an aperture size greater than 2.5–3.5 cm is a risk factor for parastomal hernia and that every millimeter increase in aperture diameter increases risk of hernia by 10 % [1, 7]. However, in obese patients and those with a very thick mesentery, the anterior and posterior rectus sheaths should be divided widely in a vertical fashion and the rectus muscle split widely in a muscle-sparing fashion; only the skin aperture should be left small enough to accommodate the bowel alone. This allows for easy passage of the stoma without damage to the vascular supply, and the large incision can accommodate the fatty mesentery of the left colon without causing external compression of the mesentery and vascular compromise. Once the bowel is mobilized such that 3–4 cm of bowel is easily and freely externalized without tension, the anterior and posterior sheaths can be partially closed around the bowel on the antimesenteric side of the aperture. Care should be taken during externalization of the bowel and closure of the abdominal wall defect around the stoma that no twisting or kinking of the bowel or volvulization can occur.

Parastomal herniation is a particular concern for this patient given the patient's risk factors of obesity, the original emergent nature of the procedure, and that it is colostomy, as these have higher rates of hernia formation compared to ileostomies [1, 3, 7]. Other risk factors for hernia formation include advanced age, poor nutrition, malignancy, steroid use, and end stomas. In addition to localizing the stoma exit to the rectus sheath and limiting the size of the aperture if possible, consideration should be given to placement of preperitoneal or sublay mesh in order to reduce the risk of hernia formation. There is good evidence including 3 randomized controlled trials demonstrating a significant risk reduction in hernia formation (RR 0.23, $p = 0.02$) and need for surgical hernia repair (RR 0.13, $p = 0.05$) when using either biological or prosthetic mesh reinforcement of the stoma aperture [8]. These studies also demonstrated no increase in rates of infections or other stoma-related morbidity and mortality. Because of the patient's risk factors, the need for early revision, and because it is the experience at our medical center that follow up for stoma closure in our patient population is unreliable, in this case I advised reinforcement with biological mesh. Although rates of infections have not been shown to be increased with prosthetic mesh when compared to bioprosthetics [1, 7], we feel that risk of infection in frankly contaminated fields and in patients who are immunocompromised because of critical illness is too great to use prosthetic material and favor biological mesh such as FlexHD®, AlloDerm®, Strattice™, or Permacol®. When utilized, it should ideally be placed in the preperitoneal space, although if coagulopathy makes extensive dissection undesirable, an underlay position can be used. The mesh should be large enough to create a 4- to 5-cm overlap and a keyhole configuration or crosscut aperture can be used to accommodate the stoma. The mesh should be secured circumferentially around the lateral borders. I recommend #1 or 0 Ethibond and space the sutures approximately 2–3 cm apart.

Once the stoma has been brought out through the skin and the aperture reinforced, the midline fascia can be closed with or without retention sutures. In the rare clean cases, the skin can be closed then the incision dressed with an occlusive dressing; in all other cases the skin incision should be left open. Application of a negative-pressure dressing is ideal as this prevents frequent painful dressing changes that occur with traditional wet to dry gauze dressings, and reduces the chances of disruption of the nearby stoma wafer and appliance by those performing wound care. Negative-pressure dressings are also occlusive and prevent contamination of the open midline wound while stoma maturation is performed. Once the midline wound has been dressed, stoma maturation can occur. First, the bowel should be secured at the four corners to the anterior fascia of the rectus sheath using absorbable seromuscular sutures. This helps prevent retraction of the stoma and may reduce risk of prolapse and hernia [6]. Next, the bowel must be opened if staplers were used for transection. This is best performed sharply with Metzenbaum scissors to avoid tissue damage and to allow assessment of the bowel perfusion. Bright pulsatile blood flow should be noted at the stoma edges. Bowel should be serially resected until healthy blood supply is encountered. Care should be taken to avoid over trimming adjacent mesentery as this may reduce perfusion to the stoma edges. The bowel should then be everted in the Brooke fashion, and this is assisted during maturation to the skin by application of eversion sutures. Absorbable suture such as chromic or vicryl is used for the eversion sutures passing through the deep dermis, full-thickness bowel at the stoma edge, and the seromuscular layer of the bowel 2–4 cm from the bowel opening. These assist with elevation of the stoma above the level of the skin which prevents retraction, improves ostomy appliance fit, and reduces risk of skin complications. Three to four eversion sutures should be placed evenly around the stoma. Eversion and bowel externalization should result in an ideal stoma height of 2–3 cm for ileostomies and 0.5–1 cm for colostomies. Elevation of the stoma less than 1 cm from the skin within 48 h of surgery has been associated with skin complications in 35 % of patients [1, 3, 4]. The remainder of the stoma edges should be matured in simple fashion to the skin edges again using small absorbable sutures such as 3-0 vicryl or chromic. Full-thickness bowel and deep dermal bites should be placed every 2–3 mm until there are no areas of skin retraction from the edge of the stoma.

In this case, I was able to assist my colleague during the take-back procedure and we were able to resect the ischemic bowel and after further mobilization were able to mature a healthy end colostomy. The patient did well, recovered from sepsis, and was discharged without further event. Unfortunately, I was then consulted several months later when, after having not shown up for any scheduled clinic visits, the patient presented to the emergency department (ED) with complaints of the stoma "not looking right." Upon examination, moderate stoma prolapse was noted (Fig. 21.3a). Stoma prolapse is relatively uncommon occurring in 3 % of ileostomies and 2 % of colostomies [1]. Risk factors for prolapse include loop stomas, advanced age, obesity, lack of preoperative stoma site marking, bowel distension, and increased intra-abdominal pressure such as chronic constipation [1, 5]. In the

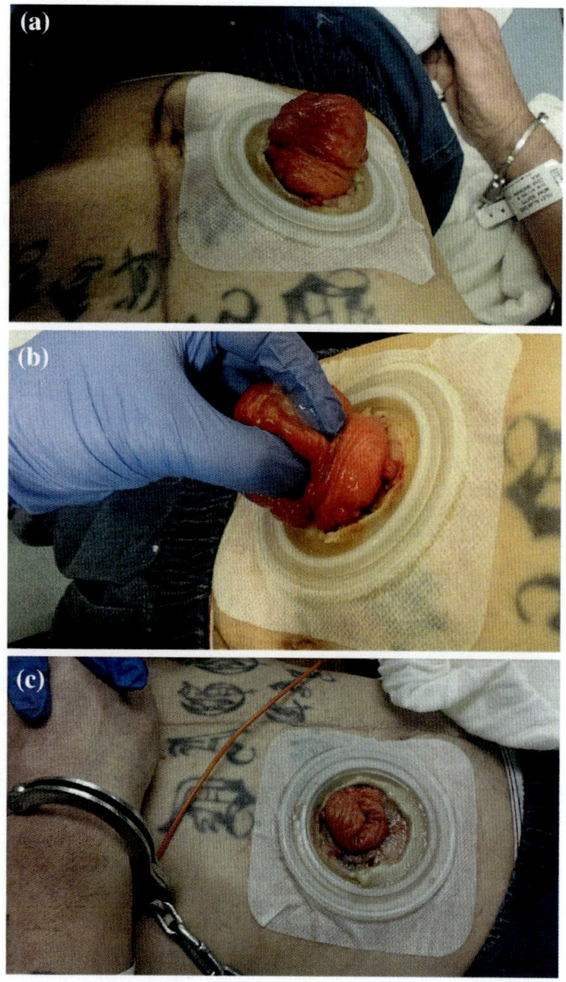

Fig. 21.3 Stoma prolapse **a** before treatment, **b** during reduction, and **c** after application of sugar and manual reduction

presence of necrosis, obstruction or incarceration operative management is required; if none are present, medical management with attempts at manual reduction can be undertaken (Fig. 21.3b). Reduction can be augmented by appropriate patient analgesia and sedation as well as application of desiccants such as granulated sugar to reduce bowel wall edema [1]. After successful reduction of the prolapsed bowel (Fig. 21.3c), the patient was discharged with instructions to follow up in clinic to initiate preoperative workup in anticipation of possible takedown and restitution of the fecal stream.

However, the patient once again failed to follow up and presented to the ED several months later with complaints of nausea, vomiting, and bulging around the stoma. Computed tomography scan in the ED revealed a parastomal hernia with omental (Fig. 21.4a) and small bowel contents (Fig. 21.4b) causing a small bowel obstruction.

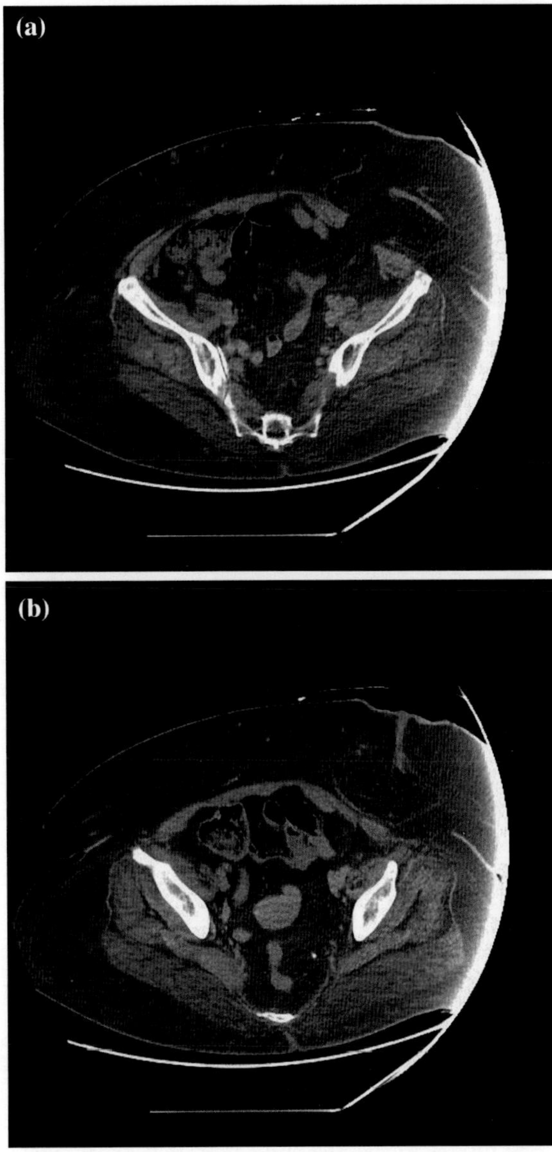

Fig. 21.4 a, b Parastomal hernia containing fat and small bowel causing small bowel obstruction

Parastomal hernia occurs in 4–50 % of stomas with higher rates seen in colostomies than ileostomies and in end stomas compared to loop stomas [1, 3, 7]. As previously discussed, technical risk factors for parastomal hernia include emergency surgery and a wide aperture for the stoma. Patient factors include obesity, pathologies that increase intra-abdominal pressure, and diseases or medications that impede wound healing. Parastomal hernias can present with a range of symptoms from relatively asymptomatic bulging to painful large abdominal masses.

Symptoms of obstruction, strangulation, or incarceration require immediate operative intervention, but in the absence of these findings parastomal hernias may be managed symptomatically with hernia support belts with or without abdominal binders. The support belt should be fitted and applied with the hernia reduced and the patient in the supine position [5]. Difficulties with stoma appliance application and skin irritation can often be resolved with flexible or convex appliances and skin protectants and barrier creams [1].

Surgery to address the hernia is required in 20–30 % of patients [1, 7]. When surgical repair is necessary, options include primary repair, open repair with mesh, laparoscopic repair with mesh, relocation of the stoma, and restoration of bowel continuity with stoma closure. Restoration of bowel continuity and elimination of the stoma, if feasible, is the preferred choice as it eliminates the need for stoma and minimizes risk of recurrence. However, when restoration of bowel continuity is not an option, repair with mesh reinforcement in the underlay or sublay locations is the preferred technique due to unacceptably high risk of recurrence with primary tissue repair and mesh onlay techniques [1, 3, 9, 10]. Relocation of the stoma is an option and may be a good choice in patients whose current stoma location is suboptimal and would benefit from relocation in a planned optimized location with the assistance of an enterostomal technician. However, repair often requires generous laparotomy and recurrence rates vary from 0 to 76 %, although this may be reduced with the use of prophylactic mesh reinforcement in the new stoma location as previously described [1, 3]. Repair of the original site with mesh reinforcement either open or laparoscopic in the sublay or underlay position has the best outcomes with low rates of surgical site and mesh infections and relatively low rates of hernia recurrence with rates ranging from 7 to 33 % with open repairs and 7–56 % in laparoscopic repairs [1, 3, 10]. In frankly infected fields and high-risk patients, reinforcement can be performed with biological mesh, with very low rates of infection; however, recurrence rates are slightly higher compared to similar mesh repairs utilizing a prosthetic material (15 % vs. 10 %) [1]. In this case, after ruling out distal obstruction with a digital rectal examination and rapid barium enema, we elected to restore bowel continuity and close the original colostomy site and reinforce the fascial closure with a mesh in the underlay position.

Clinical Scenario

54 yo obese, diabetic man is 2 months s/p total abdominal colectomy with ileostomy for c.diff colitis and toxic megacolon that occurred secondary to antibiotic treatment for lower extremity cellulitis. His ileostomy was always poorly protruding given a foreshortening of his mesentery, and now it is flat, somewhat retracted, with a poorly fitting appliance, excoriation at the skin, and the suggestion of parastomal bulge.

Complications associated with stomas are common. Early complications include stoma necrosis, retraction, wound infections, and dermatitis. Later complications include high output/dehydration, skin irritation/leakage, stenosis, prolapse, and parastomal hernias. Patient-associated risk factors for complications include emergency surgery, presence of active infection/inflammation, obesity, advanced age, poor nutrition, diabetes, malignancy, and other pre-existing comorbidities. Technical risk factors for complications include tension on the stoma due to shortened mesentery/inadequate mobilization, overly large aperture size, and suboptimal stoma placement.

This patient demonstrates common complications of retraction, leakage/skin irritation, and likely parastomal hernia. These complications are not unexpected given the risk factors of advanced age, diabetes, obesity, foreshortened mesentery, and the emergent nature of his original surgery due to active infection. Some of these complications can be addressed by careful wound care by an experienced enterostomal technician and medical management of dehydration, active infection, electrolyte imbalances, and control of stoma output. Failure to respond to conservative treatment may require surgical intervention to re-establish either bowel continuity, if possible, or stoma revision if not. During stoma revision, meticulous surgical technique including adequate mobilization of the bowel, optimal placement and sizing of the stoma aperture, and use of either biological or prosthetic mesh reinforcement of the stoma aperture are essential in reducing further complications.

This clinical scenario is unfortunately quite common, and we hope that this chapter has given the reader some helpful tips as to identifying the risk factors for complications, how to ameliorate these risk factors, and the technical considerations that should be addressed during stoma creation and postoperative care to minimize the risk and resolution of these common stoma-related complications.

Key Questions

1. *Are there any special technical tricks to bring up a difficult stoma?*
2. *Which high-risk stomas are better left alone as opposed to being revised?*

References

1. Bafford AC, Irani JL. Management and complications of stomas. Surg Clin North Am. 2013;93(1):145–66.
2. Parmar KL, Zammit M, Smith A, Kenyon D, Lees NP. A prospective audit of early stoma complications in colorectal cancer treatment throughout the Greater Manchester and Cheshire colorectal cancer network. Colorectal Dis. 2011;13(8):935–8.
3. Shabbir J, Britton DC. Stoma complications: a literature overview. Colorectal Dis. 2010;12(10):958–64.
4. Persson E, Berndtsson I, Carlsson E, Hallen AM, Lindholm E. Stoma-related complications and stoma size—a 2-year follow up. Colorectal Dis. 2010;12(10):971–6.

5. Maidl L, Ohland J. Care of stomas. In: Fischer JE, Bland KI, editors. Master of Surgery 5th Edition. 2. 5 ed. Philadelphia PA: Lippincott Williams & Wilkins; 2007. p. 1449–64.
6. Lavery IC. Technique of colostomy construction and closure. In: Fischer JE, Bland KI, editors. Mastery of surgery 5th edition. 2. 5 ed. Philadelphia PA: Lippincott Williams & Wilkins; 2007. p. 1439–49.
7. Hotouras A, Murphy J, Thaha M, Chan CL. The persistent challenge of parastomal herniation: a review of the literature and future developments. Colorectal Dis. 2013;15(5):e202–14.
8. Wijeyekoon SP, Gurusamy K, El-Gendy K, Chan CL. Prevention of parastomal herniation with biologic/composite prosthetic mesh: a systematic review and meta-analysis of randomized controlled trials. J Am Coll Surg. 2010;211(5):637–45.
9. Hotouras A, Murphy J, Power N, Williams NS, Chan CL. Radiological incidence of parastomal herniation in cancer patients with permanent colostomy: what is the ideal size of the surgical aperture? Int J Surg. 2013;11(5):425–7.
10. Hansson BM, Slater NJ, van der Velden AS, Groenewoud HM, Buyne OR, de Hingh IH, et al. Surgical techniques for parastomal hernia repair: a systematic review of the literature. Ann Surg. 2012;255(4):685–95.

Chapter 22
The Immunosuppressed Patient

Sergio E. Hernandez, Eric W. Etchill and Brian S. Zuckerbraun

Introduction

Surgery in the immunosuppressed patient poses unique challenges and considerations. In the elective surgical setting, the opportunities to optimize conditions and to thoroughly explore alternative options exist. However, when there is an urgent or emergency indication for surgery in the immunosuppressed patient, which itself may be pathophysiology secondary to the immunosuppressed state, optimization is likely not possible and there is a predisposition to the development of postoperative complications and worse outcomes. It is necessary to understand the challenges associated with different immunocompromised states, in consideration of differential diagnoses, as well as to integrate this into decision making in and out of the operating theater. This chapter focuses on challenges in the immunosuppressed patient, with a focus on HIV and pharmacological immunosuppression in the setting of therapy for malignancies, autoimmune diseases, or organ transplantation. Particular emphasis on commonly utilized therapeutic agents and their adverse effects are described. These groups of patients present unique challenges to the surgeon in perioperative and intraoperative decision making.

S.E. Hernandez · E.W. Etchill · B.S. Zuckerbraun (✉)
Department of Surgery, University of Pittsburgh, 200 Lothrop St.,
F1200 PUH, Pittsburgh, PA 15213, USA
e-mail: zuckerbraunbs@upmc.edu

S.E. Hernandez
e-mail: Hernandez.sergio@medstudent.pitt.edu

E.W. Etchill
e-mail: Etchill.eric@medstudent.pitt.edu

B.S. Zuckerbraun
VA Pittsburgh Healthcare System, Pittsburgh, PA, USA

J.J. Diaz and D.T. Efron (eds.), *Complications in Acute Care Surgery*,
DOI 10.1007/978-3-319-42376-0_22

Surgical diseases among immunocompromised patients are presented along with the surgical considerations and their medical optimization to provide a broader understanding of complex clinical scenarios. These diseases were selected to support the diagnostic challenge that is often encountered prior to obtaining a surgical consultation. The focus of this discussion will center on commonly encountered pathogens and particular considerations in the immunosuppressed. Finally, we will conclude our discussion with an analysis of preoperative management to highlight preventable complications.

Immunosuppression: Background and Challenges

Human Immunodeficiency Virus

The CDC estimates more than 1.2 million people in the USA are living with HIV [1]. Although the disease incidence has decreased, the prevalence continues to rise as a result of improved survival antiretroviral therapy (ART). Elective and urgent surgical management of HIV-positive patients is expected to grow as this population ages and surgeons must be equipped for the challenges ahead.

HIV is a RNA retrovirus with predilection toward T lymphocyte, particularly CD4 cells, resulting in chronic immunosuppression and deficiency in cell-mediated immunity [2]. Potent adaptive immune response against HIV-infected cells selects for key mutations and immune escape. HIV Infection predisposes to opportunistic infections and specifically gastrointestinal infections by depletion of gastrointestinal lymphoid cells, enterocyte apoptosis, and permeability [2]. The CDC has established guidelines to assess HIV infection status based on CD4 count. Immunocompetent hosts have CD4 counts greater than 500cell/μl while those with CD4 less than 200 cell/μl have progressed to acquired immune deficiency syndrome (AIDS) [3]. Opportunistic infections can occur during any stage of the disease but prophylactic antimicrobials are only recommended when CD4 counts fall below 250 cell/μl [3]. CD4 measurement is of particular importance to consider when timing elective operations and risk of developing certain infections (Table 22.1).

Another consideration in the management of the HIV-positive patient is the development of multiorgan dysfunction associated with the infection. For instance, chronic vascular inflammation and elevated cytokine levels leads to cardiovascular disease and thrombosis [4]. HIV nephropathy and drug-induced kidney damage is a known cause of chronic kidney disease, and transplantation has emerged as a viable option [5]. Furthermore, direct invasion of gastrointestinal (GI) tract affects GI motility. Coviral infection with HPV increases incidence of anogenital disease. Clostridium difficile colitis is of special concern in this population due to chronic antimicrobial use affecting the GI flora. Chronic liver disease due to associated HBV/HCV infection, steatosis, and hepatocellular carcinoma has emerged as the leading cause of morbidity and mortality [6]. Liver transplantation is considered a

Table 22.1 Opportunistic HIV infections and recommended treatment [3]

CD4 count (cell/ml)	Opportunistic infection	Primary regimen
<250	Coccidioidomycosis	Fluconazole/itraconazole
<200	Pneumocystis pneumonia	TMP-SMX
	Histoplasmosis	Amphotericin B
<150	*H. capsulatum*	Itraconazole
<100	*T. gondii* encephalitis	Pyrimethamine
	Cryptococcal meningitis	Amphotericin B
	CMV retinitis	Ophthalmology consult
<50	*M. tuberculosis*	INH + RIF + PZA + EMB
	MAC	Clarithromycin/azithromycin
	Candida spp	Fluconazole
	Aspergillosis	Voriconazole
	CMV esophagitis/colitis	Ganciclovir
	HPV warts	Podophyllotoxin, imiquimod, sinecatechin

CMV Cytomegalovirus; *MAC* Mycobacterium avium complex; *INH* Isoniazid; *RIF* Rifampin; *PZA* Pyrazinamide; *EMB* Ethambutol

possible alternative for liver failure in this population. Additionally, antiviral drugs affect proper endocrine function yielding insulin resistance, dyslipidemia, and lipodystrophy [6]. This multitude of disorders experienced by HIV infection often confounds perioperative management.

The side effect profile from the antiviral regimen is profound. Drug therapy often utilizes a combination of medications addressing different stages of the HIV infection pathway [7]. Initiation of ART leads to replenishment of CD4+ count with associated viral suppression [8]. Some patients develop an immune reconstitution inflammatory syndrome (IRIS) characterized by acute local and systemic inflammatory that is associated with clinical exacerbation [9]. This reaction has been linked to antigenic load of preexisting illnesses and opportunistic infections [9]. Dose- and agent-related toxicities of ART are numerous implicating mitochondrial dysfunction, metabolic derangements, myelosuppression, and allergic reactions [10]. For a summary of adverse effects with surgical implications refer to Table 22.2. Of particular importance to the surgeon is the direct nephrotoxic, hepatotoxic, and myelosuppression effects that may affect preoperative planning.

Surgical indications in HIV/AIDS patients include elective and urgent indications as would be for any particular disease, as well as for HIV disease complications intended for prophylaxis or palliation. Malignancies more prevalent in HIV population includes Kaposi's sarcoma or non-Hodgkin's lymphoma and opportunistic infection such as cytomegalovirus (CMV), cryptosporidium, and mycobacterium avium complex (MAC) are well-documented causes of bowel obstruction, perforation, and peritonitis [11]. Additionally, anorectal pathologies such as hemorrhoids, ulcers, fissures, and anal condyloma occur relatively more

Table 22.2 Side effect of antiretroviral therapy

Mechanism	Side effect
Mitochondrial dysfunction	Lactic acidosis, hepatic toxicity, pancreatitis, peripheral neuropathy, cardiomyopathy, pancreatitis, hepatic steatosis, lipodystrophy, proximal myopathy, polymyositis
Metabolic abnormalities	Fat maldistribution (lipodystrophy), dyslipidemia, hyperglycemia, glucose intolerance, insulin resistance, osteopenia, osteoporosis, osteonecrosis, arthritis
Bone marrow suppression	Anemia, neutropenia, thrombocytopenia
Allergic reactions	Rashes, hypersensitivity responses
Immune reconstitution inflammatory syndrome	Mycobacterium avium abscesses, *Mycobacterium leprae* lesions, sarcoidosis, Grave's disease, PML, SLE, antiphospholipid syndrome, vasculitis, primary biliary cirrhosis, hepatitis, polymyositis, uveitis, ITP

ITP Immune thrombocytic purpura; *PML* Progressive multifocal leukoencephalopathy; *SLE* Systemic lupus erythematosus

frequently and palliative surgery can be performed safely. However, surgery should be individualized due to decreased wound healing rates. Prevention of anorectal disease is encouraged with HPV vaccination, conservative management, and avoidance of anorectal trauma or injury. When concerns for intraepithelial neoplasia are present, a biopsy helps identify HPV serotype to guide management [12].

Active HIV virus replication has distinct effects on surgical outcomes. Patients with CD4 count <200 cells/μl or viral load exceeding 30,000 copies/ml experience higher rate of complications [13]. Preoperative hypoalbuminemia (<3.5 g/dl), age, and decreased functional status have been associated with an increased 30-day postsurgical mortality among HIV patients [14]. These patients tend to be nutritionally deficient, chronically ill, and in poor state of health. Surprisingly, elective procedures for low-risk surgeries such as hernia repair, appendectomy, and cholecystectomy do not require extensive perioperative planning and can be performed safely [13]. Emergent surgery has higher mortality and complication rates due to impaired wound healing and surgical site infections [15].

Preoperative assessment of HIV patients requires an assessment of HIV disease status, medication history, nutritional, and functional status. Preoperative laboratories should include complete blood count (CBC) and comprehensive metabolic panel (CMP) to rule out myelosuppression, HIV nephropathy, or coagulopathy. Maximizing ART to improve viral suppression and CD4 counts is of particular importance and has to be addressed in preoperative planning, but caution must be employed if IRIS occurs.

In summary, HIV is a complex multisystem disease with multiple considerations affecting surgical evaluation and outcomes. Antiretroviral treatment has dramatically delayed disease progression; however, the side effect profile of these drugs, as well as complications of patients with chronic immunosuppression secondary to HIV, presents various challenges in the surgical setting. Low-risk and elective surgeries appear to present no additional risks, while emergent and high-risk surgeries endure complications mainly dependent on the individual's state of health. Improvement of CD4 count and reduction of viral load with ART are effective methods to reduce complication rates.

Chemotherapy

Neoplastic disease is one of the leading causes of death worldwide with an incidence of 14 million in 2012, resulting in 8.2 million deaths [16]. Oncological management is complex and multimodal, often requiring combination of chemotherapy, radiation, and surgical intervention for definitive or palliative treatment. Aside from their role in solid tumor diagnosis and management, surgeons manage acute surgical interventions either separate from or influenced by the primary disease. Thus, basic knowledge of chemotherapy and its effect on immunosuppression is of utmost importance.

Chemotherapy ideally reduces disease burden by decreasing tumor size, halting disease progression, and abolishing micrometastases. In general, antineoplastic drugs act at the cellular level to reduce rapidly proliferating cells [17]. As a result, these drugs damage healthy cells with similar characteristics residing in the bone marrow, gastrointestinal tract (GI) and skin tissue. Immunosuppression and myelosuppression are of particular interest in perioperative management. This section will focus on common perioperative presentations and surgical implications of side effects encountered during antineoplastic therapy.

Chemotherapy agents are divided into alkylating agents, antitumor antibiotics, antimetabolites, plant alkaloids, hormonal therapy, and targeted tissue therapy [17]. Many of these agents function to inhibit the cell cycle in a phase-specific (antimetabolite, vinca alkaloid, and bleomycin) or non-specific manner (alkylating agents and antibiotics) [17]. A summary of side effects is found in Table 22.3.

Chemotherapy regimens are often used as combination therapies to target different pathways in the neoplastic process. Each medication's metabolism, half-life, and excretion pathway influence its toxicity profile. Further, toxicities may contribute to or exacerbate coexistent comorbidities and polypharmacy exacerbates these issues [18]. For instance, cardiotoxicity and cardiac injury are common adverse effects of antimetabolites such as doxorubicin. Thus, preoperative cardiac evaluation must be enforced. Pulmonary toxicity is common with bleomycin, methotrexate, and mitomycin C therapy resulting in early plain radiological findings of fine, reticular bibasilar infiltrates. Clinically, these findings may affect anesthesia delivery and hemodynamic response. Methotrexate and azathioprine have been linked to hepatic fibrosis and intrahepatic cholestasis, respectively [18]. Renal toxicity is common among platinum compounds, methotrexate, and streptozocin but can be avoided with adequate hydration and avoidance of simultaneous use of renal toxic compounds such as aminoglycoside antibiotics. Nitrogen mustards such as cyclophosphamide and ifosfamide often cause hemorrhagic cystitis. This is a self-limiting effect and cease after discontinuation of therapy. Treatment with mesna

Table 22.3 Chemotherapy agents and their common adverse effects

Class	Agent	Adverse effects
Alkylating agent		
Nitrosurea	Carmustine, lomustine	Pulmonary fibrosis
Methylating agent	Procarbazine	Edema, tachycardia
	Dacarbazine	Hepatic necrosis, obstruction and hepatic vein obstruction
	Temozolomide	Seizure, gait abnormality, peripheral edema
Platinum	Cisplatin	Acute renal tubular necrosis
	Carboplatin	Magnesium wasting
	Oxaliplatin	Peripheral sensory neuropathy, ototoxicity
Nitrogen mustard	Cyclophophomide	Pericarditis
	Ifosfomide	Pericardial effusions, pulmonary fibrosis, hemorrhagic cystitis, anemia, edema
	Melphalan	SIADH
	Chlorambucil	SIADH, seizure
Antimetabolite		
Anthracycline/anthraquinolone	Doxorubicin	Cardiomyopathy
	Daunorubicin, epirubicin, idarubicin, mitoxantrone	Electrocardiogram changes
Antitumor antibiotic	Bleomycin	Pulmonary fibrosis
	Mitomycin C	Pneumonitis, pulmonary hypertension
Antimetabolite: pyrimidine analogue	Capecitabine	Myocardial ischemia
	Cytarabine	Coronary vasospasm
	5-Fluorouracil	
	Gemcitabine	Proteinuria
Antimetabolite: purine analogue	Pentostatin	Pulmonary toxicity, deep vein thrombosis, chest pain, arrhythmia, AV block
	Thioguanine	Hepatotoxicity
	Cladribine	Thrombosis, tachycardia, ARF, tumor lysis syndrome
	Fludarabine	CVA, TIA, CHF, arrhythmia, ARF, tumor lysis syndrome
	Mercaptopurine	Intrahepatic cholestasis and centrilobular necrosis

(continued)

Table 22.3 (continued)

Class	Agent	Adverse effects
Antimetabolite: folate antagonist	Methotrexate	Elevated LFTs, pulmonary edema, pleural effusions, meningismus, encephalopathy, myelosuppression
Urea substitute	Hydroxyurea	Seizure, edema
Microtubule assembly inhibitor		
Taxane	Paclitaxel	Peripheral neuropathy
	Docetaxel	Bradycardia, autonomic dysfunction
Alkaloid	Vinblastine	Hypertension, MI, CVA, Raynaud's phenomenon, SIADH, GI bleeding
	Vincristine	Paresthesia, laryngeal nerve palsy, autonomic dysfunction, orthostasis, SIADH
Vascular endothelial growth factor inhibitor		
Tyrosine kinase	Imatinib	Edema, LV dysfunction
	Sorafenib	Hypertension, MI
	Sunitinib	MI, thromboembolism, adrenal insufficiency, hypothyroidism, cardiomyopathy, QT prolongation and torsade de pointes
	Dasatinib	Edema, cardiomyopathy, QT prolongation, pulmonary hemorrhage, platelet dysfunction
	Nilotinib	QT prolongation, edema, hypertension
Epidermal growth factors receptor inhibitor		
	Erlotinib	DVT, CVA, MI, arrhythmia, pulmonary toxicity, syncope, edema
	Lapatinib	Cardiomyopathy, QT prolongation, pulmonary hemorrhage
	Panitunab	Pulmonary fibrosis and edema
Angiogenesis inhibitor		
Immunomodulation	Thalidomide	Thromboembolism
	Lenalidomide	Bradycardia, edema

ARF Acute renal failure; *CVA* Cerebrovascular accident; *DVT* Deep vein thrombosis; *SIAD* Syndrome of inappropriate antidiuretic hormone; *MI* Myocardial ischemia; *TIA* Transient ischemic attack

for hemorrhagic cystitis is useful, but definite treatment may require cystoscopy-assisted hemostasis through electrocautery or sclerosis with formalin [18]. Early manifestations of neurotoxicity include neuropathy and hyporeflexia. However, neurotoxicity may progress to SIADH, tinnitus, hearing loss, autonomic instability, cranial nerve palsies, and emesis related to alkaloids, antimetabolites, or platinum agents. Emesis is a common ailment and should be readily anticipated and treated prior to chemotherapy induction.

Myelosuppression is dose limiting in many antineoplastic regimens, yielding reduced production of blood cell precursors approximately 2 weeks after induction. This cytopenia is commonly transient, lasting several days, but marked by neutropenia and absolute neutrophil count (ANC) <1000 cell/mm^3 [19]. Neutropenic patients lack the classic signs of infection (erythema and elevated cell counts) and most frequently present with fever as the sole complaint in 25–40 % of patients. Hypotension, weakness, and confusion may also occur. The source of the fever is rarely found, warranting implementation of antimicrobial therapy per Infectious Diseases Society of America (IDSA) guidelines for neutropenic patients [20]. These guidelines recommend expanded broad-spectrum coverage for gram-negative and anaerobic organisms with piperacillin–tazobactam or a carbapenem [20]. Combination therapy with antipseudomonal cephalosporins plus metronidazole is also appropriate. Therapy should be continued until resolution of symptoms and objective signs of improved neutrophil count (ANC >500 cell/mm^3) [20]. Antifungal coverage should be started with amphotericin B in the setting of continued fever, neutropenia, and clinical deterioration or lack of improvement after 5 days of adequate antimicrobial coverage. Addition of colony-stimulating factor (CSF) to boost immune response can be considered in septic patients or if ANC falls below 100 cell/mm^3 [20].

Achieving the ideal chemotherapeutic regimen includes a balance between maximizing tumor suppression and local control, and minimizing toxicity and immunosuppression. Surgeons must be able to recognize and properly evaluate antineoplastic drug toxicities in preoperative planning to reduce surgical complications. Appropriate treatment for neutropenia should focus on antimicrobial therapy and boosting the immune system prior to surgical intervention.

Biologic Therapy for Rheumatic and Autoimmune Disease

The use of targeted biologic therapy has emerged as a suitable approach for patients with rheumatic and autoimmune diseases. The mechanism of action of these agents includes reduction of chronic inflammatory changes by targeting cytokines, inflammatory cells, and costimulation molecules [21]. Considering risk and benefits of primary disease flare with serious infections from surgical complications is an important distinction.

Cytokines such as tumor necrosis factor (TNF-α), Interleukin-1 (IL-1), and Interleukin-6 (IL-6) have major roles in endothelial cell activation, promoting inflammation, coagulation, wound healing, and hepatic synthesis of acute phase reactants [21]. IL-6 is also known for B-cell activation and antibody proliferation. Additionally, cluster of identification (CD) molecules are cell surface molecules involved in activation of B and T lymphocytes particularly CD 20, 22, and 28 [22]. Drugs that target these pathways are of particular importance for the management of chronic inflammatory and autoimmune conditions. Table 22.4 includes a list of currently FDA-approved agents and indications for use.

Table 22.4 Biologic therapy and indications for use

Target	Agent	Indications and uses
TNF-a	Etarnecept	RA, PsA, JIA, plaque psoriasis
	Infliximab	RA, CD, UC, plaque psoriasis, PsA, Takayasu's vasculitis
	Adalimumab	RA, CD, UC, AS, PsA
	Golimumab	RA, PsA, AS, UC
	Certolizumab	RA, AS, Crohn's disease, PsA
IL-1	Anakinra, rilonacept, Canakinumab	RA, CAPS
IL-6	Tocilizumab	RA, JIA
INF-B1α	Avonex	Multiple sclerosis
CD-20	Rituximab	RA, MPA, pemphigus vulgaris, leukemia, lymphoma, Wegener's granulomatosis
	Ofatumumab	RA, leukemia
CD-22	Epratuzumab	SLE, Sjögren's syndrome
CD-28	Abatacept	RA, JIA

AS Ankylosing spondylitis; *CAPS* Cryopyrin-associated periodic syndrome; *CD* Crohn's disease; *INF* Interferon; *ILK* Interleukin; *JIA* Juvenile idiopathic arthritis; *MPA* Microscopic polyangiitis; *PsA* Psoriatic arthritis; *RA* Rheumatoid arthritis; *SLE* Systemic lupus erythematosus; *TNF* Tumor necrosis factor; *UC* Ulcerative colitis

The initiation of biologic treatment requires screening for previous or current tuberculosis infection, serological evidence of viral hepatitis, and previous or current malignancy. This is important as therapy with biologics can induce reactivation of latent infections [23]. Risks of myelosuppression and decreased wound healing are also prominent [24]. This infection risk is heightened by the inherent risk of autoimmune diseases. For instance, RA patient have been found to have a 13-fold increase in infection risk when compared to healthy controls in the absence of immunosuppressive regimen [25]. Interestingly, there is a lack of recommendations regarding continued use of biologics in the perioperative period but most supports cessation of therapy should be practiced when possible.

Anti-TNF-α agents have emerged as effective therapies for inflammatory bowel disease. Rituximab, originally used in the treatment of lymphoma, is a monoclonal antibody against CD 20 cells, which represses a subset of B cells via apoptosis [24]. It is approved for use in autoimmune disorders and lymphocytic malignancies but is also used off label for auto-autoimmune disorders (idiopathic thrombocytopenic purpura), desensitization of ABO blood groups in transplant incompatible patients, and dermatologic disorders [24]. IL-1 inhibitors, such as Anakinra, have few clinical indications and a short half requiring daily injections and common development of skin tissue infections at site of injection. Surgical implications of biologic are discussed separately in this chapter.

Transplant

The total number of transplants performed in the USA in 2011 reached over 29,000 [26]. Many transplant recipients are experiencing longer survival in part due to better understanding of pathophysiology involved in rejection, improvements in immunosuppressive therapy, and more efficient immunosuppressive agents combination strategies. Post-transplant immunosuppression is typically achieved with glucocorticoids, calcineurin inhibitors, antiproliferative, and/or antimetabolic drugs [18]. Surgeons must have an understanding of these immunosuppressive therapies for appropriate management of acute and elective interventions (Table 22.5).

Table 22.5 Transplant immunosuppressive agents, indications, and common adverse effects

Class	Agent	Indication	Toxicity
Corticosteroids	Prednisone, methylprednisolone, hydrocortisone	Maintenance for most transplants, high doses for acute rejection, preoperative "stress dose"	*Early*: Hyperglycemia, avascular necrosis of the hip, serious infections *Late*: Impaired wound healing, muscle wasting, osteoporosis, Cushing's syndrome, adrenal insufficiency during stress
Calcineurin inhibitors (CNI)	Tacrolimus and cyclosporine	Maintenance therapy for cardiac, renal, and hepatic transplants	Nephrotoxicity, CNS effects (seizure, coma, tremors, and headache), hyperglycemia, hypomagnesemia, hypertension, dyslipidemia, ischemic events (CVA, MI)
Antimetabolite	Sirolimus and Everolimus	Maintenance, preferred in renal transplants over CNI	Anemia, leukopenia, thrombocytopenia, impaired wound healing, hypo/hyperkalemia
Antiproliferative	Azathioprine	Chemotherapy, transplant maintenance immunosuppression	Myelosuppression, hepatotoxicity, pancreatitis, depressed neuromuscular blockade from anesthetics
	Mycophenolic acid, mycophenolate mofetil	Transplant maintenance immunosuppression	Leukopenia, CMV sepsis

Glucocorticoids are the oldest medications used in transplant immunosuppression. Immunosuppression is achieved by reducing T-cell proliferation, inflammatory cytokines, vasodilatory molecules, tissue permeability, and preventing monocyte migration [27]. They exert their role by binding to intracellular receptors and modulating cellular transcription [27]. Initial administration results in neutrophilic leukocytosis, eosinophilia, and lymphocytopenia. Interestingly, while there is a reduction in total number of B cells, immunoglobulin production is preserved [28]. Additionally, T-cell apoptosis results in impaired cell-mediated immunity [27]. The side effect profile of corticosteroid depends on amount, steroid potency, mineralocorticoid profile, and the length of treatment. Major side effects include hypertension, cardiovascular disease, hypokalemia, adrenal insufficiency, diabetes, visceral perforation, and higher risk of infection. Surgical complications and perioperative management in the setting of steroid use deserve further consideration and will be addressed later in this chapter.

Calcineurin inhibitors (CNI) are the most commonly used agents post-transplantation and include tacrolimus and cyclosporine (CsA). These agents substantially decreased organ rejection and revolutionized transplant immunosuppression when first introduced. Their mechanism of action involves blockage of NFAT (nuclear factor of activated T cells) transcription reducing cytokine release from T cells [29]. Dosage requires close monitoring due to narrow therapeutic range contingent on type of organ transplant. Oral administration requires GI absorption, P450 hepatic metabolism and bile excretion [29]. Thus, any metabolic (P450 inducer/inhibitor), physiological (alteration of GI flora, diarrhea, inflammation), or mechanical process can affect CNI metabolism. CNIs have nephrotoxic, neurotoxic, metabolic, and endocrine side effects [29]. The nephrotoxic effects are particularly important after renal transplant often requiring dosing reduction or selection of different agents. Avoiding concomitant use of nephrotoxic drugs such aminoglycosides is strongly encouraged. Neurotoxicity presents as seizure, confusion, coma, tremors, or headache [30]. Multiple electrolyte and metabolic derangements also occur including hyperglycemia, hypomagnesemia, and hypercholesterolemia [31]. Tacrolimus-induced hyperglycemia occurs by establishing insulin resistance that is further exacerbated by surgical stress. Postoperative treatment with a sliding insulin regimen may be required in a patient with otherwise adequate intrinsic glucose control [31]. Higher incidence of ischemic events (CVA and MI) complicates preoperative planning and places these patients at higher risk [31].

Antiproliferative and antimetabolic drugs include azathioprine, mycophenolic acid, mycophenolate mofetil (MMF), sirolimus, and everolimus. Azathioprine, often used in chemotherapy, interferes with DNA synthesis by incorporating false nucleotides (6-thio-GTP) into replicating strand of rapidly proliferative cells such as B and T lymphocytes [32]. Main adverse effects of azathioprine include hepatotoxity, pancreatitis, and dose-limiting myelosuppression [32]. MMF and mycophenolic acid inhibit purine synthesis and have similar preference for fast replicating cells, thus sharing side effects of azathioprine. Sirolimus (Rapamycin) and everolimus, similar to tacrolimus, reduce lymphocytic activation by inhibition of mTOR (mechanistic Target of Rapamycin) and IL-2 signaling [33]. Sirolimus has a preferred renal profile over CNI and is often used as maintenance in renal transplant. However, these agents induce severe leukopenia and thrombocytopenia. Sirolimus also decreases wound healing resulting in dehiscence and incisional hernias particularly in obese patients with BMI >32 kg/m^2 [33]. In this group, it is beneficial to switch to CNI therapy for elective surgeries for two to four months prior and restarting 6-week postoperatively to improve wound healing.

Mucosal injury and ulceration are common ailments among transplant immunosuppressive therapy. Diarrhea and GI side effects are more common with tacrolimus, CsA, and MMF in a dose-dependent fashion [34]. A proposed mechanism for MMF-associated diarrhea includes inhibition of cryptcell division and loss of duodenum villous structure [34]. Ulceration of the GI tract is multifactorial, but has been associated with utilization of NSAIDs, surgery stress, and impaired cytoprotection of mucosal defenses from decreased cell turnover [34]. GI bleeding, when it occurs, is often secondary to undiscovered ulceration. Lung transplant patients may acquire giant gastric ulcers, defined as ulcers with diameter >3 cm, resulting in high mortality secondary to bleeding [34]. Identifying patients with risk factors for GI ulcers is difficult and low threshold for routine endoscopy with biopsy in symptomatic patients is endorsed. Standard practice should include ulcer prophylaxis with PPI or H2 blockers. Perforations can occur throughout the GI tract secondary to steroids, diverticular disease, and concomitant NSAIDs use. Transplant recipients are also at increased risk for biliary tract disease from calculi influenced by cell turnover, resulting in emergent cholecystectomies with high mortality rates. In renal transplant recipients, cyclosporine has resulted in reduced bile flow and increased incidence of cholelithiasis [34]. Therefore, elective surgery for eradication of biliary pathology and ultrasound screening should be practiced during the post-transplantation period to improve outcomes. Acute pancreatitis, although uncommon, carries increased mortality rates of 64 % in liver transplants and 100 % in renal transplant patients [33]. Risk factors for acute pancreatitis include immunosuppressive agents, CMV, HBV, hypercalcemia, alcohol, cholelithiasis, and malignancy [34]. Follow-up with CT at regular intervals to identify unusual inflammation, pseudocyst formation, edema, or necrosis is beneficial. Treatment for acute pancreatitis must focus on aggressive intravenous fluid resuscitation, fasting, identification, and cessation of inciting agent followed by surgery when clinically indicated [33].

Infectious complications are of particular importance in transplant patients due to the nature of chronic immunosuppression. As previously addressed, atypical presentation of infection is common among this group of patients and the clinician must be alert and cautious during preoperative planning. Lung transplant recipients experience invasive early and late fungal infections with coccidiomycosis and aspergillus, respectively [35]. Prophylactic treatment with fluconazole is recommended for the former [36]. Cutaneous and anogenital lesions should raise concern for HPV infections and marked immunosuppression requiring biopsy and surveillance [37]. Finally, CMV infection is the most common infection among post-transplant recipients and is associated with allograft rejection, EBV post-transplantation proliferative disorder (PTLD), and high rate of mortality in the first 6 months [38].

Transplant patients represent a complex mixture of pathologies requiring multidisciplinary collaboration between physicians (transplant, infectious diseases, PCP, and surgeons) for appropriate management and risk reduction. When appropriate, termination or substitution of immunosuppressive regimen improves surgical outcomes.

Surgical Diseases

Gastrointestinal Diseases

The gastrointestinal tract is susceptible to disease from immunosuppression for multiple factors. First, antineoplastic agents are cytotoxic and affect GI cell turnover. Drug immunomodulation modifies components of innate immunity such as barrier protection, neutrophil migration, and resident dendritic cells reducing host defenses. Antibiotic regiments often used in immunocompromised patients alter the inhabitant flora selecting for virulent organisms. Finally, tissue inflammation and ischemia affect the GI tract requiring appropriate management to avoid exacerbation.

Typhlitis/Neutropenic Enterocolitis

Typhlitis describes a syndrome of gastrointestinal inflammatory conditions characterized by segmental ulceration and necrotizing inflammation of the terminal ileum, cecum, and/or ascending colon in neutropenic patients [39]. This syndrome, also referred to as neutropenic enterocolitis, ileocecal syndrome, cecitis, necrotizing enterocolitis, and agranulocytic colitis, was initially described as necrotizing cecal enteropathy in children undergoing chemotherapy for leukemia or lymphoma [40]. Typhlitis is the most common gastrointestinal infection involving neutropenic patients with incidence reaching 5.3 % in patients undergoing systemic chemotherapy and in aplastic anemia [41]. Pathogenesis of this syndrome is related to cytotoxic mucosal injury during chemotherapy that affects the immunological surface barriers resulting in bacterial and toxin translocation into the submucosa with corresponding inflammation, ulceration, and transmural necrosis [42]. This is complicated by multiple factors including neutropenia, poor host defenses against gastrointestinal flora, and superimposed infection [43]. Regional preference for the cecum is related to decreased vascularity and increased concentration of lymphatic tissue.

Clinical presentation in a subset of patients includes the triad of right lower quadrant abdominal pain, fever and neutropenia along with non-specific symptoms of nausea, vomiting, abdominal distention, and watery or bloody diarrhea [44]. Physical examination is often non-specific with abdominal distention and pain localization to the right lower quadrant in 40–69 % of patients [45]. An acute abdomen is rarely the presenting symptom and high index of suspicion should be practiced to prevent complications in neutropenic patients presenting with abdominal pain. As clinical presentation is often vague, imaging studies such as computed tomography (CT) and ultrasound (US) increase the likelihood of diagnosis.

Transmural bowel wall thickening >10 mm has been associated with increased mortality and some authors have proposed thickening >4 mm as a diagnostic criteria in the setting of neutropenia, fever, and abdominal pain [46]. CT delivers the best evaluation of bowel wall thickening. CT with oral and intravenous contrast provides a detailed picture of bowel integrity, pneumatosis intestinalis, free air, and surrounding edema or hemorrhage [47]. Ultrasound can expedite diagnosis of typhlitis by demonstrating a doughnut-like, hypoechoic fluid filled intestinal lumen separated by a thickened hyperechoic mucosal wall [48]. Early inflammatory changes identified by ultrasound can expedite medical management and reduce operative indications especially in the pediatric population where radiation exposure is of concern. Plain radiography rarely provides additional information. The mortality rates of neutropenic patients necessitating surgery have been reported as high as 57 %; thus, medical management is often the recommended initial approach focusing on improving neutropenia, decreasing inflammation, and antibiotic therapy [43]. Further medical management includes bowel rest, nasogastric tube decompression, fluid resuscitation, and antipyretic therapy. Bone marrow stimulation should be considered per Infectious Disease Society of America guidelines for all neutropenic patients who fail to improve on initial broad-spectrum antibiotics, or have worsening neutropenia [49]. Surgical intervention is considered as a last resort therapy.

Surgical management is indicated for severe cases demonstrating free intraperitoneal air, uncontrolled sepsis based on large volume fluid resuscitation, continued gastrointestinal bleeding notwithstanding improvement of neutropenia, thrombocytopenia or coagulopathy, and overall clinical deterioration despite appropriate medical management [50]. Diagnostic laparoscopy has been reported to rule out other abdominal pathologies such as appendicitis and diverticulitis [42]. However, the value of diagnostic laparoscopy has yet to be established as normal serosa is often present despite mucosal necrosis [42]. If surgery is inevitable, then normalization or improvement of neutrophilic count must be sought preoperative to prevent and reduce surgical complications [51]. A right hemicolectomy with end ileostomy is generally the indicated procedure based upon the normal distribution of disease [52].

Cytomegalovirus (CMV) Gastrointestinal Manifestations

CMV is a DNA virus member of the herpes family with a 50–80 % prevalence in the general US population before age 40, with most of the infections occurring before age 20 and with the index infectious disease usually manifesting as a mild mononucleosis like illness [53]. In developing countries, CMV infection is almost universal. Initial acute systemic illness caused by CMV may be more severe in an immune compromised individual (e.g., in a CMV-negative transplant recipient who receives an organ from a CMV-positive donor). Following initial infection, the virus persists in a chronic latent state, with infection suppressed by an intact immune system [53]. Immunosuppressed states can lead to reactivation and infection [54], most often associated with HIV infection and pharmacologically immunosuppressed transplant recipients. Reactivation also occurs with rheumatologic and inflammatory bowel disease (IBD). Early diagnosis and treatment can expedite medical management and limit the progression of disease and the possible need for surgical management.

The clinical manifestation of CMV commonly includes the gastrointestinal tract, but the particular pattern of presentation is highly dependent on the particular immunosuppressed state. In HIV, patients frequently present with diarrhea due to CMV colitis [54]. HIV patients can also present with symptoms of esophagitis including odynophagia, dysphagia, or heartburn, as well as symptoms and complications of enteritis, such as abdominal pain, nausea, vomiting, GI bleeding, perforation, or diarrhea [54]. After solid organ transplantation, the incidence of CMV reaches 75 % within the first 6–12 months [55]. In this group, donor CMV seropositivity and recipient seronegativity are the most important risk factor for infection [55]. Symptoms suggestive of CMV commonly overlap with symptoms of organ rejection, leukopenia, or constitutional symptoms. Transplant patients also suffer from colitis and gastritis that can range from asymptomatic to hemorrhagic manifestations and/or perforation [52, 53]. In cancer patients, gastrointestinal CMV infection has an attributable mortality of 42 % [56]. Another group of patients that may be susceptible to superimposed CMV infection are those with IBD who may be refractory to medical treatment [57].

Diagnosis of CMV colitis can be challenging, as the presentation is often non-specific. Endoscopy with biopsy and histopathological identification remains the gold standard for diagnosis of CMV. The classic histological appearance is that of intranuclear inclusions with a surrounding halo, commonly having an "owl eye" appearance [58]. Intranuclear inclusions represent active viral replication. Sometimes, however, the endoscopy is normal requiring blind biopsy of multiple segments if the clinical suspicion is high. The CMV DNA test, quantitative PCR, and antigen testing, pp65, are used as markers of active infection [59]. PCR testing is preferred in immunocompromised patients for its ability to test patients with leukopenia, and the reliability as a diagnostic modality [59]. Although consensus about cutoffs for diagnosis with PCR and pp65 has not been achieved, viral culture of blood and urine is universally accepted to have minimal diagnostic value [59]. Imaging studies in CMV are often non-specific with CT revealing prominent circumferential bowel wall thickening with mesenteric stranding and deep ulcerations [60]. Regardless of the tests used to confirm CMV infection, accurate and timely diagnosis begins with consideration of the disease process.

Cytomegalovirus colitis can be focal, segmental, or generalized showing endoscopic findings of edematous mucosa, well-demarcated linear ulcerations, patchy erythema, or subepithelial hemorrhage [58]. On the other hand, CMV enteritis usually appears as a focal problem. Some reports of CMV enteritis have included small bowel perforation and severe hemorrhage [61, 62]. Failure to identify CMV enteritis can result in local and systemic disease such as viral syndrome and invasive disease including pneumonitis, retinitis, and CNS involvement (myelitis, encephalitis). CMV esophagitis occurs primarily in AIDS patients with CD count less than 50 cells/μl and patients with malignancies undergoing concurrent chemotherapy [63].

The primary treatment for gastrointestinal CMV should be prompt initiation of intravenous ganciclovir (5 mg/kg for 14–21 days) if disease is severe [64]. Oral valganciclovir (900 mg BID) has been shown to be as effective as IV ganciclovir for systemic treatment, but decreased bioavailability of 60 %, oral formulation variations and decreased absorption in GI disease limit its uses. Oral ganciclovir can be used as oral prophylaxis in solid organ transplant patients [59]. In transplanted patients, preemptive therapy has been shown to be as efficient as prophylaxis in CMV prevention. Preemptive therapy focuses on screening with CMV pp65 antigen or CMV viral load, and initiating treatment when evidence of viral replication is identified prior to symptom manifestation [64]. CMV resistance to ganciclovir can be identified by assays for resistance mutations. CMV ganciclovir resistance should prompt use of IV foscarnet therapy (90 mg/kg BID) [64]. Currently, several clinical trials are underway to assess the efficacy of CMV vaccines [59].

Acute abdominal presentations such as perforations and fulminant colitis are rare but share similarities to other etiologies of infectious colitides, including *C. difficile* colitis. The diagnosis can be particularly challenging in the setting of inflammatory bowel disease. Imaging, stool samples, and laboratories are inconclusive and should be avoided. Colonic perforation due to CMV infection has been associated with 87 % mortality [65, 66]. Given CMV's multifocal nature, surgical management must be individualized depending on gastrointestinal segment involvement. For instance, resection of distal small bowel perforation can be treated with end ostomy and mucus fistula or a right colectomy. Subsequent confirmatory laparotomies and imaging are helpful in excluding further gastrointestinal involvement [67]. High rates of complications are expected in these patients and emphasis on early detection is critical. Many surgical interventions can be avoided with timely and effective antiviral management.

Clostridium Difficile Infection

Clostridium difficile infection (CDI) is a major cause of acquired gastrointestinal disease and is the most common nosocomial pathogen in all patients. In the USA, CDI incidence in 2011 was estimated at 453,000, with 61,400 first recurrences, and 29,000 mortalities [68]. Clostridium difficile is an anaerobic, spore forming, toxin-producing, gram-positive bacillus that colonizes the GI tract [69]. Outside of the colon it exists in a spore form that is resistant to heat, acid, and antibiotics. *C. difficile* releases two toxins, an enterotoxin (toxin A) and the more potent and virulent cytotoxin (toxin B). These toxins affect intracellular cytoskeleton proteins, signaling pathways, and extracellular junctional proteins leading to inflammation, mucosal injury, and fluid secretion [69]. This leads to the clinical manifestations of diarrhea, often associated with elevated white blood cell counts. Host factors protecting against CDI include colonization by non-toxic producing species, antitoxin A antibody and IL-8 production [70]. Risk factors associated with CDI include antibiotic exposure, the use of proton pump inhibitors, GI surgery, and immunosuppression [71].

There are several diagnostic strategies available to determine CDI in the setting of the clinical diarrheal illness. Most recent guidelines for CDI diagnosis recommend using nucleic acid amplification tests (NAAT) to detect *C. difficile* toxin genes via PCR in symptomatic patients because of the relatively high sensitivity, specificity, and quick turnaround time [72]. NAAT are preferred over toxin A+B enzyme immunoassay (EIA) as these fail to capture certain strains that only produce toxin B. Immunocompromised patients should be screened for CDI at the earliest sign of diarrheal illness.

The classical presentation for CDI is a diarrhea illness ranging from mild to severe. Patients report anywhere from 10 to 15 episodes of daily watery diarrhea associated with abdominal pain, low-grade fever, and leukocytosis. Mild disease has been defined as CDI with diarrhea as the only presenting complaint [72]. Several attempts at developing severity-scoring criteria for CDI have been performed including the Hines VA, UPMC index, and Beth Israel, but validation is lacking [73]. Recent recommendations classify severe CDI as hypoalbuminemia (<3 g/dl), plus either white blood cell (WBC) counts >15,000 cell/mm^3 or abdominal distention. Additionally, complicated CDI or fulminant colitis is characterized by sepsis, fever ≥38.5 °C, WBC ≥35,000 cells/mm^3 or <2000 cell/mm^3, and serum lactate >2.2 mmol/l [72].

Medical treatment for CDI is largely dependent on severity (Table 22.6). Treatment for non-severe CDI should constitute of oral metronidazole for initial presentation or oral vancomycin for those patients who fail to respond after 5–7 days [72]. Randomized clinical trials have consistently demonstrated equivalent efficacy between both therapies for non-severe disease. Oral/enteral/rectal vancomycin is not absorbed and achieves maximal concentration locally, while metronidazole may be delivered by oral or parenteral routes. Repeat stool assays to track progress of disease are not warranted as assays can remain positive up to 6 weeks after treatment completion [72].

Severe disease presents with signs of systemic toxicity, hypoalbuminemia, and abdominal distention with the presence or absence of diarrhea. The standard of therapy in severe disease is oral vancomycin [72]. Vancomycin enemas are advised for patients unable to tolerate an oral regimen, or with significant abdominal distention. In the case of ileus, patients have delayed passage of oral antibiotics, thereby reducing efficacy of treatment. Fidaxomicin (200 mg BID for 10 days) can be used as alternative treatment to vancomycin in patients with severe disease who fail to respond to initial management and those patients with suspected higher rate of recurrence [74, 75].

Table 22.6 CDI severity criteria and recommended treatment [72]

CDI severity	Criteria	Treatment
Mild–moderate	Diarrhea	Metronidazole 500 mg PO TID for 10d or vancomycin 125 mg PO QID for 10d
Severe disease	Serum albumin <3 g/dl and WBC >15,0000 cells/ml or abdominal distention	Vancomycin 125 mg PO QID for 10d
Complicated (fulminant)	CDI with any of the following: ICU admission for CDI hypotension (±vasopressor), temperature >38.5, abdominal distention or ileus, end organ dysfunction, or AMS WBC >35,000 or <2000 cells/ml, and serum lactate >2.2 mmol/l	Vancomycin 500 mg PO QID + metronidazole 500 mg IV q8h + vancomycin enemas (500 mg vancomycin in 500 ml saline) +surgical consultation
Recurrent	CDI within 8 weeks of therapy	Repeat metronidazole, pulse vancomycin consider FMT after 3 recurrences

AMS Altered mental status; *CDI* Clostridium difficile infection; *ICU* Intensive care unit; *PO* Per os; *TID* Ter in die; *QID* Quarter in die

Colonoscopy can reveal a non-specific or pseudomembranous colitis described as raised and adherent yellow plaques. Pseudomembranous formation occurs from toxin-related endothelial damage resulting in local epithelial necrosis, neutrophil migration, and collection of cellular debris [76]. CT imaging, showing thickened colonic wall, is of limited diagnostic value but can be used in severe CDI for disease monitoring [77].

Recurrent CDI (RCDI) is a well-established problem, usually occurring within 8 weeks of initial therapy in up to 35 % of patients who present with an initial episode of CDI [78]. The etiology of recurrence is unknown, but change in the colonic microbiota or infection with another clostridium species has been hypothesized [78]. Management of first recurrence should be treated with vancomycin. A second relapse should be treated with pulsed vancomycin regimen (standard dosing followed by 125 mg vancomycin every 3 days for 10 doses). Fidaxomicin has an emerging role in the treatment of recurrences. In the setting of a third recurrence, fecal microbiota transplant (FMT) should be considered. FMT therapy consists of repopulating the microbiome using healthy donor stool into gastrointestinal tract of patients with RCDI [79].

Immunocompromised patients are at high risk of CDI particularly due to frequent hospitalizations, as well as chronic antibiotic and cytotoxic drug treatment. Any evidence of diarrhea should prompt immediate testing for CDI and institution of empiric treatment in the setting of high clinical suspicion. A recent study demonstrated that FMT therapy in the immunocompromised patient resulted in effective management with no serious adverse effects [80]. However, skepticism exists about the transfer of pathogens into immunosuppressed patients.

Surgical consultation for CDI is recommended for complicated disease. Indications for surgery include clinical deterioration despite appropriate treatment after 5 days, hypotension requiring vasopressor support, sepsis, WBC ≥50,000 cells/mm^3, or lactate >5 mmol/l as these patients have shown to have mortality ranging from 35 to 80 % [72]. Fulminant CDI usually involves the entire colon and subtotal colectomy with end ileostomy has been the standard of care. Alternatively, recent evidence evaluated the effect of laparoscopic loop ileostomy with intraoperative lavage (polyethylene glycol 3350/balanced electrolyte solution) and postoperative anterograde colonic vancomycin flushes through ileostomy, which resulted in reduced mortality when compared to colectomy and colon preservation in 93 % of cases [81]. Predictors of postoperative mortality after surgery for fulminant colitis include Age ≥80, thrombocytopenia (<150,000 cells/ mm^3), INR >2, BUN >40 mg/dl, severe COPD, preoperative shock, dialysis dependence, and cardiac arrest [82]. In these patients, aggressive medical management and careful preoperative counseling are advised.

Lastly, prevention and infection control of CDI are the cornerstone of incidence reduction. All patients with suspected CDI must undergo screening and confirmatory testing as previously discussed. Patients testing positive should be placed in contact precautions and isolation [83]. Additionally, healthcare professionals must practice hand hygiene, barrier precautions, and disinfection of the patient environment to prevent dispersion [84]. Alcohol-based hand hygiene does not eradicate *C. diff* spores; thus, use of soap and water is the only proven method to decrease spreading the disease.

Bacterial Infections: Staphylococcus, Klebsiella, and Yersinia

Several pathogens may result in acute diarrheal illness in the inpatient setting including, *Staphylococcus aureus*, *Clostridium perfringens*, *Klebsiella oxytoca,* and enteropathogenic species such as *Salmonella*, *Campylobacter*, enterohemorrhagic *Escherichia coli*, and *Yersinia* [85]. These species are an important source of morbidity among the immunocompromised patients. However, clinicians must be aware that many causes of diarrhea in these immunocompromised populations are non-infectious in nature and causes include antineoplastic agents, medications, enteral feeding and underlying disease and must be considered in addition to pursuing infectious causes [86]. Reports validating guidelines for stool culture testing recommend individualized management in immunosuppressed patients.

Diarrhea from gastrointestinal flora imbalance is common among immunosuppressed patients [85]. In neutropenic patients, gram-negative bacteremia from presumed gastrointestinal sources is common. Prophylactic use of fluoroquinolones can be beneficial for patients who have recently undergone allogeneic hematopoietic stem cell transplants (HSCT). Chemotherapy-induced viridian-group streptococcal infection can present as a toxic shock syndrome. While fluoroquinolones have been demonstrated to be effective at controlling GI flora, some centers have instituted parenteral vancomycin treatment in attempts to reduce the incidence of infection [85]. Vancomycin-resistant enterococcus (VRE) is rising as the most common blood stream infection in preengraftment stem cell transplant neutropenic patients. In these patients, careful selection of antibiotics that minimizes antianaerobic activity may be effective [85].

Staphylococcus aureus produces enterotoxins (A, C, D, and leucotoxins) and is an important cause of food poisoning [87]. Colonization levels with *S. aureus* rise during hospitalizations and are associated with procedures such as nasogastric tube feeding. A study reported *S. aureus* as a cause of nosocomial diarrhea in 7.3 % of cases, with *Clostridium difficile* coinfection and oxacillin-resistant species occurring in 14.6 % [88]. Similarities to CDI were also seen under endoscopy, with a yellow green pseudomembrane that was easily removed from the mucosa [88]. Interestingly, S. aureus was more commonly isolated from the small bowel, but reports of colitis are not uncommon. Other reports investigating MRSA-associated diarrhea have isolated MRSA from stool cultures in the absence of common enteropathogens (viruses, parasites, and *C. difficile*). This report concluded that testing stool cultures for *S. aureus* in cases of negative CDI may be warranted in immunosuppressed patients [89]. More studies are needed to validate this conclusion.

Klebsiella oxytoca is a gram-negative bacterium implicated in cases of antibiotic-associated hemorrhagic colitis in the absence of CDI [90]. Patients present with abdominal pain and bloody diarrhea in the setting of recent exposure to β-lactam antibiotics and NSAIDs. This organism is most commonly found in the ascending colon, similar to enterohemorrhagic *E. coli* and induces cytotoxin-mediated mucosal damage [91]. Endoscopic findings reveal mucosal edema without evidence of pseudomembranes and segmental hemorrhagic colitis with rectal sparing [90]. *Klebsiella oxytoca* produces β-lactamases resulting in resistance to penicillin and cephalosporins. Simultaneous use of NSAIDs is often reported with development of K. *oxytoca* diarrhea, but the implications of this finding are not known. Treatment for *K. oxytoca*-associated diarrhea includes cessation of antibiotics and NSAIDs. Patients presenting with hemorrhagic colitis with negative screen for CDI should undergo testing for *K. oxytoca.*

Yersinia enterocolitica is an uncommon gastrointestinal pathogen, presenting with abdominal tenderness and diarrhea. *Y. enterocolitica* has been associated with erythema nodosum, Reiter's syndrome, myocarditis, pneumonia, acute renal failure, meningitis, and sepsis [92]. The presence of high-iron environment, low temperature, and high pH stimulates *Yersinia* growth [92]. Not surprisingly, *Y. enterocolitica* septicemia has been associated with iron overload, hemochromatosis, elevated aluminum, chronic liver disease, and diabetes which are frequently present in immunocompromised patients [92]. In transplant patients, treatment with high-dose steroids and OKT3 for steroid-resistant rejection has also been implicated with *Yersinia* infection [92].

Parasitic Infections

Microsporidia are obligated intracellular and spore forming parasites with fungal characteristics that represent a common cause of chronic diarrhea [93].

Pathogenesis involves a spore with the capacity of forming a polar filament and transferring cellular contents to achieve local and systemic infection [93]. Transmission occurs via fecal–oral, waterborne, or airborne route. There are 14 microsporidium pathogenic to humans, of which *Encephalitozoon* and *Enterocytozoon* are the most common.

Microsporidia-induced illness presents with watery diarrhea, wasting, and abdominal pain. In HIV patients, the parasite has a predilection for villous epithelial cells of the small intestine causing atrophy and crypt hyperplasia, reducing the surface area [94]. Disseminated infection may manifest as encephalitis, pneumonitis, hepatitis, myositis, or nephritis [94]. Infection in renal transplant patients and disseminated disease in hematopoietic transplant has been reported. Microsporidium can be detected as spores in feces, body fluids, or biopsy specimens. Less specific detection can be achieved by serology, trichome stain, or immunofluorescence [94]. Treatment with albendazole (400 mg twice daily) is effective against most species, but fumagillin (60 mg/day) should be used in cases of *E. bieneusi* infection [95].

Strongyloides stercoralis is another opportunistic parasite that may cause serious repercussions in solid organ transplant recipients [96]. The parasite migrates through the skin, it is transported through the circulatory system as a larvae, establishes itself in the lungs, ascends through the tracheobronchial tree, and it is swallowed and migrates to the small intestine where it invades the mucosa [96]. Infection screening guidelines for *S. stercoralis* is only recommended for living and high-risk patients who have traveled to endemic area in the Caribbean, Central America, Southeast Asia, Africa, Europe, UK, and southeastern USA [96]. Donor patients can be asymptomatic, but *S. stercoralis* infection can induce hyperinfection and disseminated disease in recipients affecting the skin, cardiovascular and CNS [96]. Respiratory infection and distress are often common. A positive pretransplant screen for *S. stercoralis* with enzyme immunoassay has a sensitivity of 90 % and specificity of 99 % [96]. Testing for stool ova and parasite is only effective during larval shedding and may otherwise yield false-negative results. Diagnosis should prompt treatment with thiabendazole or ivermectin [96]. Subsequent immunosuppression with cyclosporin has been shown to reduce hyperinfection.

Helicobacter Pylori

Helicobacter pylori is a gram-negative, microaerophilic, spiral-shaped organism that uses adhesion proteins, flagella, cellular toxins, and urease to invade the gastric mucosa [97]. *H. pylori* has been implicated in numerous of gastrointestinal disorders including gastritis, peptic ulcer disease, gastric adenocarcinoma, and mucosa-associated lymphoid tissue (MALT) lymphoma. Global prevalence of *H. pylori* is associated with low socioeconomic status, and initial infection often occurs in childhood [97]. *H. Pylori* seropositive transplant patients have an increased risk for developing peptic ulcer disease [98]. Prevalence in renal transplant patients ranges from 29 to 70 % depending on the country of origin [98]. However, evidence of spontaneous conversion to seronegative status has been reported in part due to chronic antibiotic use, chemotherapy agents or both [98]. Incidence of gastrointestinal complications has been reported at 20 % after renal transplantation. Nonetheless, screening for H. pylori infection with noninvasive testing such as urea breath test (UBT), fecal antigen test, or serology is recommended for all transplant patients [98]. Appropriate treatment with antibiotics (clarithromycin 500 mg BID and amoxicillin 1000 mg BID or metronidazole 500 mg BID if penicillin allergy exists) and proton pump inhibitor (esomeprazole 40 mg QD) should be instituted followed by confirmation of eradication [99]. *H. pylori* eradication can be confirmed with UBT, fecal antigen test, or upper endoscopy performed four weeks after treatment completion [99]. Serology testing should be avoided for confirmation as antigens may remain positive for up to 6 months after treatment.

Infectious Esophagitis

Odynophagia is the most common presentation of esophagitis, but retrosternal chest pain, reflux, and fever have also been reported [100]. Both Herpes and Candida are causes of esophagitis in the immunocompromised host.

Herpes simplex virus (HSV) is a DNA virus with predilection for mucosal surfaces. The two described viruses, HSV-1 and HSV-2, show tropism for specific tissue types and generally have different transmission routes [101]. HSV-1 affects mostly the oral mucosa and infection is established early in life. Its prevalence has reached approximately 90 % in the general population. On the other hand, HSV-2 has 20 % prevalence in the USA and produces most cases of genital herpes [101]. Both viruses establish a latent infection in the dorsal root ganglion. During reactivation, the virus has predilection for squamous epithelia, which is problematic in the immunocompromised host.

Of the HSV viruses, HSV-1 is the most commonly isolated from esophagitis in transplant and HIV patients, but HSV-2 has occasionally been reported [100]. Esophagitis in HIV qualifies as an AIDS defining diagnosis and occurs prominently when CD4 count falls below 50 cells/μl. HSV esophagitis in AIDS patients has been complicated by esophageal perforation and transesophageal fistulas [100]. In transplant patients, HSV presents within the first 6-week post-transplantation as a complication of pharmacological management of acute rejection, often with immunosuppression with high-dose steroids and antilymphocyte agents.

Candida is a yeast and is considered a normal component of gastrointestinal flora. Candida infection most often occurs as a result of bacterial flora eradication due to antibiotics. CD4 T-cell reduction plays an important role in gastrointestinal defense against Candida species. Patients with AIDS have a lifetime incidence of 10–15 % [102]. Patients on chronic inhaled steroids or those with hematologic malignancies are also at an increased risk for infection [103, 104]. *Candida albicans* remains the most commonly isolated species in esophagitis, but increased frequency of non-albicans species has been isolated from HIV-infected individuals [102]. Patients often present with odynophagia, dysphagia, and retrosternal pain, but asymptomatic presentation is not uncommon. Frequently, candida esophagitis rises from oropharyngeal spread, but the esophagus may be the only site involved in 10 % of cases. Esophageal infection of the distal esophagus is the most commonly involved segment. Reports of severe infections with necrotizing component, perforations, and fistulas are concerning and emphasize the need for early diagnosis [105].

Endoscopy with tissue biopsy is the gold standard for diagnosis of esophagitis as well as establishing the pathogen associated with the clinical disease. In HSV infection, esophagoscopy often reveals well-circumscribed ulcers with a superficial, "volcano-like" appearance, as well as white exudates and intervening friable mucosa often localizing to the distal esophagus [106]. Biopsy must be obtained from the edge of the ulcer as the center lacks squamous epithelium and histopathology reveals the characteristic Cowdry type A inclusion bodies [106]. HSV viral cultures of samples and polymerase chain reaction (PCR) can reliably detect infection from tissue samples, but more research is needed to identify their utility.

Treatment for HSV esophagitis consists of oral acyclovir (400 mg) for 14–21 days [107]. Patients with severe odynophagia may require admission for alimentation and hydration. Parenteral acyclovir (5 mg/kg) for 7–14 days should be administered [107]. Failure to improve with the previous therapy may indicate antiviral resistance. If this is the case, treatment with foscarnet can be implemented.

Endoscopic biopsy is the gold standard for diagnosing candida esophagitis. Endoscopic findings include white mucosal plaques, and biopsy reveals yeast with pseudohyphae invading the mucosal cells. An alternative practical approach routinely utilized in AIDS patients, due to the invasive nature of endoscopies, includes initiation of systemic antifungal treatment with expected symptomology improvement in 3–5 days [102]. A lack of improvement requires esophagogastroduodenoscopy (EGD) and biopsy. Antifungal treatment reduces the signs and symptoms of infection; however, this therapy often does not lead to complete eradication leading to common recurrences and resistance among immunocompromised patients. Fluconazole (200–400 mg) for 3 weeks is preferred for its increased clinical response and reduced relapse rates [102]. In refractory cases, other preparations and antifungals can be used such as ketoconazole and voriconazole. Topical agents such as nystatin, clotrimazole, and miconazole are not effective in esophageal candidiasis and must be avoided.

Gastrointestinal Complications of Antivascular Endothelial Growth Factor Therapy

Angiogenesis plays a critical role in tumor development, progression, and metastases. Rapidly progressive tumors activate pro-angiogenic factors such as vascular endothelial growth factor (VEGF) [108]. Anti-VEGF agents such as bevacizumab increase survival and reduce metastases progression of oncologic pathologies such as colorectal, breast, ovarian, renal, and advanced non-small cell lung cancer. The effectiveness of these medications results from decreased vasculature, tumor regression, and more effective chemotherapy agent delivery [108]. Bevacizumab carries a dose- and tumor-dependent risk for gastrointestinal (GI) perforation with incidence reaching 1.5 % [109]. Mortality is higher if perforation occurs in patients on anti-VEGF therapy [109]. Perforations can occur throughout the GI tract and are related to tumor necrosis, diverticulitis, ulceration, obstruction, and colitis [110]. Increased incidence of perforation may result from inhibition of nitric oxide leading to vasoconstriction, impaired healing of inflammatory processes (ulcers, colitis, etc.) and wound healing resulting in microperforations. Risk factors resulting in perforation include recent instrumentation (colonoscopy, sigmoidoscopy), gastrointestinal obstruction, radiation exposure, surgery, tumor resection, and diverticulitis. The Food and Drug Administration recommends stopping anti-VEGF agents in the setting of intestinal perforation; however, findings from multiple studies favor an individualized approach considering risks and benefits on a case-by-case basis.

Skin and Soft Tissue Infections

Skin and soft tissue infections (SSTIs) are superficial infections involving the skin, subcutaneous tissue, muscle, and fascia. SSTIs range from simple and localized disease to deep infections with the ability to spread systemically causing widespread necrosis, septic shock, and death [111].

Cellulitis and Abscess

The IDSA classifies all immunocompromised patients presenting with skin and soft tissue infections (SSTIs) as severely infected and requiring hospitalization [111]. These patients may harbor an infection without appropriately mounting an immune response; thus, blood cultures, empiric antimicrobial therapy, and early surgical intervention are essential early management strategies [111]. Early incision and drainage of abscesses to obtain culture and sensitivity data are essential for identification and appropriate treatment of the causative bacterial, fungal, or viral organisms. Unlike in immunocompetent hosts where antibiotic therapy for simple abscesses is not necessary, treatment with antibiotics in immunosuppressed patients is recommended [111]. Among neutropenic patients, fungal infections with *Candida, Aspergillus, and Mucor/Rhizopus* are common entities of SSTIs. These infections can present with persistent or recurrent fever and empiric antifungal therapy with echinocandin or amphotericin B plus fluconazole should be instituted.

Polymerase chain reaction for viral entities (VZV, HSV) is recommended for unexplained lesions and negative cultures.

The astute clinician must keep a broad differential in the setting of immunosuppressed patients presenting with symptoms suggestive of an SSTI. Consideration of drug eruption or adverse reaction, cutaneous infiltration of malignancy and radiation-induced reaction may manifest as skin changes that may appear similar to superficial infections [111]. Graft-versus-host disease (GVHD) in patients with allogeneic transplant can present similarly. Sweet syndrome or acute febrile neutrophilic dermatosis develops in patients with leukemia [111]. This syndrome is characterized by erythematous skin lesions, easily mistaken for cellulitis, following chemotherapy or treatment with methylating agents [112]. Sweet syndrome responds to systemic corticosteroid therapy and does not require surgical intervention. In patients with immunodeficiency, a prompt biopsy and histological evaluation along with specialist consultation can yield a diagnosis of unclear skin findings.

Necrotizing Soft Tissue Infections

Necrotizing soft tissue infections (NSTI) are characterized by rapidly progressive fulminant soft tissue destruction and symptoms of systemic infection. NSTI are uncommon infections with a high incidence of mortality requiring prompt recognition, surgical intervention, and broad antibiotic management.

Classification of NSTI based on the tissue involvement includes necrotizing cellulitis, fasciitis, myositis, or Fournier's gangrene, which involves the perineum and genitals. Necrotizing fasciitis most commonly affects the lower extremities in 58 % of cases and has a mortality ranging from 6 to 76 % [113]. Similarly, Fournier's gangrene has a mortality ranging from 20 to 50 %. Fournier's gangrene can spread to the rectum, retroperitoneum, abdominal wall, lower extremities, and gluteal areas and is often polymicrobial in nature [113].

In addition to location, causal microorganisms can be used to classify NSTIs. Type 1 infections are most common and polymicrobial. Type 2 infections involve colonization by group β-hemolytic streptococci or community acquired MRSA, and type 3 infections are the result of gram-negative bacilli [113]. The release of bacterial toxins in a closed compartment results in necrosis, ischemia, and septic shock once toxins are released systemically. Laboratory values and CT scoring systems have been developed for earlier recognition of NSTIs. CT findings with high specificity for NSTIs include perifascial air, muscle/fascial edema, fluid tracking, lymphadenopathy, and subcutaneous edema [114]. Ultrasound can be effectively used to diagnose soft tissue infections, with findings of cobble stones and fluid accumulation greater than 4 mm may be indicative of NSTI [115].

Time to surgical debridement has been consistently found to be a key prognostic factor of morbidity and mortality in the setting of NSTI. Surgical debridement should be extensive enough to encompass all necrotic tissue, generally requiring an initial incision that extends beyond indurated or cellulitic skin changes [115].

Aggressive initial debridement with subsequent "second look" surgeries for follow-up and final debridement are often required [115]. Notably, postoperative clinical deterioration suggests that the infection has not been eradicated and frequently mandates emergent surgery. In the setting of Fournier's gangrene, fecal diversion through diverting colostomy minimizes bacterial load and reinfection. This, in turn, reduces the number of debridements required to achieve infection control. Alternatively, rectal diversion devices such as silicon catheters may reduce the need for surgical diversion and colostomy [115]. Broad-spectrum antibiotics should be initiated as soon as infection is suspected.

Detecting NSTI's in immunosuppressed patients can be clinically challenging and confounding physical examination findings may delay diagnosis. NSTI's in immunosuppressed patients can present with classic findings of erythema, fluctuance, and crepitus. However, they are frequently afebrile, lack purulent discharge, and fail to mount an appropriate immune response resulting in decreased WBC counts [116]. Multiple comorbidities in immunosuppressed patients may result in medical rather than surgical admission, delaying the diagnosis of NSTI and time to surgical debridement which has been demonstrated to increase mortality by up to 20 % [116]. High suspicion for NSTI in immunocompromised patients should encourage prompt surgical consultation to increase the likelihood of timely intervention.

Surgical Considerations in Immunosuppressed Patient

Perioperative Management of Immunosuppression

Preoperative planning in immunosuppressed patients is an important first step in identifying operative risk factors such as comorbidities, functional status, and medication information including side effect profile, dosage and length of treatment that may ultimately alter perioperative course.

Steroids

Appropriate perioperative management of steroids in patients receiving chronic systemic steroids is essential for avoiding steroid-related intraoperative and postoperative complications. As previously discussed, early side effects of chronic corticosteroid therapy includes glucose intolerance, avascular necrosis, immunosuppression, and subsequent heightened infection risk. Late manifestations include cushingoid changes, hypertension, cardiovascular disease, muscle wasting, and osteoporosis. Preoperative assessment of patients receiving glucocorticoid therapy should take into consideration the amount and duration of steroid treatment, clinical

Table 22.7 Recommended intraoperative steroid dosing for patients with HPA suppression

Surgical Stress	Intraoperative	Postoperative
Minor procedures, surgery under local anesthesia, EBL <500 ml (IHR, I&D, arthroscopy)	Continue morning dosing, no extradosing	Continue current regimen
Moderate stress, EBL 500–1500 ml (hysterectomy, orthopedic procedures, laparoscopic procedures, GI resection)	Continue morning dose + 50 mg; hydrocortisone IV preoperative	25 mg hydrocortisone IV q8h for 24 h, no taper, continue regular dosing
Major stress, EBL >1500 ml (GI cancer resection, CPB, intracranial, major vascular procedure, expected ICU)	Continue morning dose + 100 mg; hydrocortisone IV preoperative	50 mg hydrocortisone IV q8h for 24 h, taper by half per day until maintenance level

CPB Surgery on cardiopulmonary bypass; *EBL* Estimated blood loss; *GI* Gastrointestinal; *ICU* Intensive care unit; *I&D* Incision and debridement; *IHR* Inguinal hernia repair

evidence of hypothalamus–pituitary axis (HPA) dysfunction and the anticipated surgical stress and length of procedure [117].

Stress doses of steroids (25–100 mg) are considered the standard of practice in the prevention of adrenal insufficiency postoperative. Recent evidence suggests simply restarting the prescribed dosage for patients on chronic steroid regimens in specific situations [118]. For instance, patients taking prednisone (5 mg daily or 10 mg every other day) or equivalent steroids are considered to have a normal HPA axis and should be continued on regular schedule throughout perioperative period [119]. Conversely, patients with a suppressed HPA axis would benefit from supplemental perioperative steroids. These patients include anyone taking 20 mg prednisone daily (or equivalent), as well as those with Cushing's syndrome [119]. The recommended stress dose depends on procedure length and anticipated surgical stress (Table 22.7). Patients with an intermediate risk of HPA suppression may benefit from a formal evaluation of HPA axis. Obtaining morning cortisol levels or ACTH stimulation tests are the recommended screening methods [119]. In the setting of perioperative hypotension, adrenal insufficiency should be suspected as the cause and treated accordingly with steroids if other causes of hypotension have been ruled out. Additionally, preoperative assessment of cardiovascular risk factors is beneficial to avoid postoperative acute coronary syndromes induced by surgical stress [120].

Biologic Therapies

Biologic therapy is often considered second line in RA and other autoimmune disorders, and the clinical utility of this drug class continues to rise with pharmaceutical advancement and drug development. Knowledge of biologic therapy indications, half-life, adverse effects, and length of treatment is important to avoid surgical complications. Surgeons are encouraged to delay surgery and develop a high index of suspicion for atypical signs of infection as it may be masked in this patient population.

The major side effect of anti-TNF-α therapy is increased risk of infection including bacterial, opportunistic infection and tuberculosis reactivation. Incidentally, the risk of gram-positive sepsis is increased. Evidence regarding perioperative management of TNF antagonists suggests that procedure complexity may influence surgical outcomes, with low-risk orthopedic procedures considered safe and extensive abdominal surgery experiencing anastomotic leaks, dehiscence, and impaired wound healing. Thus, TNF antagonists should be stopped at least 4 weeks prior to surgery whenever possible [121].

Interleukin-1 inhibitors like Anakinra are associated with fairly common injection site soft tissue infections. Preclinical models of IL-1 inhibitor show inhibition of angiogenesis, collagen deposition, and fibrosis, which may impact wound healing. Interleukin inhibitors have few clinical utilities and should be stopped at least one week prior to surgery [122]. Rituximab is implicated in reactivations of HBV and JC virus infection [122]. When possible, surgery should be delayed until B cell counts (CD 19+ cell counts) improve but rituximab therapy is not a contraindication to surgery [122].

Risk of Infectious Complications

Surgical Site Infection

Surgical site infections (SSI) are any infections occurring within 30 days of surgical intervention or 90 days of prosthetic implant. The incidence of SSI's varies with incisional depth and whether the surgical procedure is superficial or deep [123]. The CDC has established guidelines for the management and treatment of SSI [123]. Predictors of SSI include wound classification, as well as patient and operative risk factors that are summarized in Table 22.8 [124]. SSI is among the most common form of hospital-acquired infections with an incidence as high as 17 % of all nosocomial infections [124]. Appropriate interventions to reduce risk factors must be undertaken to improve surgical outcomes.

In the immunosuppressed patient, the risk of SSI can be reduced by optimizing immunosuppression status, considering the dosing and length of immunosuppressive agents, and appropriately managing comorbidities such as diabetes and obesity. In cancer patients, increased incidence of SSI has been associated with duration of surgery beyond 5 h, presence of remote infection at time of surgery, use of abdominal drains, and a duration of prehospital stay longer than 22 days [125]. In renal transplant patients, BMI >30 kg/m^2 at the time of surgery has been found to be a strong indicator of SSI. Other studies in renal transplant patients have identified

Table 22.8 Patient and operative risk factors influencing surgical site infections [124]

Patient risk factors	Operative risk factors
Age: >65	Duration of surgery
Malnutrition	Infection control strategies
Diabetes: glucose >200 mg/dl 48 h preoperative	Preoperative hair removal: shaving
Coexisting infection: remote site, skin	Preoperative preparation: skin antisepsis, surgical scrub
Obesity	Length of surgery
Smoking	Inadequate instrument sterilization
Microbe colonization: nasal *S. aureus*	Surgical drains: separate incision
Immunosuppression	Surgical site foreign body
Preoperative length of stay	Operating room environment: ventilation
Preoperative transfusion	Surgical technique: poor hemostasis, tissue trauma, failure to obliterate dead space, excessive electrocautery

a possible link with acute graft rejection, diabetes, and sirolimus regimens as indicators of SSI [126]. Immunosuppression in HIV patients has been associated with increased postoperative infections as previously discussed. Among HIV-positive patients, the incidence of SSI can reach as high as 47.5 % and up to 88 % in cases involving contaminated wounds. Risk factors associated with SSI in HIV patients include a low CD4 count (CD <200 cells/mm^3), preoperative hypoalbuminemia, and postoperative anemia [127]. Preoperative hypoalbuminemia has also been found as independent risk factor for SSI in women undergoing abdominal hysterectomy [128]. Finally, appropriate antibiotic coverage depending on wound classification should be implemented.

Steroid immunosuppression is formulated through inhibition of cytokine release resulting in substandard inflammatory and febrile response. The associated risk infections with steroid use are proportional to dose and length of use [129]. Viral, bacterial, and fungal infections are common, but opportunistic infections should not be expected unless simultaneous immunosuppression through another process is present.

Anastomotic Complications

Anastomotic complications are a known complication of gastrointestinal and colorectal surgery and are associated with increased morbidity and mortality. Anastomosis breakdown results in complications such as bleeding, strictures, fistulas, dehiscence, and leaks. Anastomotic leakage incidence has ranged from 3 to 19 % with a mortality reaching 20 % in some cases [130]. Features of a successful anastomosis include appropriate blood flow, lack of tension, and decreased risk of infection source. Additionally, low-lying anastomosis at the anal verge and extraperitoneal anastomosis carry an increased risk of complications [130]. Risk factors for anastomosis break down include male sex, smoking, radiotherapy, blood transfusion, and obesity [130]. The role or association of immunosuppressive medications regimen have not been thoroughly investigated in the setting of anastomotic complications.

The effect of corticosteroids on wound healing is a well-known side effect, mainly due to reduction of inflammatory cells such as macrophages and polymorphonuclear cells as well as reduction of cytokine responsible for activating collagen synthesis [131]. Chronic steroid use for longer than 30 days has been shown to impair wound healing from two- to fivefold, but acute high doses taken for less than 10 days appear to be safe [132]. Similarly, steroids have an increased risk of anastomotic leaks when compared to steroid naive patients (6.8 % vs. 3.3 %) [131]. Other agents implicated in wound healing include antiproliferative agents such as sirolimus. These agents appear to have an increased incidence of wound dehiscence with high-dose regimens [33]. Cessation or reduction of dosing is recommended two to four months prior to surgery; however, more studies are needed to arrive at concrete recommendations [33].

Immunosuppressed patients must be carefully evaluated for anastomotic complications in the immediate and late postoperative period. Clinicians must be vigilant for clinical signs of anastomotic break down such as pain, fever, peritonitis, and radiographic evidence of fluid or gas collections.

Summary

The immunosuppressed patient represents a heterogeneous population with chronic comorbidities. The immunocompromised state may profoundly influence surgical outcomes. When possible, medical optimization of immunosuppressed patients will decrease surgical burden. Surgical complications can be reduced or avoided with appropriate perioperative planning and optimization.

Surgical diseases in the immunosuppressed patients are inclusive of those in immune-competent patients plus the additional risks associated with compromise of the immune system. Many of the infectious diseases associated with the immunocompromised state can be managed medically, but a key to successful management, both medically and surgically, is early consideration and diagnosis.

Clinical Scenario

A 43-year-old woman at 2 weeks s/p starting induction chemotherapy for AML develops severe right-sided and right lower quadrant pain with WBC 0.5 and ANC of 1. Computerized tomography demonstrates severe cecal thickening and stranding.

The scenario represents a real challenge in the immunosuppressed patient. The leading differential diagnoses include typhlitis or neutropenic enterocolitis, or other infectious colitides such as Clostridium difficile infection, other bacterial infections, or CMV colitis. However, given the neutropenia and localization of the disease process to the cecum, the diagnosis of typhlitis should be the leading differential diagnosis.

This should be considered an oncologic emergency and requires multimodal management between medical and surgical teams. The initial management is mainly supportive and would include transfer to a medical unit that would allow for close observation and neutropenic contact precautions, intravenous fluids, bowel rest, nasogastric tube suction if there is abdominal distention, and rapid initiation of empiric antibiotics. Intravenous antibiotic regimens should include coverage of enteric gram-negative and anaerobic bacterial organisms, including clostridium species. Due to the prevalence of Clostridium difficile infection, inclusion of intravenous metronidazole or oral vancomycin should be added until this disease is ruled out. Avoidance of agents that suppress gastrointestinal motility should be considered. Blood cultures should be obtained for bacteria and fungus. If there is a lack of response to antibacterial agents, antifungal regimens should be added early.

These patients often require support with blood component transfusions including packed red blood cells and platelet transfusions. The use of granulocyte colony-stimulating factor (GCSF) is not proven; however, many advocate for the use in these patients as resolution of the disease often mirrors the resolution of neutropenia. There is a hypothetical concern about increasing inflammation and exacerbating obstruction with the use of GCSF.

Surgery is not often required in these patients and is only utilized when medical management fails. However, surgical consultation should be obtained immediately in patients with typhlitis, as early recognition of failure of medical therapy and surgical resection is associated with improved outcomes versus surgical consultation and therapy as a late salvage approach. Indications for surgery include gross perforation, ongoing hemorrhage despite correction of thrombocytopenia and coagulopathies, ongoing obstruction, peritonitis with sepsis, or fistula formation with sepsis. Typical surgical management involves segmental resection of the involved segment, most often an ileocecal resection or right hemicolectomy, and creation of an end ileostomy. Restoration of gastrointestinal continuity with anastomosis should be deferred in this setting. In some cases, where resection may not be indicated, proximal diversion of the fecal stream with loop ileostomy may be of benefit.

References

1. Hall HI, An Q, Tang T, Song R, Chen M, Green T, et al. Prevalence of diagnosed and undiagnosed HIV infection-United States, 2008–2012. MMWR Morb Mortal Wkly Rep. 2015;64(24):657–62.
2. Maartens G, Celum C, Lewin SR. HIV infection: epidemiology, pathogenesis, treatment, and prevention. Lancet. 2014;384(9939):258–71.
3. Kaplan JE, Benson C, Holmes KK, Brooks JT, Pau A, Masur H. Guidelines for prevention and treatment of opportunistic infections in HIV-infected adults and adolescents: Recommendations from CDC, the National Institutes of Health, and the HIV Medicine Association of the Infectious Diseases Society of America. PsycEXTRA Dataset: American Psychological Association (APA); 2009.
4. Khunnawat C, Mukerji S, Havlichek D, Touma R, Abela GS. Cardiovascular manifestations in human immunodeficiency virus-infected patients. Am J Cardiol. 2008;102(5):635–42.
5. Hilton R. Human immunodeficiency virus infection and kidney disease. J Roy Coll Phys Edinburgh. 2013;43(3):236–40.
6. Chu C, Selwyn PA. Complications of HIV infection: a systems-based approach. Am Fam Phys. 2011;83(4):395–406.
7. Günthard HF, Aberg JA, Eron JJ, Hoy JF, Telenti A, Benson CA, et al. Antiretroviral treatment of adult HIV infection. JAMA. 2014;312(4):410.
8. Hofman P, Nelson AM. The pathology induced by highly active antiretroviral therapy against human immunodeficiency virus: an update. CMC. 2006;13(26):3121–32.
9. Littlewood KE. The immunocompromised adult patient and surgery. Best Pract Res Clin Anaesthesiol. 2008;22(3):585–609.
10. Hannaman MJ, Ertl MJ. Patients with immunodeficiency. Med Clin North Am. 2013;97 (6):1139–59.
11. Saltzman DJ. The surgeon and AIDS. Arch Surg. 2005;140(10):961.
12. Weledji EP, Nsagha D, Chichom A, Enoworock G. Gastrointestinal surgery and the acquired immune deficiency syndrome. Ann Med Surg. 2015;4(1):36–40.
13. Deneve JL, Shantha JG, Page AJ, Wyrzykowski AD, Rozycki GS, Feliciano DV. CD4 count is predictive of outcome in HIV-positive patients undergoing abdominal operations. Am J Surg. 2010;200(6):694–700.
14. King JT Jr, Perkal MF, Rosenthal RA, Gordon AJ, Crystal S, Rodriguez-Barradas MC, et al. Thirty-day postoperative mortality among individuals with HIV infection receiving antiretroviral therapy and procedure-matched, uninfected comparators. JAMA Surg. 2015;150(4):343–51.
15. Tran HS, Moncure M, Tarnoff M, Goodman M, Puc MM, Kroon D, et al. Predictors of operative outcome in patients with human immunodeficiency virus infection and acquired immunodeficiency syndrome. Am J Surg. 2000;180(3):228–33.
16. Cancer. 2014;120(14).
17. Sahai SK. Perioperative assessment of the cancer patient. Best Pract Res Clin Anaesthesiol. 2013;27(4):465–80.
18. Desai DM, Kuo PC. Perioperative management of special populations: immunocompromised host (cancer, HIV, transplantation). Surg Clin North Am. 2005;85(6):1267–82.
19. Steele TA. Chemotherapy-induced immunosuppression and reconstitution of immune function. Leuk Res. 2002;26(4):411–4.
20. Freifeld AG, Bow EJ, Sepkowitz KA, Boeckh MJ, Ito JI, Mullen CA, et al. Executive summary: clinical practice guideline for the use of antimicrobial agents in neutropenic patients with cancer: 2010 update by the infectious diseases society of America. Clin Infect Dis. 2011;52(4):427–31.
21. Nishimoto N. Cytokine signal regulation and autoimmune disorders. Autoimmunity. 2005;38 (5):359–67.

22. Zola H. Human leukocyte differentiation antigens as therapeutic targets: the CD molecules and CD antibodies. Expert Opin Biol Ther. 2001;1(3):375–83.
23. Singh JA, Furst DE, Bharat A, Curtis JR, Kavanaugh AF, Kremer JM, et al. 2012 update of the 2008 American College of Rheumatology recommendations for the use of disease-modifying antirheumatic drugs and biologic agents in the treatment of rheumatoid arthritis. Arthritis Care Res. 2012;64(5):625–39.
24. Rosman Z, Shoenfeld Y, Zandman-Goddard G. Biologic therapy for autoimmune diseases: an update. BMC Med. 2013;11(1):88.
25. Doran MF, Crowson CS, Pond GR, O'Fallon WM, Gabriel SE. Predictors of infection in rheumatoid arthritis. Arthritis Rheum. 2002;46(9):2294–300.
26. Organ procurement and transplantation network and scientific registry of transplant recipients 2010 data report. Am J Transplant. 2011;12:1–156.
27. Fauci AS, Dale DC, Balow JE. Glucocorticosteroid therapy: mechanisms of action and clinical considerations. Ann Intern Med. 1976;84(3):304–15.
28. Settipane GA, Pudupakkam RK, McGowan JH. Corticosteroid effect on immunoglobulins. J Allergy Clin Immunol. 1978;62(3):162–6.
29. Naesens M, Kuypers DRJ, Sarwal M. Calcineurin inhibitor nephrotoxicity. Clin J Am Soc Nephrol. 2009.
30. Gijtenbeek JMM, van den Bent MJ, Vecht CJ. Cyclosporine neurotoxicity: a review. J Neurol. 1999;246(5):339–46.
31. Danovitch GM. Immunosuppressant-induced metabolic toxicities. Transpl Rev. 2000;14 (2):65–81.
32. Connell WR, Kamm MA, Ritchie JK, Lennard-Jones JE. Bone marrow toxicity caused by azathioprine in inflammatory bowel disease: 27 years of experience. Gut. 1993;34(8):1081–5.
33. Nashan B, Citterio F. Wound healing complications and the use of mammalian target of rapamycin inhibitors in kidney transplantation. Transpl J. 2012;94(6):547–61.
34. Helderman JH, Goral S. Gastrointestinal complications of transplant immunosuppression. J Am Soc Nephrol. 2002;13(1):277–87.
35. Singh N, Limaye AP, Forrest G, Safdar N, Muñoz P, Pursell K, et al. Late-onset invasive aspergillosis in organ transplant recipients in the current era. Med Mycol. 2006;44(5):445–9.
36. Keckich DW, Blair JE, Vikram HR, Seville MT, Kusne S. Reactivation of coccidioidomycosis despite antifungal prophylaxis in solid organ transplant recipients. Transplantation. 2011;92(1):88–93.
37. Euvrard S. External anogenital lesions in organ transplant recipients. A clinicopathologic and virologic assessment. Arch Dermatol. 1997;133(2):175–8.
38. Hodson EM, Barclay PG, Craig JC, Jones C, Kable K, Strippoli GFM, et al. Antiviral medications for preventing cytomegalovirus disease in solid organ transplant recipients. Cochrane Database Syst Rev Wiley-Blackwell. 1996.
39. Shamberger RC, Weinstein HJ, Delorey MJ, Levey RH. The medical and surgical management of typhlitis in children with acute nonlymphocytic (myelogenous) leukemia. Cancer. 1986;57(3):603–9.
40. Amromin GD. Necrotizing enteropathy. JAMA. 1962;182(1):23.
41. Gorschluter M, Mey U, Strehl J, Ziske C, Schepke M, Schmidt-Wolf IGH, et al. Neutropenic enterocolitis in adults: systematic analysis of evidence quality. Eur J Haematol. 2005;75 (1):1–13.
42. Urbach DR, Rotstein OD. Typhlitis. Can J Surg. 1999;42(6):415–9.
43. Glenn J, Funkhouser WK, Schneider PS. Acute illnesses necessitating urgent abdominal surgery in neutropenic cancer patients: description of 14 cases and review of the literature. Surgery. 1989;105(6):778–89.
44. Ullery BW, Pieracci FM, Rodney JRM, Barie PS. Neutropenic enterocolitis. Surg Infect. 2009;10(3):307–14.
45. T-f Hsu, Huang H-H, Yen DH-T, Kao W-F, Chen J-D, Wang L-M, et al. ED presentation of neutropenic enterocolitis in adult patients with acute leukemia. Am J Emerg Med. 2004;22 (4):276–9.

46. Cardona AF, Ramos PL, Casasbuenas A. From case reports to systematic reviews in neutropenic enterocolitis. Eur J Haematol. 2005;75(5):445–6.
47. Frick MP, Maile CW, Crass, Goldberg ME, Delaney JP. Computed tomography of neutropenic colitis. Am J Roentgenol. 1984;143(4):763–5.
48. Dietrich CF, Hermann S, Klein S, Braden B. Sonographic signs of neutropenic enterocolitis. World J Gastroenterol. 2006;12(9):1397–402.
49. Ozer H, Armitage JO, Bennett CL, Crawford J, Demetri GD, Pizzo PA, et al. 2000 update of recommendations for the use of hematopoietic colony-stimulating factors: evidence-based, clinical practice guidelines. American society of clinical oncology growth factors expert panel. J Clin Oncol. 2000;18(20):3558–85.
50. Wade DS. Abdominal pain in neutropenic patients. Arch Surg. 1990;125(9):1119.
51. Badgwell BD, Cormier JN, Wray CJ, Borthakur G, Qiao W, Rolston KV, et al. Challenges in surgical management of abdominal pain in the neutropenic cancer patient. Ann Surg. 2008;248(1):104–9.
52. Machado NO. Neutropenic enterocolitis: a continuing medical and surgical challenge. North Am J Med Sci. 2010;2(7):293–300.
53. Boppana SB, Fowler KB. Persistence in the population: epidemiology and transmisson. In: Arvin A, Campadelli-Fiume G, Mocarski E, Moore PS, Roizman B, Whitley R, et al., editors. Human Herpesviruses: biology, therapy, and immunoprophylaxis. Cambridge: Cambridge University Press Copyright (c) Cambridge University Press 2007; 2007.
54. Baroco AL, Oldfield EC. Gastrointestinal cytomegalovirus disease in the immunocompromised patient. Curr Gastroenterol Rep. 2008;10(4):409–16.
55. Razonable RR. Management strategies for cytomegalovirus infection and disease in solid organ transplant recipients. Infect Dis Clin North Am. 2013;27(2):317–42.
56. Torres HA, Kontoyiannis DP, Bodey GP, Adachi JA, Luna MA, Tarrand JJ, et al. Gastrointestinal cytomegalovirus disease in patients with cancer: a two decade experience in a tertiary care cancer center. Eur J Cancer. 2005;41(15):2268–79.
57. Kandiel A, Lashner B. Cytomegalovirus colitis complicating inflammatory bowel disease. Am J Gastroenterol. 2006;101(12):2857–65.
58. Peter A, Telkes G, Varga M, Sarvary E, Kovalszky I. Endoscopic diagnosis of cytomegalovirus infection of upper gastrointestinal tract in solid organ transplant recipients: hungarian single-center experience. Clin Transpl. 2004;18(5):580–4.
59. Kotton CN, Kumar D, Caliendo AM, Asberg A, Chou S, Danziger-Isakov L, et al. Updated international consensus guidelines on the management of cytomegalovirus in solid-organ transplantation. Transplantation. 2013;96(4):333–60.
60. Murray JG, Evans SJ, Jeffrey PB, Halvorsen RA. Cytomegalovirus colitis in AIDS: CT features. Am J Roentgenol. 1995;165(1):67–71.
61. Morunglav M, Theate I, Bertin G, Hantson P. CMV enteritis causing massive intestinal hemorrhage in an elderly patient. Case Report Med. 2010;2010:1–4.
62. Michalopoulos N, Triantafillopoulou K, Beretouli E, Laskou S, Papavramidis TS, Pliakos I, et al. Small bowel perforation due to CMV enteritis infection in an HIV-positive patient. BMC Res Notes. 2013;6(1):45.
63. Wang HW, Kuo CJ, Lin WR, Hsu CM, Ho YP, Lin CJ, et al. The clinical characteristics and manifestations of cytomegalovirus esophagitis. Dis Esophagus. 2015;n/a-n/a.
64. Tan BH. Cytomegalovirus treatment. Curr Treat Options Infect Dis. 2014;6(3):256–70.
65. Kram HB, Shoemaker WC. Intestinal perforation due to cytomegalovirus infection in patients with AIDS. Dis Colon Rectum. 1990;33(12):1037–40.
66. Wexner SD, Smithy WB, Trillo C, Hopkins SB, Dailey TH. Emergency colectomy for cytomegalovirus ileocolitis in patients with the acquired immune deficiency syndrome. Dis Colon Rectum. 1988;31(10):755–61.
67. Arnold M, Itzikowitz R, Young B, Machoki SM, Hsiao NY, Pillay K, et al. Surgical manifestations of gastrointestinal cytomegalovirus infection in children: clinical audit and literature review. J Pediatr Surg. 2015.

68. Lessa FC, Mu Y, Bamberg WM, Beldavs ZG, Dumyati GK, Dunn JR, et al. Burden of clostridium difficile infection in the United States. N Engl J Med. 2015;372(9):825–34.
69. Kuehne SA, Cartman ST, Heap JT, Kelly ML, Cockayne A, Minton NP. The role of toxin A and toxin B in clostridium difficile infection. Nature. 2010;467(7316):711–3.
70. Jiang ZD, Garey KW, Price M, Graham G, Okhuysen P, Dao-Tran T, et al. Association of Interleukin-8 polymorphism and immunoglobulin G anti-toxin A in patients with clostridium difficile–associated diarrhea. Clin Gastroenterol Hepatol. 2007;5(8):964–8.
71. Kwok CS, Arthur AK, Anibueze CI, Singh S, Cavallazzi R, Loke YK. Risk of clostridium difficile infection with acid suppressing drugs and antibiotics: meta-analysis. Am J Gastroenterol. 2012;107(7):1011–9.
72. Surawicz CM, Brandt LJ, Binion DG, Ananthakrishnan AN, Curry SR, Gilligan PH, et al. Guidelines for diagnosis, treatment, and prevention of clostridium difficile infections. Am J Gastroenterol. 2013;108(4):478–98.
73. Fujitani S, George WL, Murthy AR. Comparison of clinical severity score indices for Clostridium difficile infection. Infect Control Hosp Epidemiol. 2011;32(3):220–8.
74. Sartelli M, Malangoni MA, Abu-Zidan FM, Griffiths EA, Di Bella S, McFarland LV, et al. WSES guidelines for management of clostridium difficile infection in surgical patients. World J Emerg Surg. 2015;10(1).
75. Cornely OA, Crook DW, Esposito R, Poirier A, Somero MS, Weiss K, et al. Fidaxomicin versus vancomycin for infection with Clostridium difficile in Europe, Canada, and the USA: a double-blind, non-inferiority, randomised controlled trial. Lancet Infect Dis. 2012;12 (4):281–9.
76. Farooq PD, Urrunaga NH, Tang DM, von Rosenvinge EC. Pseudomembranous colitis. Dis Mon. 2015;61(5):181–206.
77. Valiquette L, Pépin J, Do XV, Nault V, Beaulieu AA, Bédard J, et al. Prediction of complicated clostridium difficile infection by pleural effusion and increased wall thickness on computed tomography. Clin Infect Dis. 2009;49(4):554–60.
78. Barbut F, Petit JC. Epidemiology of clostridium difficile-associated infections. Clin Microbiol Infect. 2001;7(8):405–10.
79. Bakken JS, Borody T, Brandt LJ, Brill JV, Demarco DC, Franzos MA, et al. Treating clostridium difficile infection with fecal microbiota transplantation. Clin Gastroenterol Hepatol. 2011;9(12):1044–9.
80. Kelly CR, Ihunnah C, Fischer M, Khoruts A, Surawicz C, Afzali A, et al. Fecal microbiota transplant for treatment of clostridium difficile infection in immunocompromised patients. Am J Gastroenterol. 2014;109(7):1065–71.
81. Neal MD, Alverdy JC, Hall DE, Simmons RL, Zuckerbraun BS. Diverting loop ileostomy and colonic lavage. Ann Surg. 2011;254(3):423–9.
82. Lee DY, Chung EL, Guend H, Whelan RL, Wedderburn RV, Rose KM. Predictors of mortality after emergency colectomy for clostridium difficile colitis. Ann Surg. 2014;259 (1):148–56.
83. Cohen Stuart H, Gerding Dale N, Johnson S, Kelly Ciaran P, Loo Vivian G, McDonald LC, et al. Clinical practice guidelines for clostridium difficile infection in adults: 2010 update by the society for healthcare epidemiology of America (SHEA) and the infectious diseases society of America (IDSA). Infect Control Hosp Epidemiol. 2010;31(5):431–55.
84. Landelle C, Verachten M, Legrand P, Girou E, Barbut F, Buisson CB. Contamination of healthcare workers' hands with clostridium difficile spores after caring for patients with C. difficile infection. Infect Control Hosp Epidemiol. 2014;35(01):10–5.
85. Taur Y, Pamer EG. The intestinal microbiota and susceptibility to infection in immunocompromised patients. Curr Opin Infect Dis. 2013;26(4):332–7.
86. Polage CR, Solnick JV, Cohen SH. Nosocomial diarrhea: evaluation and treatment of causes other than Clostridium difficile. Clin Infect Dis. 2012;55(7):982–9.
87. Le Loir Y, Baron F, Gautier M. Staphylococcus aureus and food poisoning. Genet Mol Res. 2003;2(1):63–76.

88. Flemming K, Ackermann G. Prevalence of enterotoxin producing staphylococcus aureus in stools of patients with nosocomial diarrhea. Infection. 2007;35(5):356–8.
89. Boyce JM, Havill NL. Nosocomial antibiotic-associated diarrhea associated with enterotoxin-producing strains of methicillin-resistant staphylococcus aureus. Am J Gastroenterol. 2005;100(8):1828–34.
90. Gorkiewicz G. Nosocomial and antibiotic-associated diarrhoea caused by organisms other than Clostridium difficile. Int J Antimicrob Agents. 2009;33:S37–41.
91. Högenauer C, Langner C, Beubler E, Lippe IT, Schicho R, Gorkiewicz G, et al. Klebsiella oxytoca as a causative organism of antibiotic-associated hemorrhagic colitis. N Engl J Med. 2006;355(23):2418–26.
92. Fakir M, Wong T, Toupance O, Lavaud S, Wynckel A, Chanard J. Yersinia enterocolitica septicemia in a renal transplant recipient on oral iron supplementation. Transplantation. 1995;60(2):206–8.
93. Anane S, Attouchi H. Microsporidiosis: epidemiology, clinical data and therapy. Gastroenterol Clin Biol. 2010;34(8–9):450–64.
94. Didier ES, Weiss LM. Microsporidiosis. Curr Opin Infect Dis. 2011;24(5):490–5.
95. Champion L, Durrbach A, Lang P, Delahousse M, Chauvet C, Sarfati C, et al. Fumagillin for treatment of intestinal microsporidiosis in renal transplant recipients. Am J Transpl. 2010;10 (8):1925–30.
96. Le M, Ravin K, Hasan A, Clauss H, Muchant DG, Pasko JK, et al. Single donor-derived strongyloidiasis in three solid organ transplant recipients: case series and review of the literature. Am J Transpl. 2014;14(5):1199–206.
97. Stabile BE, Smith BR, Weeks DL. Helicobacter pylori infection and surgical disease—part I. Curr Probl Surg. 2005;42(11):756–89.
98. Ueda Y, Chiba T. Helicobacter pylori in solid-organ transplant recipient. Curr Opinion Organ Transpl. 2008;13(6):586–91.
99. Chey WD, Wong BC. American college of gastroenterology guideline on the management of helicobacter pylori infection. Am J Gastroenterol. 2007;102(8):1808–25.
100. Lavery EA, Coyle WJ. Herpes simplex virus and the alimentary tract. Curr Gastroenterol Rep. 2008;10(4):417–23.
101. Steiner I, Kennedy PGE, Pachner AR. The neurotropic herpes viruses: herpes simplex and varicella-zoster. Lancet Neurol. 2007;6(11):1015–28.
102. Vazquez J. Optimal management of oropharyngeal and esophageal candidiasis in patients living with HIV infection. HIV. 2010;89.
103. Kanda N, Yasuba H, Takahashi T, Mizuhara Y, Yamazaki S, Imada Y, et al. Prevalence of esophageal candidiasis among patients treated with inhaled fluticasone propionate. Am J Gastroenterol. 2003;98(10):2146–8.
104. Samonis G, Skordilis P, Maraki S, Datseris G, Toloudis P, Chatzinikolaou I, et al. Oropharyngeal candidiasis as a marker for esophageal candidiasis in patients with cancer. Clin Infect Dis. 1998;27(2):283–6.
105. Patel R, Paya CV. Infections in solid-organ transplant recipients. Clin Microbiol Rev. 1997;10(1):86–124.
106. Wong RCK, Abdul-Karim FW. Atypical herpes simplex esophagitis. Gastrointest Endosc. 2005;61(2):291–2.
107. Brady RC, Bernstein DI. Treatment of herpes simplex virus infections. Antiviral Res. 2004;61(2):73–81.
108. Folkman J. Role of angiogenesis in tumor growth and metastasis. Semin Oncol. 2002;29 (6Q):15–8.
109. Hapani S, Chu D, Wu S. Risk of gastrointestinal perforation in patients with cancer treated with bevacizumab: a meta-analysis. Lancet Oncol. 2009;10(6):559–68.
110. Kozloff M, Yood MU, Berlin J, Flynn PJ, Kabbinavar FF, Purdie DM, et al. Clinical outcomes associated with bevacizumab-containing treatment of metastatic colorectal cancer: the BRiTE observational cohort study. Oncologist. 2009;14(9):862–70.

111. Stevens DL, Bisno AL, Chambers HF, Dellinger EP, Goldstein EJC, Gorbach SL, et al. Practice guidelines for the diagnosis and management of skin and soft tissue infections: 2014 update by the infectious diseases society of America. Clin Infect Dis. 2014;59(2):e10–52.
112. Guhl G, García-Díez A. Subcutaneous sweet syndrome. Dermatol Clin. 2008;26(4):541–51.
113. Sartelli M, Malangoni MA, May AK, Viale P, Kao LS, Catena F, et al. World society of emergency surgery (WSES) guidelines for management of skin and soft tissue infections. World J Emerg Surg. 2014;9(1):57.
114. McGillicuddy EA, Lischuk AW, Schuster KM, Kaplan LJ, Maung A, Lui FY, et al. Development of a computed tomography-based scoring system for necrotizing soft-tissue infections. J Trauma Inj Infect Crit Care. 2011;70(4):894–9.
115. Hakkarainen TW, Kopari NM, Pham TN, Evans HL. Necrotizing soft tissue infections: review and current concepts in treatment, systems of care, and outcomes. Curr Probl Surg. 2014;51(8):344–62.
116. Keung EZ, Liu X, Nuzhad A, Adams C, Ashley SW, Askari R. Immunocompromised status in patients with necrotizing soft-tissue infection. JAMA Surg. 2013;148(5):419.
117. Salem M, Tainsh RE Jr, Bromberg J, Loriaux DL, Chernow B. Perioperative glucocorticoid coverage. A reassessment 42 years after emergence of a problem. Ann Surg. 1994;219 (4):416–25.
118. Kelly K, Domajnko B. Perioperative stress-dose steroids. Clin Colon Rectal Surg. 2013;26 (03):163–7.
119. Axelrod L. Perioperative management of patients treated with glucocorticoids. Endocrinol Metab Clin North Am. 2003;32(2):367–83.
120. Wei L, MacDonald TM, Walker BR. Taking glucocorticoids by prescription is associated with subsequent cardiovascular disease. Ann Intern Med. 2004;141(10):764–70.
121. Chang MI, Cohen BL, Greenstein AJ. A review of the impact of biologics on surgical complications in crohn's disease. Inflamm Bowel Dis. 2015;1.
122. Mushtaq S, Goodman SM, Scanzello CR. Perioperative management of biologic agents used in treatment of rheumatoid arthritis. Am J Ther. 2011;18(5):426–34.
123. Mangram AJ, Horan TC, Pearson ML, Silver LC, Jarvis WR. Guideline for prevention of surgical site infection, 1999. centers for disease control and prevention (CDC) hospital infection control practices advisory committee. Am J Infect Control. 1999;27(2):97–132; quiz 3–4; discussion 96.
124. Klevens RM, Edwards JR, Richards CL Jr, Horan TC, Gaynes RP, Pollock DA, et al. Estimating health care-associated infections and deaths in U.S. hospitals, 2002. Public Health Rep. 2007;122(2):160–6.
125. Guinan JL, McGuckin M, Nowell PC. Management of health-care–associated infections in the oncology patient. Oncology (Williston Park, NY). 2003;17(3):415–20; discussion 23–6.
126. Harris AD, Fleming B, Bromberg JS, Rock P, Nkonge G, Emerick M, et al. Surgical site infection after renal transplantation. Infect Control Hosp Epidemiol. 2015;36(4):417–23.
127. Zhang L, Liu BC, Zhang XY, Li L, Xia XJ, Guo RZ. Prevention and treatment of surgical site infection in HIV-infected patients. BMC Infect Dis. 2012;12:115.
128. Coleman JS, Green I, Scheib S, Sewell C, Lee JM, Anderson J. Surgical site infections after hysterectomy among HIV-infected women in the HAART era: a single institution's experience from 1999–2012. Am J Obstet Gynecol. 2014;210(2):117.e1–7.
129. Stuck AE, Minder CE, Frey FJ. Risk of infectious complications in patients taking glucocorticosteroids. Rev Infect Dis. 1989;11(6):954–63.
130. Slieker JC, Komen N, Mannaerts GH, Karsten TM, Willemsen P, Murawska M, et al. Long-term and perioperative corticosteroids in anastomotic leakage: a prospective study of 259 left-sided colorectal anastomoses. Arch Surg. 2012;147(5):447–52.
131. Eriksen TF, Lassen CB, Gogenur I. Treatment with corticosteroids and the risk of anastomotic leakage following lower gastrointestinal surgery: a literature survey. Colorectal Dis. 2014;16(5):O154–60.
132. Wang AS, Armstrong EJ, Armstrong AW. Corticosteroids and wound healing: clinical considerations in the perioperative period. Am J Surg. 2013;206(3):410–7.

Chapter 23
Management of Anastomotic Leaks—Early <7 Days and Late >7 Days

Jason A. Snyder and Martin A. Croce

Introduction

Anastomotic leaks are among the most dreaded and challenging complications encountered by acute care surgeons. Despite technical advances, anastomotic leaks remain a major source of postoperative morbidity and mortality [1]. Predicting anastomotic leaks in patients can be difficult, as can be seen in the occasional patient that leaks despite the absence of common risk factors. Leak rates of 2–5 % have been reported [1, 2]. Mortality rates as high as 24 % can be seen, with worse outcomes for foregut surgery [2]. Maintaining a high index of suspicion in all patients with anastomoses and a clear understanding of the signs and symptoms of anastomotic leak is critical in early identification of patients with this problem.

Assessment of Anastomotic Leaks

Hypervigilance in the care of postoperative patients with gastrointestinal anastomoses is the surest way to identify leaks early and minimize morbidity. Thorough history and physical is critical in identifying patients at risk for anastomotic leak. Clinical suspicion should promptly lead to further investigation via radiographic or operative assessment. Often the first indication of an early leak may be an abnormal postoperative period with delayed return of bowel function. Early perturbations in the patient's heart rate with isolated tachycardia can hint at possible anastomotic

J.A. Snyder · M.A. Croce (✉)
Department of Surgery, Elvis Presley Memorial Trauma Center, University of Tennessee Health Science Center, 910 Madison Ave. #220, Memphis, TN 38163, USA
e-mail: mcroce@uthsc.edu

J.A. Snyder
e-mail: snyderj@wudosis.wustl.edu

J.J. Diaz and D.T. Efron (eds.), *Complications in Acute Care Surgery*,
DOI 10.1007/978-3-319-42376-0_23

complications. Worsening abdominal pain, oliguria, or fevers while non-specific can also allude to the presence of a leak. Obvious findings such as stool or succus draining from wounds or drains provide a clear indicator of anastomotic failure. This finding may be heralded by skin changes at the incision site.

In the absence of irrefutable evidence of an anastomotic leak, radiographic examinations are often invaluable to provide objective evidence of the leak as well as anatomic localization of the leak. Computerized tomography (CT) is the most commonly utilized imaging modality given the ability to identify non-luminal pathology such as abscesses as well as the GI tract which can aid in planning interventions. The upper gastrointestinal (UGI) study is another commonly performed study in patients undergoing gastric surgery. This study can provide both anatomic and functional information. Water-soluble enema studies are of particular benefit in assessing the distal colon and rectal anastomoses and can be more sensitive than CT. In a retrospective study, Nicksa et al. [3] found that CT missed 80 % of colorectal anastomotic leaks seen on water-soluble enema. One study found clinical assessment to have 82 % accuracy, water-soluble enema to have 93 % accuracy, and CT to have 94 % accuracy [4]. Given barium's propensity for inducing an inflammatory reaction in the peritoneum, iodinated water-soluble contrast is the medium of choice when imaging for anastomotic leaks.

Gastric Anastomotic Leaks

As acid suppression therapy has flourished in the treatment of peptic ulcer disease, the frequency with which surgeons operate on the stomach for ulcer disease has significantly decreased. While the need for ulcer operations have decreased, gastric surgery for morbid obesity is becoming increasingly common and the acute care surgeon is increasingly finding himself caring for patients with complications following Roux-en-Y gastric bypass or sleeve gastrectomy. Leaks from Roux-en-Y gastric bypasses most commonly occur at the gastrojejunostomy site [5]. Sleeve gastrectomy leak rates are reported from 1.4 to 5.8 % [6–8]. Pickleman [2] found a leak rate of 4.8 % in total gastrectomy versus 1.3 % in partial gastrectomy.

Several techniques exist to mitigate anastomotic leakage. Drain placement following gastric surgery can lead to early detection of possible leaks. However, drains adjacent to anastomoses can also become self-fulfilling prophecies; the foreign body can also precipitate anastomotic leaks. Early signs of leak can be isolated tachycardia, fever, elevated white blood cell count, or PO intolerance. The identification of turbid, purulent or bilious fluid, or food particles in the drain can provide early identification of a leak. High amylase content in drain fluid can also be an indicator that there may be an anastomotic disruption. Lee et al. [9] reviewed nearly 2000 patients undergoing gastric cancer surgery and found increased need for postoperative percutaneous drainage in patients who did not receive prophylactic drains (9.1 vs. 1.9 %). Risk factors for percutaneous drainage included age, open surgery, and longer operative times. The authors suggested a selective approach based on the above risk factors when deciding upon prophylactic drains.

Staple line reinforcement is a frequently performed procedure during sleeve gastrectomy. Utilization of running absorbable sutures or coapplication of glycolide trimethylene carbonate copolymer (Gore Seamguard) with the linear stapler is frequently employed to reinforce the gastric staple line. Dapri et al. [10] performed a prospective randomized clinical trial comparing no reinforcement, suture reinforcement, and Seamguard reinforcement and found no difference in leak rates.

Management of gastric anastomotic leaks is dependent upon the time of diagnosis, the size of the leak, and the clinical appearance of the patient. A number of validated minimally invasive procedures exist for managing leaks at the gastric anastomosis. Despite this, operative treatment is still frequently required. Floridly septic patients or patients with peritonitis are not the appropriate candidate for non-operative management.

Early leaks (<7 days) are often managed surgically. Laparoscopic or open approaches are both appropriate options. Primary suture closure of the defect can provide temporary relief of peritoneal contamination though is rarely successful in isolation. Complete revision of the anastomosis can be considered if the proposed sites of the new anastomosis are free of inflammation and edema. Placement of omental patch over the defect can also minimize leakage. Reduction in bacterial burden in the peritoneal cavity also improves chances of closure, and therefore, peritoneal toilet is important. Placement of closed suction drains around the anastomosis can also mitigate peritoneal contamination and facilitate closure of the anastomosis. Even if the repair fails, the drain may provide a path of egress for gastric contents, permitting a controlled fistula. The surgeon's clinical assessment of the severity of the leak should be used when deciding upon distal feeding access (i.e., feeding jejunostomy).

Small leaks detected early as well contained abscesses can often be managed non-operatively with percutaneously placed drains (or maintenance of surgically placed drains), NPO, and intravenous antibiotics. Endoluminal therapies including fibrin glue, covered stents, fistula plugs, or clips have been shown to be effective in small case series though robust evidence is still lacking. Covered stents have the added benefit of permitting oral intake assuming a postplacement UGI is negative for continued leak. Eubanks et al. reported 16 of 19 patients (84 %) successfully treated for anastomotic leaks by covered stents. Stent migration required three patients to undergo surgical retrieval [11].

Late leaks (>7 days) will typically present as contained abscesses or fistulae rather than free contamination of the peritoneal cavity. The non-operative endoluminal therapies mentioned above can be especially useful in these patients, as the adhesive burden in the late postoperative period can be prohibitive. NPO and parenteral nutritional support is critical in facilitating closure of gastrocutaneous fistulae.

Reoperation for late leaks should only occur after non-operative modalities have been exhausted. The failure rate for this problem is much higher than with early leaks and should be carefully planned out with thorough preoperative imaging via

UGI or CT with oral contrast. Simple re-anastomosis is an option in healthy tissue. On the other hand, simply observing a gastric fistula should not be entertained. Creation of a gastrojejunostomy directly over an anastomotic leak can provide internal drainage of a fistula. Another option is formation of a Roux limb of jejunum to a proximal gastric remnant or to the esophagus. This can isolate the affected portion of stomach and facilitate closure [12].

Small Intestine Anastomotic Leaks

Anastomotic leaks of the small bowel occur in approximately 5.5 % of anastomoses [1]. The failure of these anastomoses has been shown to be associated with corticosteroid use, malnutrition (albumin <3.0 g/L), bowel obstruction, peritonitis, COPD, and perioperative transfusion of more than 2 U PRBC [13]. Open surgery appears to confer a higher rate of intestinal leak versus laparoscopic procedures. Chemotherapy, anticoagulation, and intra-operative blood loss are all associated with increased leak rates [14]. Table 23.1 lists risk factors associated with anastomotic leaks [15].

The technical details associated with small bowel anastomosis such as stapled versus hand-sewn or end-to-end versus side-to-side have been extensively studied and reveal that there is no unmistakably superior method. The best tactic to decrease leak rates is meticulous attention to the technical details in whichever technique is preferred by the surgeon. Tension-free anastomosis with a healthy blood supply is critical in a successful anastomosis. The creation of the suture line should be

Table 23.1 Risk factors for anastomotic leak

Risk factors
Technical error
Emergency surgery
Prolonged operative time
Blood loss
Use of vasopressors
Tension on anastomosis
Suture line tension
Poor blood supply
Steroids
Obesity
Smoking
Advanced age
COPD
Reoperative surgery
Malnutrition
Radiation

performed while avoiding overtightening. Excessively tight suture lines may lead to focal ischemia and subsequent leak.

Identification of anastomotic leaks in the small intestine is typically identified by CT with oral contrast [1]. Dependent upon the clinical situation, fluoroscopic studies can be of benefit; small bowel follow through can provide dynamic information, while fistulogram can help delineate the precise loop of bowel associated with an enterocutaneous fistula.

Early anastomotic leaks in the small intestine will typically present in a dramatic fashion and should typically be managed operatively, notably in the setting of peritonitis, sepsis, or hemodynamic instability. The presentation of an early anastomotic leak typically indicates a technical failure and should usually be addressed surgically. The limited presence of adhesions early in the postoperative course can make resection of a failed anastomosis and fresh anastomosis an often successful course of management. The distance from typical endoscopic routes of entry makes endoluminal therapies less feasible in small bowel fistulae.

Late anastomotic leaks in the small intestine can be very difficult to manage operatively given the dense adhesive burden in a postoperative abdomen. Factors leading to late development of anastomotic leaks include anastomoses under tension, deserosalized bowel, and suture hematomas. Factors preventing spontaneous closure of leaks are remembered by the mnemonic FRIENDS: Foreign bodies, Radiation, Infection/inflammatory bowel disease, Epithelialization of the tract, Neoplasm, Distal obstruction, Short fistula tracts less than 2 cm. The presence of abscesses adjacent to an anastomotic leak can further prevent spontaneous closure of fistulae.

Imaging can be indispensable in the patient with late anastomotic leakage in delineating anatomy and identifying drainable collections. Intra-luminal and intravenous contrast enhanced CT scans can identify abscesses as well as fistula anatomy. Contrast enhanced fluoroscopy studies such as UGI or fistulograms can provide additional information if CT imaging is not clear.

Late anastomotic leaks often present as enterocutaneous fistulae (ECF) and can manifest in several ways. The finding of an intra-abdominal abscess requiring percutaneous drainage can then begin draining enteric contents. Postoperative wound infections, opened at bedside, can also begin leaking succus. Spontaneous drainage through the skin may occur in leaks that occur near the abdominal wall. Given that non-operative management is often attempted first, patients may undergo significant daily fluid and electrolyte losses, notably potassium, sodium, phosphate, and magnesium. Proximal fistulae can lead to metabolic acidosis due to loss of bicarbonate. Fistula output can be classified as low (<500 cc/day) or high output (>500 cc/day).

NPO, parenteral nutrition, antibiotics, and percutaneous drainage are the first line of treatment in management of late anastomotic leaks. Percutaneous drainage can be invaluable in the management of late anastomotic leaks of the intestine. Serial CT scanning to assess adequacy of drainage should be undertaken with drain upsizing as needed to accomplish source control. The addition of octreotide can also reduce fistula output though with no proven effect on outcomes. One early study blinded octreotide administration and found that patients off octreotide had output averaging 698 ml/day with a reduction to 246 ml/day after two days of octreotide [16]. Octreotide has also been demonstrated to shorten the time to closure of fistula [17]. Low output fistulae will often respond to these measures alone. Enteral nutrition may be considered in patients with low output fistulae. If PO intake is tolerated and the output does not increase, then enteral feeding may be used in lieu of TPN. Nutritional support is critical to the success of spontaneous fistula closure, and requirements are typically closer to 30 kcal/kg/d in patients with high output fistulae [18]. In patients who are severely malnourished, gradual initiation of nutritional support should be undertaken to prevent refeeding syndrome.

Fistula output is typically caustic and can lead to significant skin complications. Early utilization of drainage management systems, ideally with the assistance of a stomal therapist, should be attempted. Vacuum-assisted dressings are frequently used to isolate fistulas and reduce soilage of adjacent skin.

Closure of enterocutaneous fistulae will ideally occur spontaneously. This can require a great deal of patience from both the patient and the surgeon. A wide range of spontaneous closure rates for intestinal fistulae are reported from 20 to 90 % [19–22]. The above-mentioned modalities should be exhausted in the interim while waiting a minimum of three months before attempting surgical control of ECF. This will permit reduction in the dense adhesions often seen in this setting and reduce the risk of serosal injuries or enterotomies. Early operation can lead to life-threatening blood loss from highly vascular adhesive tissue that can be difficult to control due to the dense fused visceral block.

Undertaking surgical correction of ECF requires a great deal of planning and patience. Ideally, mobilization of the entirety of bowel is crucial to eliminate points of obstruction. Once the bowel is mobilized, resection of the affected segment is undertaken. Ensuring that there is healthy tissue covering the entirety of the bowel is critical to prevent further leaks. Meticulous repair of the inevitable serosal tears or enterotomies encountered during adhesiolysis is mandatory.

Anastomotic leaks can also manifest in the open abdomen as enteroatmospheric fistulae (EAF). Management of EAF is extremely challenging to even the most experienced surgeon and close attention should be paid to techniques that can minimize risk of fistula formation. Wound care of the open abdomen should not be relegated to junior members of the surgical team as aggressive dressing changes or missed subtle findings can lead to months of further complications. Placement of the omentum over exposed bowel can protect the bowel from overlying dressings. Avoiding the placement of gauze or vacuum sponges directly on bowel is important to prevent fistula formation. We use polyglactin (Vicryl) mesh if unable to close an open abdomen. Eventual placement of autologous skin grafts allows formation of a suitable barrier that minimizes desiccation of the underlying bowel. Placement of the skin graft should only be undertaken once a suitable bed of granulation tissue forms—typically around 10–14 days.

EAF present a challenge from a wound care standpoint. Given that the fistula is often in the midst of fused loops of bowel, applying ostomy appliances directly to the loop of bowel is undesirable and preventing spillage of enteric contents across the visceral block can be challenging. Proximal diversion, while appealing, can be difficult due to foreshortening of the mesentery preventing an ostomy from reaching the skin. The initial goal of wound care in EAF should be attainment of granulation or coverage of the surrounding open abdomen. This can be accomplished several ways. Vacuum-assisted closure can be attempted, though care must be taken to cover the exposed bowel with a barrier such as petrolatum gauze or plastic sheets. Some concerns exist about this technique increasing fistula output due to negative pressure. The floating stoma, as originally described by Subramaniam et al. [23], entails placement of a plastic sheet over the exposed bowel with a hole cut overlying the fistula. This opening is then sutured to the bowel, encircling the fistula and preventing effluent from spilling onto the exposed bowel. A stoma appliance can then be applied to the fistula and changed as needed.

After a suitable containment solution has been found for the fistula, the surrounding bowel should be covered with a split thickness skin graft. Once the skin graft incorporates, a simple stoma appliance can be applied over the fistula and then treated as an ileostomy. Eventual closure of the abdominal wall can be undertaken once the skin graft passes the "pinch test"; once the grafted skin can be pinched up and off the underlying bowel, it is ready for resection and abdominal wall closure with attendant resection of fistula and anastomosis in a non-inflamed field.

Colorectal Anastomotic Leaks

Anastomotic leaks within the colon (6.0 %) and rectum (7.0 %) occur with greater frequency than small bowel (5.5 %) [1]. Reasons for the higher rate of failure may be due to the potential for anastomotic tension and a more tenuous blood supply. Notably, the larger bacterial load in the colon may contribute to the higher rate of intra-abdominal infections when compared to other sites of surgery within the abdomen. The higher risk of infection may contribute to the greater risk of anastomotic failure. One study found colorectal anastomotic leaks to carry a 13 % mortality and therefore require a great deal of vigilance in monitoring for their presence [24]. Risk factors for anastomotic leaks of the colon include albumin <3.5 g/dL, operative time of >200 min, intra-operative blood loss of >200 ml, intra-operative transfusion requirements, and positive histologic margin involvement in inflammatory bowel disease [25]. Adding insult to injury, anastomotic leaks after resections for colon cancer carry a higher risk of local cancer recurrence [26].

A number of techniques are utilized to mitigate the risk of anastomotic leaks in colorectal surgery. Pelvic drains are theorized to eliminate abscess formation adjacent to rectal anastomoses; though as previously noted, drains may be a double-edged sword. Definitive data regarding this benefit are lacking [27]. Air leak testing of left-sided and rectal anastomoses has not been definitively shown to be of benefit, but is often performed [27]. Given the lack of harm and potential for benefit, testing for air leaks should be strongly considered. Protective diverting stomas have been shown to decrease the incidence of anastomotic leak and reduce the need for urgent operation [28]. Understanding of the preoperative and intra-operative risk factors for anastomotic leaks should guide the surgeon's decision to perform a protective diverting ostomy.

Management of early colorectal anastomoses should typically be managed by proximal diversion. Patients with generalized peritonitis after a recent colorectal anastomosis should be promptly resuscitated and taken to the OR. Delaying definitive treatment for imaging should be avoided. Resection of a leaking anastomosis with diversion by an end colostomy has the least risk of further anastomotic complications, while anastomotic revision with proximal diverting loop ostomy is often performed if the patients is stable and there is minimal contamination. Proximal diversion and drainage of the anastomotic site is of particular value in low pelvic anastomoses where the distal rectal cuff length is short and may preclude resection and re-anastomosis. The omentum can be invaluable in covering anastomotic sites of concern.

Late colorectal anastomotic leaks usually present as abscesses or fistulae with often minimal systemic disturbances. The drainage of purulence per rectum or vagina can herald an anastomotic leak and abscess after low rectal anastomoses [29]. Given the consistency of stool versus succus, late colonic leaks are typically low output. Most management algorithms do not require NPO status. Antibiotics and percutaneous drainage of abscesses can often be adequate treatment. Spontaneous closure can occur in about a third of patients [2]. Rectovaginal or rectovesical fistulae will typically require fistulectomy and revision of the anastomosis with a diverting colostomy proximal to the anastomosis. Leaks recalcitrant to drainage may require reexploration with resection of the anastomosis and possibly permanent diversion for more distal leaks.

Pancreatic Anastomotic Leaks

As surgical subspecialization continues, pancreatic anastomoses are performed less commonly by the emergency general surgeon. By far, the most common procedure involving a pancreatic duct anastomosis is the pancreaticoduodenectomy. The vast majority of data pertaining to leaks is based on experience derived from this procedure. Anastomotic leaks of pancreaticojejunostomies following pancreaticoduodenectomy are common complications ranging from 8 to 17 % [30–33]. Mortality following anastomotic leak has a wide range [1, 30, 32, 33] with some case series reporting rates approaching 20 % [1, 32]. Postoperative pancreatic fistulas were defined by a consensus of the International Study Group on Pancreatic Fistula; drain output of any measurable volume of fluid on or after postoperative day 3 with an amylase content greater than 3 times the serum amylase activity [34].

Risk factors associated with pancreatic anastomotic leaks include normal, soft pancreatic texture, small ducts <2 mm [35], advanced age, prolonged period of jaundice, and increased intra-operative blood loss [32]. Technical aspects involved in creating pancreaticojejunostomies have been investigated extensively. Duct to mucosa versus invagination of the pancreatic remnant has been compared with some evidence that invagination has a lower risk of fistula [36], though other studies appear to show no difference [37–39]. Surgeon experience appears to play a greater role in the development of pancreatic leaks than the particulars of the anastomosis [40, 41].

Drainage of pancreatic anastomoses has been used routinely to minimize the effect of pancreatic leaks. A prospective randomized trial from Memorial Sloan Kettering found that drains failed to reduce complication rates and actually found a higher rate of leaks in the drained group [42]. Somatostatin analogues have also been used to minimize pancreatic exocrine secretions in the perioperative period with the thought that it should mitigate the risk of leakage, prospective randomized trials have yielded mixed results on its efficacy [43–45]. Temporary occlusion of the pancreatic duct with fibrin plugs also does not appear to reduce leak rates [46]. Reviewing management of pancreatic trauma at our institution, stapled versus oversewing for distal pancreatectomy does not appear to significantly effect pancreatic leak rates (12 vs. 11 %) [47].

Early pancreatic leaks should be suspected when patients have abnormal recovery, worsening abdominal pain, PO intolerance, fevers, or sepsis. Stable, afebrile patients with drain output concerning for pancreatic leaks may not require any further imaging. Pancreatic protocol CT can be helpful in assessing the duct and adjacent abscesses if the patient is showing clinical signs of infection. Typically, the management of anastomotic leaks of the pancreas is non-operative with continued tube drainage. Spontaneous closure rates are typically high with one study reporting around 80 % [33]. Surgical intervention with wide drainage with or without closure of the leaking site can be considered if drain placement is ineffective as evidenced by uncontrolled leaks or abscesses unreachable by percutaneous drainage.

Late pancreatic leaks or early leaks persisting despite conservative management may need to be addressed surgically. Placement of a Roux limb to internally drain the fistula can be effective, but should only be considered if the pancreas is firm. Re-resection of the cut end with oversewing of the duct is usually sufficient. Omentum should be secured to the resected edge. Completion pancreatectomy is also an option that can be undertaken for recalcitrant pancreatic fistulae, but should be reserved for severe cases [33].

Summary

Identifying patients at risk of anastomotic leaks and vigilance in the postoperative period for early detection of anastomotic leaks can have a significant effect on long-term outcomes. A thorough understanding of the non-operative and operative management options is equally important in providing a higher rate of success for patients who develop anastomotic leaks. While both frustrating and challenging, the vast majority of anastomotic leaks can have successful outcomes if managed appropriately.

Clinical Scenario

18 yo man underwent right hemicolectomy and liver repair following gunshot wound to the abdomen. The patient initially presented with peritonitis and received 3 uPRBC transfusion intra-operatively. Primary anastomosis was performed. On PO day 7, he demonstrates feculent drainage from his midline wound.

Basically, there are only two possibilities for the feculent drainage—a missed injury (less likely) or anastomotic leak (more likely). Both would need operation in this scenario. There may be some concern about reoperation due to adhesions, but the adhesions should be quite manageable at 7 days post-operatively. Care must be taken especially when using finger fracture, however, since the bowel will be somewhat friable.

If the drainage is from a missed injury to the colon, simple repair will not suffice. The bowel will likely be inflamed and not hold suture well. The segment should be resected. Depending on the quality of the bowel, anastomosis may be performed with proximal diverting ostomy. If the bowel is too inflamed, proximal end ostomy should be performed. If the drainage is from an anastomotic leak, the anastomosis should be resected. The surgeon must avoid the temptation of placing a suture or two to repair the leak, since that technique is doomed to failure. Depending on the quality of the bowel, another anastomosis may be performed with diverting loop ileostomy. If this is not possible, diverting ileostomy should be performed.

Key Questions

1. *How do you manage the systemically asymptomatic (no intra-abdominal sepsis) midline enterocutaneous on post-op day 14?*
2. *Should reoperative exploration entail another full lysis of adhesions?*

References

1. Turrentine FE, et al. Morbidity, mortality, cost, and survival estimates of gastrointestinal anastomotic leaks. J Am Coll Surg. 2015;220:195–206.
2. Pickleman J. The failed gastrointestinal anastomosis: an inevitable catastrophe? J Am Coll Surg. 1999;188:473–82.
3. Nicksa GA, et al. Anastomotic leaks: what is the best diagnostic imaging study? Dis Colon Rectum. 2007;50:197–203.
4. Nesbakken A, et al. Anastomotic leak following mesorectal excision for rectal cancer: true incidence and diagnostic challenges. Colorectal Dis. 2005;7:576–81.

5. Thodiyil PA, et al. Selective nonoperative management of leaks after gastric bypass: lessons learned from 2675 consecutive patients. Ann Surg. 2008;248:782–92.
6. Stroh C, et al. Results of more than 11,800 sleeve gastrectomies: data analysis of the German bariatric surgery registry. Ann Surg. 2015; doi:10.1097/SLA.0000000000001559.
7. Spyropoulos C, et al. Management of gastrointestinal leaks after surgery for clinically severe obesity. Surg Obes Relat Dis. 2012;8:609–15.
8. Sakran N, et al. Gastric leaks after sleeve gastrectomy: a multicenter experience with 2834 patients. Surg Endosc. 2013;27:240–5.
9. Lee J, et al. Do all patients require prophylactic drainage after gastrectomy for gastric cancer? The experience of a high-volume center. Ann Surg Oncol. 2015;22:3929–37.
10. Dapri G, Cadière GB, Himpens J. Reinforcing the staple line during laparoscopic sleeve gastrectomy: prospective randomized clinical study comparing three different techniques. Obes Surg. 2010;20:462–7.
11. Eubanks S, et al. Use of endoscopic stents to treat anastomotic complications after bariatric surgery. J Am Coll Surg. 2008;206:935–8.
12. Nedelcu AM, Skalli M, Deneve E, Fabre JM, Nocca D. Surgical management of chronic fistula after sleeve gastrectomy. Surg Obes Relat Dis. 2013;9:879–84.
13. Golub R, Golub RW, Cantu R, Stein HD. A multivariate analysis of factors contributing to leakage of intestinal anastomoses. J Am Coll Surg. 1997;184:364–72.
14. Luján JJ, et al. Factors influencing the outcome of intestinal anastomosis. Am Surg. 2011;77:1169–75.
15. Hyman NH. Managing anastomotic leaks from intestinal anastomoses. Surg J R Coll Surg Edinb Irel. 2009;7:31–5.
16. Nubiola-Calonge P, et al. Blind evaluation of the effect of octreotide (SMS 201-995), a somatostatin analogue, on small-bowel fistula output. Lancet Lond Engl. 1987;2:672–4.
17. Hesse U, Ysebaert D, de Hemptinne B. Role of somatostatin-14 and its analogues in the management of gastrointestinal fistulae: clinical data. Gut. 2001;49:iv11–20.
18. Schecter WP. Management of enterocutaneous fistulas. Surg Clin North Am. 2011;91:481–91.
19. Dárdai E, Pirityi S, Nagy L. Parenteral and enteral nutrition and the enterocutaneous fistula treatment. II. Factors influencing the outcome of treatment. Acta Chir Hung. 1991;32:305–18.
20. Martinez D, et al. The outcome of intestinal fistulae: the Louisiana State University Medical Center-Shreveport experience. Am Surg. 1998;64:252–4.
21. Garden OJ, Dykes EH, Carter DC. Surgical and nutritional management of postoperative duodenal fistulas. Dig Dis Sci. 1988;33:30–5.
22. Hollington P, et al. An 11-year experience of enterocutaneous fistula. Br J Surg. 2004;91:1646–51.
23. Subramaniam MH, Liscum KR, Hirshberg A. The floating stoma: a new technique for controlling exposed fistulae in abdominal trauma. J Trauma. 2002;53:386–8.
24. Alves A, Panis Y, Pocard M, Regimbeau JM, Valleur P. Management of anastomotic leakage after nondiverted large bowel resection. J Am Coll Surg. 1999;189:554–9.
25. Telem DA. Risk factors for anastomotic leak following colorectal surgery: a case-control study. Arch Surg. 2010;145:371.
26. Branagan G, Finnis D. Prognosis after anastomotic leakage in colorectal surgery. Dis Colon Rectum. 2005;48:1021–6.
27. Davis B, Rivadeneira DE. Complications of colorectal anastomoses. Surg Clin North Am. 2013;93:61–87.
28. Montedori A, Cirocchi R, Farinella E, Sciannameo F, Abraha I. Covering ileo- or colostomy in anterior resection for rectal carcinoma. Cochrane Database Syst Rev. 2010; doi:10.1002/14651858.CD006878.pub2.
29. Morks AN, Ploeg RJ, Sijbrand Hofker H, Wiggers T, Havenga K. Late anastomotic leakage in colorectal surgery: a significant problem. Colorectal Dis Off J Assoc Coloproctol G B Irel. 2013;15:e271–5.

30. Vin Y, et al. Management and outcomes of postpancreatectomy fistula, leak, and abscess: results of 908 patients resected at a single institution between 2000 and 2005. J Am Coll Surg. 2008;207:490–8.
31. Grobmyer SR, et al. Pancreatic anastomotic failure after pancreaticoduodenectomy. Am J Surg. 2000;180:117–20.
32. Yeh TS, et al. Pancreaticojejunal anastomotic leak after pancreaticoduodenectomy–multivariate analysis of perioperative risk factors. J Surg Res. 1997;67:119–25.
33. Miedema BW. Complications following pancreaticoduodenectomy: current management. Arch Surg. 1992;127:945.
34. Bassi C, et al. Postoperative pancreatic fistula: an international study group (ISGPF) definition. Surgery. 2005;138:8–13.
35. van Berge Henegouwen MI, De Wit LT, Van Gulik TM, Obertop H, Gouma DJ. Incidence, risk factors, and treatment of pancreatic leakage after pancreaticoduodenectomy: drainage versus resection of the pancreatic remnant. J Am Coll Surg. 1997;185:18–24.
36. Berger AC, et al. Does type of pancreaticojejunostomy after pancreaticoduodenectomy decrease rate of pancreatic fistula? A randomized, prospective, dual-institution trial. J Am Coll Surg. 2009;208:738–47.
37. El Nakeeb A, et al. Comparative study between duct to mucosa and invagination pancreaticojejunostomy after pancreaticoduodenectomy: a prospective randomized study. Int J Surg. 2015;16:1–6.
38. Bassi C, et al. Duct-to-mucosa versus end-to-side pancreaticojejunostomy reconstruction after pancreaticoduodenectomy: results of a prospective randomized trial. Surgery. 2003;134: 766–71.
39. Yang Y-M, et al. Risk factors of pancreatic leakage after pancreaticoduodenectomy. World J Gastroenterol. 2005;11:2456–61.
40. Schmidt CM. Effect of hospital volume, surgeon experience, and surgeon volume on patient outcomes after pancreaticoduodenectomy: a single-institution experience. Arch Surg. 2010;145:634.
41. Gordon TA, et al. Complex gastrointestinal surgery: impact of provider experience on clinical and economic outcomes. J Am Coll Surg. 1999;189:46–56.
42. Conlon KC, et al. Prospective randomized clinical trial of the value of intraperitoneal drainage after pancreatic resection. Ann Surg. 2001;234:487–94.
43. Yeo CJ, et al. Does prophylactic octreotide decrease the rates of pancreatic fistula and other complications after pancreaticoduodenectomy?: Results of a prospective randomized placebo-controlled trial. Ann Surg. 2000;232:419–29.
44. Montorsi M, et al. Efficacy of octreotide in the prevention of pancreatic fistula after elective pancreatic resections: a prospective, controlled, randomized clinical trial. Surgery. 1995;117:26–31.
45. Allen PJ, et al. Pasireotide for postoperative pancreatic fistula. N Engl J Med. 2014;370:2014–22.
46. Suc B, et al. Temporary fibrin glue occlusion of the main pancreatic duct in the prevention of intra-abdominal complications after pancreatic resection: prospective randomized trial. Ann Surg. 2003;237:57–65.
47. Sharpe JP, et al. Impact of a defined management algorithm on outcome after traumatic pancreatic injury. J Trauma Acute Care Surg. 2012;72:100–5.

Chapter 24
The Relaparotomy in the Delayed (2–3 Week) Postoperative Period

Nicole Stassen and Michael Rotondo

Introduction

Webster defines reoperation as an operation to correct a condition not corrected by a previous operation or to correct the complications of a previous operation [1]. For the surgeon, the definition is more personal as it is often perceived as a failure or personal shortcoming. Early re-operative intervention has struck fear in the hearts of surgeons for many years [2]. In emergency surgery, outcomes are significantly worse when relaparotomy is required [3, 4]. Kim et al. [5] showed an overall mortality rate of 9 % in patients undergoing emergency surgery, with an increase to 21 % in patients who required relaparotomy. Timing of re-operation is also fraught with difficulty as re-operative surgery in the more immediate (less than 10 days) and more significantly delayed time periods (after six to eight weeks) is viewed to be less technically difficult as adhesions are thought to be less dense during those time periods [6].

The main questions when approaching a patient who potentially requires a relaparotomy in the delayed postoperative period can be split into the following categories:

N. Stassen (✉) · M. Rotondo
Department of Surgery, University of Rochester Medical Center,
601 Elmwood Ave, Box Surg, Rochester, NY 14642, USA
e-mail: nicole_stassen@urmc.rochester.edu

M. Rotondo
e-mail: michael_rotondo@urmc.rochester.edu

J.J. Diaz and D.T. Efron (eds.), *Complications in Acute Care Surgery*,
DOI 10.1007/978-3-319-42376-0_24

- Preoperative Decision-making
  - Is this an issue which truly requires relaparotomy at this time or can it be delayed to a more desirable time period?
  - Can this problem be managed in a less invasive way?
  - What, if any, diagnostic studies are necessary for operative decision-making and planning?
- Intra-operative Decision-making and Management
  - Are there challenges that are present with relaparotomy that is not present with the initial surgery and how can you best manage them?
  - What are the differences in intra-operative management in the relaparotomy patient?
- Postoperative Challenges
  - What are the differences in postoperative management in the relaparotomy patient?

In this chapter, we will seek help to guide you through these questions and their potential solutions.

Preoperative Decision-Making

The most important question to answer preoperatively is whether this patient indeed requires another laparotomy or will the cure, operative, or non-operative be worse than the situation at hand. Literature has shown that having ischemic bowel at initial laparotomy or requiring emergent surgery places a patient at a higher risk for both developing an early postoperative bowel obstruction and potentially requiring relaparotomy [5, 7]. Early postoperative bowel obstruction has a greater rate of strangulation and mortality as well as a greater rate of non-adhesive causes such as internal hernia, ischemia, fascial dehiscence, inflammatory reactions, and anastomotic technical failures when compared to more delayed bowel obstructions [8]. Fortunately, over seventy percent of early postoperative small bowel obstructions respond to conservative management with bowel rest, nasogastric suction, and intravenous fluids [9]. However, the time frame over which the bowel obstructions resolve can be quite extensive, ranging from seven to twenty-eight days [10]. Being able to more accurately predict which patient will have a more protracted or unsuccessful course of non-operative management would be quite advantageous. This would allow the surgeon to intervene in an earlier, likely safer, time period and save the patient from an extended time with inadequate nutrition, nasogastric decompression, and a protracted hospitalization. Computed tomography (CT) can be helpful in differentiating those who are more likely to have a complete obstruction, which would mandate more emergent re-operation, from those who have an incomplete obstruction that may resolve with conservative management [11]. Often times in a postoperative patient, however, the CT scan is not always as clear-cut, necessitating other methods of identifying the patient who will require a re-operation. A formal upper gastrointestinal study with small bowel follow through utilizing water-soluble contrast can help differentiate whether the obstruction is functional or mechanical [12]. Another diagnostic and potentially therapeutic intervention that has been gaining ground is a gastrografin challenge as described by Goussous et al., where a patient undergoes nasogastric tube decompression for a short interval with subsequent administration of gastrografin. The presence of contrast in the colon within eight hours or the patient having a bowel movement represents a successful challenge indicating that the obstruction will most likely resolve with non-operative management with a 94 % positive predictive value [13]. The sensitivity of a positive gastrografin challenge predicting resolution of a postoperative bowel obstruction without operative intervention is 98 % with a specificity of 63 % [14]. A negative gastrografin challenge does not have the same predictive quality as a positive challenge as in the early postoperative period a patient with an ileus may have delayed transit, yet resolve without operative intervention. If a patient has a negative gastrografin challenge and if there are no clinical or radiological signs of the obstruction improving after two weeks, the patient should undergo re-exploration as the obstruction is unlikely to resolve with conservative management [8, 14].

For the case above, another dilemma is determining whether the thickened segment of jejunum seen on CT is compromised and beyond salvage or if it will recover over time. Findings on CT that raise concern for bowel ischemia include a thickened bowel wall, mural thumb printing, pneumatosis intestinalis and/or portal venous gas, absence of bowel wall enhancement with intravenous contrast, hazy mesentery, and free fluid [15]. The patient in the scenario above has a segment of thickened bowel, but none of the other pathognomonic findings concern for bowel ischemia. At postoperative day seven could the thickening still just be resolving inflammation from having been ischemic prior to the first operation? Certainly, physical examination findings of localized or generalized peritonitis and serum studies including an elevated white blood cell count or elevated lactate level could help differentiate more simple "postoperative inflammation" from something more sinister.

What about the finding of a "transition point" seen on the CT scan of our patient is that alone enough to mandate repeat laparotomy? In all comers with small bowel obstructions, Suri et al. found that an identifiable transition point on CT was significantly associated with the need for operation in patients with a small bowel obstruction, while both Zielinski et al. and Colon et al. did not. Making the finding of a transition point in our patient is not single handedly predictive of requiring another operation [16–18].

Other common clinical scenarios encountered by acute care surgeons that can necessitate re-operation in the early postoperative period are wound dehiscence (skin and/or fascia), intra-abdominal abscess formation, and anastomotic leaks. Skin dehiscence can often be managed with local debridement and wound care either with dressing changes or in some larger wounds negative pressure wound therapy with a vacuum-assisted dressing management system (KCI, San Antonio, TX). Fascial dehiscence nearly always requires re-operation. It is important however to determine the etiology of the fascial dehiscence (technical error, fascial quality, intra-abdominal cause, etc.) so that it can be addressed in order to prevent recurrence. For a dehiscence caused by a technical error or fascial quality, the only intervention needed may be fascial reclosure. (Please see the intra-operative decision-making and management section for further details on suggestions and pitfalls of re-operative fascial closure.) Any contributing intra-abdominal cause like bowel distension or infection should be addressed prior to reclosure of the fascia.

Advances in minimally invasive percutaneous interventions have greatly decreased the need for open operative drainage of intra-abdominal collections and abscesses [19]. When percutaneous drainage fails, however, operative intervention may be necessary to control the intra-abdominal sepsis [20]. This can be performed laparoscopically or open depending on the clinical situation as well as the skill set of the surgeon. During the abdominal washout, performing as little dissection as is necessary in order to control the septic source and placing drains will help decrease the change of doing further harm.

Anastomotic leaks also require re-intervention. There is a growing body of literature regarding conservative management of controlled leaks with bowel rest and percutaneous intervention [21]. A limited trial of conservative management in a completely non-toxic patient with a truly walled-off collection with no diffuse peritoneal spillage can be considered. The danger with this approach, however, is missing early signs of organ dysfunction and thereby greatly increasing the patient's risk of developing sepsis and organ failure. For the vast majority of anastomotic leaks, re-operation, either open or laparoscopic, with drainage and most often fecal diversion either with a loop or end ostomy depending on the clinical situation is required [22].

So what should be done with the patient above with a persistent small bowel obstruction and obvious mid-jejunal transition point with a thickened segment of bowel? If she has an elevated lactate, elevated white blood cell count, peritoneal findings or a small bowel follow though study that shows a mechanical obstruction, she should undergo re-operation as her issues are unlikely to resolve with continued conservative management.

Intra-operative Decision-Making and Management

Once it is determined that the patient needs to undergo re-exploration the question of when and how comes to the forefront. Ideally, re-exploration is undertaken either prior to postoperative day ten or after six weeks. Often times this is not possible. The re-operative abdominal wall is a challenge in and of itself as repeated operation through an incompletely or minimally healed wound portends potential major complications in the abdominal wall [23]. An abdominal wall that has sustained multiple incisions is more also more likely to have altered vascularity and impaired wound healing leading to a higher risk of poor fascial healing as well as skin and soft tissue infections. Dense adhesions and scar tissue formation within the re-operative abdomen also lead to a higher risk of inadvertent intra-abdominal injuries and postoperative complications that may require yet another surgical procedure to correct [24]. The patient and their family should be counseled regarding the increased complexity and difficulty of a re-operative procedure as well as the prolonged recovery that will likely be encountered compared to a primary procedure.

Advances in imaging techniques, particularly computed tomography, have greatly enhanced not only our ability to make more educated decisions regarding the need for re-operation but have also greatly assisted our ability to preoperatively plan [25]. Prior to proceeding with the re-operation care should be taken to ensure that the patient is adequately resuscitated. Also, the surgeon should ensure that they are well prepared and rested for the procedure as it will likely be challenging and present multiple obstacles and decision points.

Determining whether to proceed with an open or laparoscopic approach depends on the initial procedure performed, the indication for re-operation, and the skill set of the surgeon. Laparoscopic re-operative surgery can be performed safely after both open and laparoscopic surgery, but the experience can be limited depending on the initial case performed and the complication that is present [26, 27]. Certainly if the original operation was performed laparoscopically, it is more likely that a re-operation will be not only initially attempted laparoscopically but will be able to be completed laparoscopically [28]. The experience of laparoscopically managing complications of certain laparoscopic procedures, particularly bariatric procedures and cholecystectomy, is much greater than other gastrointestinal surgery complications. Relaparoscopy for complications encountered after colorectal surgeries such as postoperative hemorrhage, abscess, and anastomotic leak is becoming more successful as the experience with laparoscopic colorectal surgeries is increasing [29, 30]. For postoperative bowel obstructions, the success rate of laparoscopic treatment is dependent on not just the adhesive burden within the peritoneal cavity, but also the distension and friability of the bowel.

Entry into the abdomen whether laparoscopic or open can be difficult. An extension of the existing open incision or even an alternate incision may be helpful in gaining entry into the peritoneal cavity. If the case is approaching laparoscopically, one may access the peritoneal cavity using the Hasson technique or by establishing pneumoperitoneum with a Veress needle at a site remote from previous surgery and using a trans-trocar visualization to gain access. Certainly, a more direct visualized entry into the re-operative abdomen is much safer than a blind entry. Additional ports should be placed under direct vision to allow for triangulation of the affected area of the abdominal cavity. The patient in the above case had only one surgery preceding the lysis of adhesions and on computed tomography appears to have a relatively limited area of difficulty. This makes an initial attempt at laparoscopic re-exploration a valid option if the surgeon has the technical ability to perform the procedure safely. It is unacceptable to allow a patient to suffer from unnecessary ongoing contamination or bleeding while the surgeon is struggling to preserve the tenets of minimally invasive surgery. Making a fresh assessment of the local condition and making the best selection of the possible interventions to solve the issues at hand are paramount. Certainly in re-operation for complications, conversion to an open procedure should not be considered a failure.

It is important to deal with operative issues encountered as thoroughly as is necessary to solve the issue for which you are returning without causing further harm. Preoperative imaging can help guide a more limited operative intervention in many cases whether it is with the ability to place the incision directly over the affected area or limiting exploration to the suspected area. Adhesiolysis in the early re-operative period can be much more challenging than when further delayed. Multiple techniques may be required to be successful in lysing adhesions to allow for visualization of the issues at hand. Utilizing saline-soaked laparotomy sponges or a saline-filled bulb syringe to create more edematous planes within the more dense adhesions can be quite helpful. Also moving from an area where you have no visualization of planes to another area is also important.

Common clinical scenarios seen by most acute care surgeons include anastomotic leak, intra-abdominal sepsis that has failed less invasive interventions (limited or multiple), or postoperative bowel obstruction. When re-exploring a patient with an anastomotic leak, limited evaluation of the anastomosis with drain placement, abdominal washout, and creation of a proximal diverting ostomy may be all that is truly necessary. Patient with multiple abscesses guided washout of those areas with drain placement. For the case above, identifying the affected bowel limb, adequate mobilization of the limb to allow for resection and anastomosis is what needed to alleviate the obstruction that is present on computed tomography. Further adhesiolysis is not warranted. In some more complicated cases, a staged "damage control" procedure where the surgeon takes what the abdomen gives them and limits the amount of intervention as dictated by patient illness may be required to more successfully manage the patient [31, 32]. Ensuring that the patient is adequately resuscitated before, during, and after surgery is also important and should not be overlooked.

Fascial closure in the early re-operative abdomen is a travel into Pandora's box that one would gladly avoid as the fascial edge is almost always affected by the initial closure. The first decision point when nearing the end of the relaparotomy is whether the abdomen should be closed at this time or should be left open for a return evaluation. If a staged procedure is necessary, temporary abdominal closure can be accomplished in many ways. If likely only a single return to the operating room is indicated hours, a Barker vacuum pack is the closure method of choice [33]. If more than one re-operation is needed, consideration of a Wittmann patch (Starsurgical, Burlington, WI) or an ABThera open-abdomen negative pressure system (KCI, San Antonio, TX) would be better options to help prevent the loss of fascial domain [34, 35]. When the time for abdominal closure is reached, it determines whether the integrity of the fascia is adequate for primary closure without tension. Closing with a running or interrupted suture at the fascial level is dependent on the comfort and experience of the surgeon. Utilizing internal retention sutures, particularly with a running closure, is something that should be considered and the surgeon should have a low threshold for their use. Utilizing native tissue for closure is the most desired option if at all possible. If the fascia will not close without tension, a release of just the posterior rectus fascia can assist with medial mobilization of the rectus fascia to overcome up to six-centimeter defects. If this does not accomplish a tension-free midline repair, utilizing a posterior rectus component separation and transversus abdominis muscle release as described by Petro et al. [36] can often assist with closing the defect. Buttressing the component mobilizing closure, either a posterior rectus separation alone or a more complex component separation, with an underlay of vicryl mesh or a biologic can decrease the risk of future incisional hernia formation [37, 38]. Skin closure at the conclusion of the re-operative procedure is dictated by the wound class. If significant contamination is present, the skin incision should be left open, with the potential for delayed primary closure in three to four days pending the appearance of the wound [39]. A commercial vacuum dressing (KCI, San Antonio, TX) or simple saline-soaked dressing changes can be used for treatment of the open skin incision. If there is no significant intra-abdominal contamination during the case and the patient is not septic, the skin incision may be loosely closed with interspersed wicks that can be removed or changed postoperatively. The wound should be carefully inspected daily for any signs and symptoms of a wound infection. If present, the wound should be opened expeditiously.

Peri-operative management of the re-operative patient is often more complicated than in the index operation. Communicating with anesthesia before and during the case about the patient's clinical status, the initial operative plan and intra-operative adjustments including the potential need for an abbreviated laparotomy depending on intra-operative findings can help anesthesiologist optimize their anesthetic regimen for the patient. Ensuring the patient has adequate monitoring in place (arterial line, large bore intravenous access, and intra-operative trans-esophageal) and is adequately resuscitated throughout the case is imperative. The re-operative patient is more likely to require postoperative intensive care than after the index case.

Postoperative Challenges

For the re-operative patient, ensuring adequate nutrition and wound management can be more complicated than in the non-re-operative patient. Optimizing a re-operative patient's nutritional status can be difficult as most have already been without adequate nutrition for an extended time and enteral feeding may not be possible. Early initiation of parenteral nutrition may be necessary to ensure that the patient receives adequate nutrition, in particular protein, and support during the recovery period [40]. Enteral nutrition should be started as soon as it is clinically feasible and the parenteral nutrition should be stopped at that time. Supplementation of micronutrients, such as zinc, selenium, copper, and vitamins C, E, and B is also important for wound healing and should not be overlooked [41].

Postoperatively, the re-operative patient is also at much higher risk for wound complications and fascial dehiscence than after the primary operation. If the wound is closed, it should be inspected frequently by the surgical team with a low threshold for opening with any sign of infection. If the skin incision is left open, wound management with a commercial vacuum dressing (KCI, San Antonio, TX) can assist with wound healing, but should not be used in a contaminated wound. The vacuum dressing can serve as a stent of sorts for the fascial closure; however, it should be changed at least every forty-eight hours in the early postoperative period to ensure fascial integrity. Once a granulation is established, this interval may be lengthened.

General postoperative issues including adequate analgesia, effective pulmonary toilet, instigation of deep venous thrombosis prophylaxis, ensuring adequate volume resuscitation, appropriate drain management as well as continued management of preexisting health problems should all be optimized in the re-operative patient.

Conclusion

In conclusion, relaparotomy in the delayed postoperative period can be accomplished safely depending on patient selection, preoperative preparation, and selection of the simplest effective procedure. Taking a stepwise approach to the patient is essential as there are potential pitfalls at every step.

Clinical Scenario

42 y.o woman underwent open laparotomy and adhesiolysis for acute small bowel obstruction. Her original abdominal surgery was for an ectopic pregnancy when she was 22. Intra-operatively, no bowel was resected, but a 20-cm segment of distal jejunum was dusky but felt to "pink up." Post-op day 7, she has a persistent small bowel obstruction and obvious mid-jejunal transition point with a thickened segment of bowel.

The surgeon is stuck a bit between a rock and a hard place in the above clinical scenario with regard to the decision to re-operate on the patient at this time. Is postoperative day seven long enough to truly determine whether this area of bowel will not improve on its own? So re-operating early will result in an unnecessary re-exploration. If the bowel does not recover and the re-exploration is delayed for another week will the abdomen be too hostile to resect the area without doing harm?

Given the initial operative findings of an initially dusky segment of bowel that corresponds to the transition point seen on CT, the likelihood that this could be a developing stricture at that location is high favoring early re-exploration and resection of the affected segment. Delaying the intervention for another ten to fourteen days will make the re-exploration more difficult and would not be advised.

Key Question

1. *How do you decide where it is safest to enter the relaparotomy abdomen?*

References

1. Merriam-Webster dictionary. [Internet]. Available from http://www.merriam-webster.com.
2. Harbrecht PJ, Garrison RN, Fry DE. Early urgent re-laparotomy. Arch Surg. 1984;119: 369–74.
3. Hutchins RR, Gunning MP, Lucas DN, et al. Relaparotomy for suspected intraperitoneal sepsis after abdominal surgery. World J Surg. 2004;28:137–41.
4. Lamme B, Boermeester MA, Reitsma JB, et al. Meta-analysis of re-laparotomy for secondary peritonitis. Br J Surg. 2002;89:1516–24.
5. Kim JJ, Liang MK, Subramanian A, et al. Predictors of re-laparotomy after non-trauma emergency general surgery with initial fascial closure. AJS. 2011;202:549–52.
6. Brochausen C, et al. Intraperitoneal adhesions—an ongoing challenge between biomedical engineering and the life sciences. J Biomed Mater. 2011;98:143.
7. Masoomi H, Kang CY, Chaudry O, et al. Predictive factors of early bowel obstruction in colon and rectal surgery: data from the nationwide inpatient sample, 2006–2008. JACS. 2012;214: 831–7.
8. Pickleman J, Lee RM. The management of patients with suspected early postoperative small bowel obstruction. Ann Surg. 1989;210:216–9.
9. Fazio VW, Ziv Y, Church JM, Oakley JR, Lavery IC, Milsom JW, et al. Ileal pouch–anal anastomosis complications and function in 1005 patients. Ann Surg. 1995;222:120–7.
10. Ellozy SH, Harris MT, Bauer JJ, Gorfine SR, Kreel I. Early postoperative small-bowel obstruction: a prospective evaluation in 242 consecutive abdominal operations. Dis Colon Rectum. 2002;45:1214–7.
11. Mallo RD, Salem R, Lalani T. Computed tomography diagnosis of ischemia and complete obstruction in small bowel obstruction: a systematic review. J Gastrointest Surg. 2005;9: 690–4.
12. Maung AA, Johnson DC, Piper GL, Barbosa RR, et al. Evaluation and management of small-bowel obstruction: an Eastern Association for the Surgery of Trauma practice management guideline. J Trauma Acute Care Surg. 2012;73(5 Suppl 4):S362–9.
13. Goussous N, Eiken PW, Bannon MP, Zielinski MD. Enhancement of a small bowel obstruction model using the gastrografin(R) challenge test. J Gastrointest Surg. 2013;17: 110–7.
14. Khasawneh MA, Martinez Ugarte ML, Srvantstian B, et al. Role of gastrografin challenge in early postoperative small bowel obstruction. J Gastrointest Surg. 2014;18:363–8.
15. Saini DK, Chaudhary P, Durga CK, Saini K. Role of multislice computed tomography in evaluation and management of intestinal obstruction. Clin Pract. 2013;3:51–5.
16. Suri RR, Vora P, Kirby JM, Ruo L. Computed tomography features associated with operative management for non strangulating small bowel obstruction. Can J Surg. 2014;57:254–9.
17. Zielinski MD, Eiken PW, Bannon MP, et al. Small bowel obstruction—who needs an operation? A multivariate prediction model. World J Surg. 2010;34:910–9.
18. Colon MJ, Telem DA, Wong D, et al. The relevance of transition zones on computed tomography in the management of small bowel obstruction. Surgery. 2010;147:373–7.
19. Robert B, Chivot C, Fuks D, Gondry-Jouet C, Regimbeau JM, Yzet T. Percutaneous, computed tomography-guided drainage of deep pelvic abscesses via a transgluteal approach: a report on 30 cases and a review of the literature. Abdom Imaging. 2013;38:285–9.
20. Kassi F, Dohan A, Soyer P, Vicaut E, Boudiaf M, Valleur P, Pocard M. Predictive factors for failure of percutaneous drainage of postoperative abscess after abdominal surgery. Am J Surg. 2014;207:915–21.

21. Brunner W, Rossetti A, Vines LC, Kalak N, Bischofberger SA. Anastomotic leakage after laparoscopic single-port sigmoid resection: combined transanal and transabdominal minimal invasive management. Surg Endosc. 2015;Mar 18. [Epub ahead of print].
22. Khan AA, Wheeler JM, Cunningham C, George B, Kettlewell M, Mortensen NJ. The management and outcome of anastomotic leaks in colorectal surgery. Colorectal Dis. 2008;10: 587–92.
23. Carlson MA. Acute wound failure. Curg Clin N Am. 1997;77:607–36.
24. Iqbal CW, Pham TH, Joseph A, et al. Long-term outcome of 254 complex incisional hernia repairs using the modified Rives-Stoppa technique. World J Surg. 2007;31:2398–404.
25. Harris C, Nicholson DA, Anderson ID. Computed tomography: a vital adjunct in the management of complex post operative sepsis. BJS. 1998;85:861–2.
26. McCormick JT, Papasavas PK, Caushaj PF, Gagne DJ. Laparoscopic revision of failed open bariatric procedures. Surg Endosc. 2003;17:413–5.
27. Papasavas PK, Caushaj PF, McCormick JT, et al. Laparoscopic management of complications following laparoscopic Roux-en-Y gastric bypass for morbid obesity. Surg Endosc. 2003;17: 610–4.
28. McCormick JT, Simmang CL. Reoperation following minimally invasive surgery: are the “rules” different? Clin Colon Rectal Surg. 2006;19:217–22.
29. Liu J, Bruch H, Farke S, Nolde J, Schwandner O. Stoma formation for fecal diversion: a plea for the laparoscopic approach. Tech Coloproctol. 2005;9:9–14.
30. Boulez J, Espalieu Ph, Fontaumard E, Meeus P. Laparoscopic colo-rectal surgery; analysis of 113 cases. Hepatogastroenterology. 1997;44:40–4.
31. Rotondo MF, Schwab CW, McGonigal MD, et al. ‘Damage control’: an approach for improved survival in exsanguinating penetrating abdominal injury. J Trauma. 1993;35: 375–83.
32. Sartelli M, Abu-Zidan FM, Ansaloni L, et al. The role of the open abdomen procedure in managing severe abdominal sepsis: WSES position paper. World J Emerg Surg. 2015;10:35.
33. Barker DE, Kaufman HJ, Smith LA, Ciraulo DL, Richart CL, Burns RP. Vacuum pack technique of temporary abdominal closure: a 7-year experience with 112 patients. J Trauma. 2000;48:201–6.
34. Tieu BH, Cho SD, Luem N, Riha G, Mayberry J, Schreiber MA. The use of the Wittmann Patch facilitates a high rate of fascial closure in severely injured trauma patients and critically ill emergency surgery patients. J Trauma. 2008;65:865–70.
35. Roberts DJ, Zygun DA, Grendar J, Ball CG, Robertson HL, Ouellet JF, Cheatham ML, Kirkpatrick AW. Negative-pressure wound therapy for critically ill adults with open abdominal wounds: a systematic review. J Trauma Acute Care Surg. 2012;73:629–39.
36. Petro CC, Como JJ, Yee S, Prabhu AS, Novitsky YW, Rosen MJ. Posterior component separation and transversus abdominis muscle release for complex incisional hernia repair in patients with a history of an open abdomen. J Trauma Acute Care Surg. 2015;78:422–9.
37. Wang TY, Elliott R, Low DW. Damage control abdomen: single-stage reconstruction using a vicryl mesh buttress. Ann Plast Surg. 2013;70:324–30.
38. Diaz JJ Jr, Cullinane DC, Khwaja KA, Tyson GH, et al. Eastern Association for the Surgery of Trauma: management of the open abdomen, part III-review of abdominal wall reconstruction. J Trauma Acute Care Surg. 2013;75:376–86.
39. Seamon MJ, Smith BP, Capano-Wehrle L, Fakhro A, Fox N, Goldberg M, Martin NM, Pathak AS, Ross SE. Skin closure after trauma laparotomy in high-risk patients: opening opportunities for improvement. J Trauma Acute Care Surg. 2013;74:433–40.
40. Arabi YM, Aldawood AS, Haddad SH, Al-Dorzi HM, et al. PermiT Trial Group. permissive underfeeding or standard enteral feeding in critically ill adults. N Engl J Med. 2015;372 (25):2398–408.
41. Preiser JC, van Zanten AR, Berger MM, Biolo G, Casaer MP, et al. Metabolic and nutritional support of critically ill patients: consensus and controversies. Crit Care. 2015;29(19):35.

Chapter 25
The Management of the Entero-Atmospheric Fistula (EAF)

Narong Kulvatunyou and Peter Rhee

Background

The concept of open abdomen was popularized in the era of damage control laparotomy (DCL) for trauma (Fig. 25.1). The concept has been applied to an emergency general surgery and intra-abdominal sepsis as well. In trauma, however, the pendulum has now swung toward performing less DCL. This will probably lead to a lower incidence of open abdomen-related complications, i.e., ventral hernia and enteric fistula. Prior reported incidence of open abdomen-related fistula may be as high as 21 % [1].

In this clinical presentation, the fistula presented is termed an "entero-atmospheric fistula" (EAF). It is a fistula without an epithelialized tract and the opening is exposed to air (hence the term "atmosphere") instead of skin. This type of fistula is very different from the traditionally discussed entero-cutaneous fistula (ECF), because EAF presents a much more clinical challenge in terms of patient's critical illness, controlling fistula effluence, and the unlikely spontaneous closure of the fistula. However, there have been several prior case reports of spontaneous fistula closure of the EAF using various techniques [2–4]. These will be further discussed later.

N. Kulvatunyou (✉) · P. Rhee
Division of Acute Care Surgery, Department of Surgery, University of Arizona, 1501 N. Campbell Ave., Room 5411, PO Box 245603, Tucson, AZ 85727-5063, USA
e-mail: nkulvatunyou@surgery.arizona.edu

P. Rhee
e-mail: prhee@surgery.arizona.edu

J.J. Diaz and D.T. Efron (eds.), *Complications in Acute Care Surgery*,
DOI 10.1007/978-3-319-42376-0_25

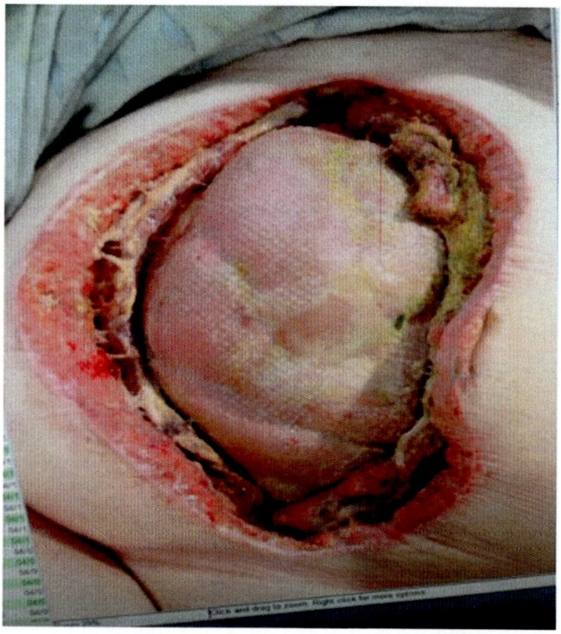

Fig. 25.1 Budding mucosa (*arrow*) below the VICRYL mesh in an open abdomen

Etiology

Etiology for EAF is somewhat different from ECF, which often discussed in terms of intrinsic versus extrinsic factors. Intrinsic factors included conditions such as an inflammatory bowel disease and diverticulitis. Extrinsic factors included postoperative anastomotic leak and iatrogenic bowel injury. On the contrary, EAF arises mostly from extrinsic factors, usually in association with open abdomen. For example, the fistula can arise from an unrecognized iatrogenic bowel injury that is delay detected during a postoperative course (Fig. 25.2), an anastomotic leak (Fig. 25.3), a significant trauma that is associated with significant loss of abdominal wall domain (Fig. 25.4), or a complication of open abdomen from desiccation (our case scenario). Therefore, whether the open abdomen is intentional or unintentional, the open abdomen is definitely a risk factor for EAF development.

Classification

In ECF, a general classification of fistula is often based on effluent output per 24 h. A high output is 500 cc per 24 h, while a low output is less than 200 cc, and a moderate output is between 200 and 500 cc. The classification can also be based on the anatomical location such as gastric versus small bowel versus large bowel. These classifications may have some predictive roles of possible spontaneous fistula

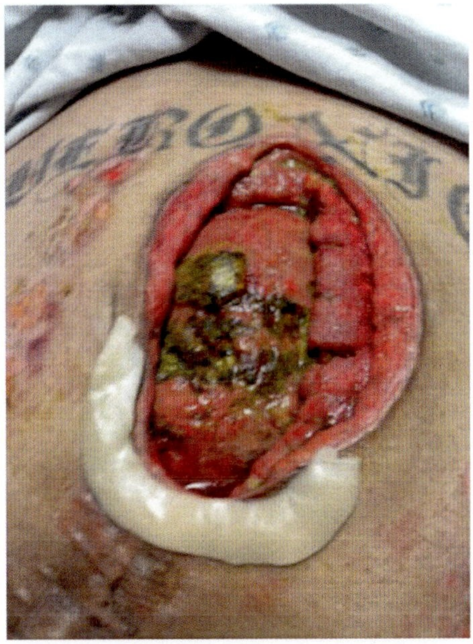

Fig. 25.2 Atmospheric small-bowel fistula arises from unrecognized iatrogenic small-bowel injury in a 46-year-old male who underwent ventral hernia repair and lysis of adhesion

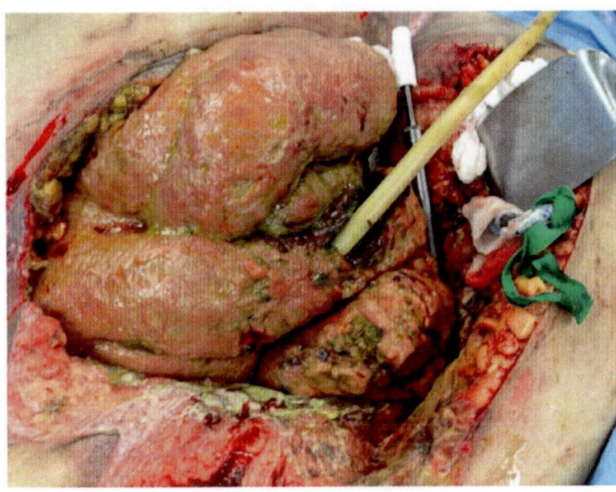

Fig. 25.3 Atmospheric small-bowel fistula arises from an anastomotic leak 10 days postoperatively in a morbidly obese patient with a body mass index of 75

closure. These two schematic classifications can certainly be applied to EAF, but the relationship of fistula classification and spontaneous fistula closure outcome has never been studied because EAF is more rare. All reports on EAF [2–10] have all been either a case report or case series with a very limited number of patients; therefore, any definitive conclusion is very difficult. Furthermore as mentioned previously, because of the lack of fistula tract in EAF, the spontaneous fistula closure is most unlikely.

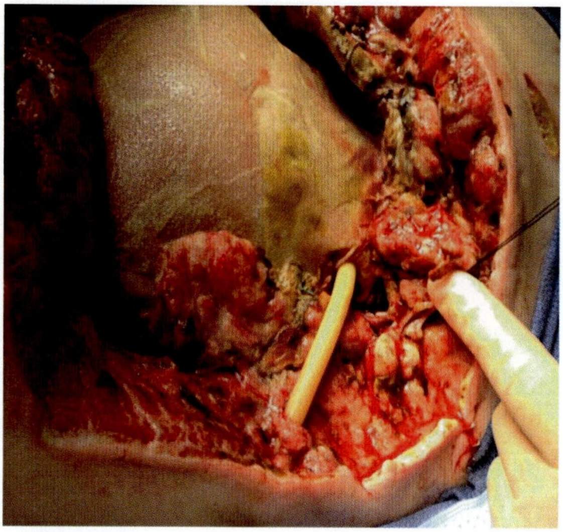

Fig. 25.4 Atmospheric (gastric and small bowel) fistula arises from open abdomen due to gunshot wound that is associated with a significant loss of abdominal domain

Management

The general principle of ECF management can still be applied to EAF. These include sepsis source control, fluid and electrolytes monitoring with appropriate replacement, nutritional support, and wound/skin care and protection. However, a general notion in ECF that the fistula might close spontaneously after ruling out distal obstruction and foreign body may not be equally applicable to EAF, because EAF has different etiologies, lacks the fistula track, and is often associated with a complex and austere intra-abdominal environment that often arises from the intra-abdominal catastrophe. EAF is also often associated with significant abdominal wall domain loss and/or defect that requires a major abdominal wall reconstruction during the reoperation.

Although the hope in managing EAF is that one would like to achieve a spontaneous fistula closure, but in reality knowing that spontaneous fistula closure is unlikely, the true goal in EAF management is to control the fistula effluence well enough that a tissue coverage; i.e., skin graft can be accomplished. Then a plan to return at a later date to deal with the fistula take-down and reconstruction of the abdominal wall defect can be implemented. Various surgical techniques [2–10] in dealing with EAF have been reported in the literature. Most cases were anecdotal author's personal case reports. Some were case series. The summary of these reports including technique is listed in the table (see Table 25.1). The main idea among these various reports can be grouped as either attempts to close the fistula primarily [2–4], or to control the effluence with tissue coverage using skin graft. Our own authors at some points have attempted all of these techniques including a recently reported "Fistula Patch" by Wang et al. [10]. The authors experienced different results (personal experience) from what has been reported. As a result,

Table 25.1 Various techniques used to close the fistula or control the effluence of the fistula

Authors	Technique	N	Comment
1. Jamshidi and Schecter [2]	Biological dressing	$N = 7$	Success closure 5/7 patients
2. Girard et al. [3]	Biological dressing + fibrin glue	$N = 1$	Success closure
3. Sarfeh and Jakowatz [4]	Primary repair + STSG	$N = 1$	Success closure
4. Al-Khoury et al. [5]	Malecot tube + VAC	$N = 1$	
5. Subramaniam et al. [6]	Floating stoma	$N = 7$	
6. Cheesborough et al. [7]	Red rubber tube + STSG	$N = 7$	
7. Gunn et al. [8]	Fistula VAC	$N = 15$	Success closure 11/15 patients
8. Layton et al. [9]	Baby nipple + VAC	$N = 1$	
9. Wang et al. [10]	Fistula patch	$N = 11$	
10. Kulvatunyou et al. (current series)	Malecot tube + advanced flap ± VAC	$N = 3$	

STSG Split thickness skin graft; *VAC* Vacuum-assisted closure

authors have also come up with our own approach, and we used a modified Hirschberg' Malecot tube technique [5] that we will further discussed later.

Several authors reported attempts to close the fistula primarily using a combination of biological dressing such as human acellular dermal matrix (Alloderm, LifeCell Corp, Branchburg, New Jersey) [2] or skin graft [4], and with the use of fibrin glue [3]. Success was anecdotal [3, 4]. Jamshidi and Schecter [2] reported success in 5 out of 7, but the factors predicting success were not detailed. In authors' personal experience, a direct closure of the fistula can be attempted, but success in our own hands has been poor. The reasons for these failures may be that our EAF had significantly high output of over 1 L per 24 h, or our fistulas were associated with a bowel motility dysfunction that may behave like a functional intestinal obstruction.

In the remaining studies, other authors have reported different techniques used to control fistula effluence. Among these techniques included the use of a Malecot tube and a wound VAC [5], a floating stoma using a sewn in plastic sheet [6], a red rubber tube and a wound VAC [7], a modified wound VAC [8], a wound VAC with a baby nipple to control the fistula [9], and a most recently reported a temporary internal stent termed a "Fistula Patch" [10]. The goal for all of these reports was to control the fistula effluence to prevent wound contamination, so that wound can be allowed to heal by contraction with the assistance of tissue coverage by skin graft.

Controlling the effluence using the modified wound VAC [8] has always been our own preference and it seems to work very well at controlling the effluence. However, the wound care and wound dressing change can be quite labor intensive as dressing needs to be changed 3–4 times per week, sometimes daily. The dressing change can be quite time consuming and often requires the help of the special wound care nurse. This implies that patient will need to remain in the hospital for a long period of time, or attempt to discharge patient to a long-term facility will be difficult due to the lack of special wound care nurse. Because of this dilemma, the authors have modified the technique to control the effluence by adapting the Malecot technique of Dr. Hirshberg's [5]. Instead of bringing the Malecot tube directly through the foam of the wound VAC device as reported by Dr. Hirshberg, we bring the Malecot tube through the skin after we have mobilized and advanced the skin flap bilaterally toward the midline (Figs. 25.5, 25.6, 25.7). The goal is to convert the EAF into the ECF.

On occasion, if the authors cannot mobilize and advance the skin flaps toward the midline and over the fistula due to a significant abdominal wall thickness and edema, then the authors will bring and exteriorize the Malecot tube toward the nearest skin (Fig. 25.8). This approach will not completely divert the fistula effluence because there will still be a leak around the fistula, but the technique helps minimize the wound bed contamination and allows the wound VAC to last longer than 48 h. Diverting fistula effluence through Malecot tube also makes wound VAC dressing change more simplified. Then after a period of wound healing by

(a) (b)

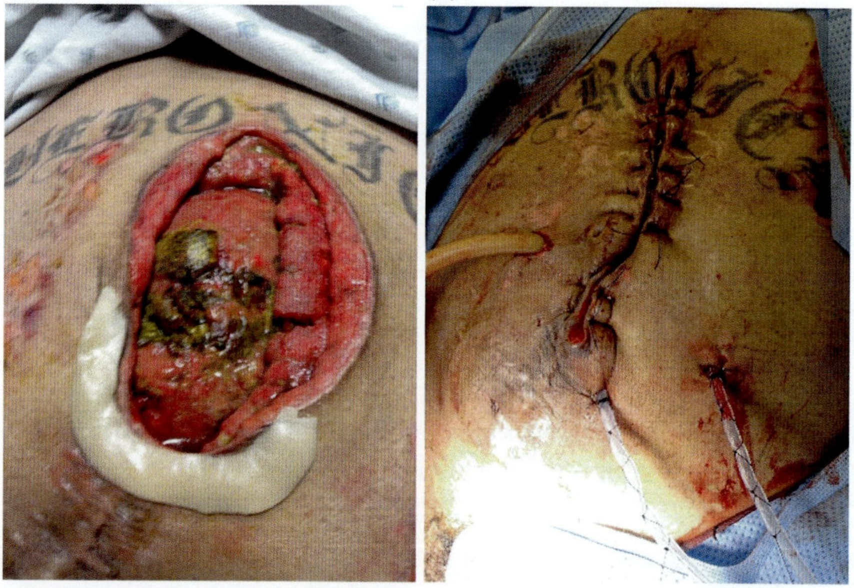

Fig. 25.5 Patient presented 1 month after ventral hernia repair that is complicated by entero-atmospheric fistula. After a thorough washout, we raised bilateral skin flaps and advanced toward midline. We then cannulated the fistula using the 32-French Malecot tube (*black arrow*) and exteriorized the tube through the skin on the right side of the abdomen. The incision was initially closed completely, but this was a mistake. Later we had to reopen the wound at the bottom of the incision to allow some drainage as Jackson-Pratt drain was not adequate

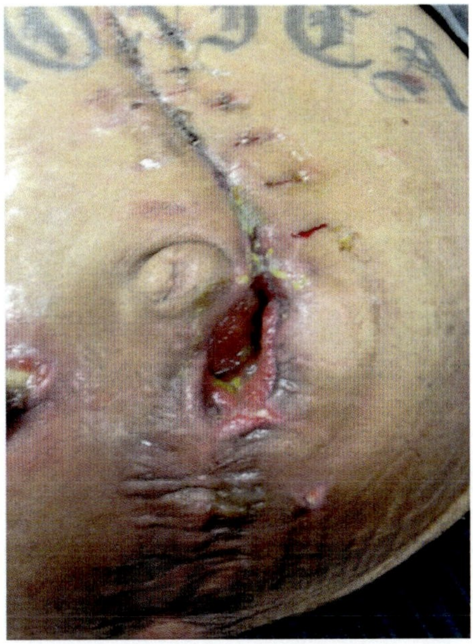

Fig. 25.6 On postoperative day 3, the bottom of the incision was reopened (*black arrow*) to allow a better drainage of fluid including the fistula effluence that leaks around the Malecot tube. The exteriorized Malecot tube (*black arrow head*) was still to the right of the incision

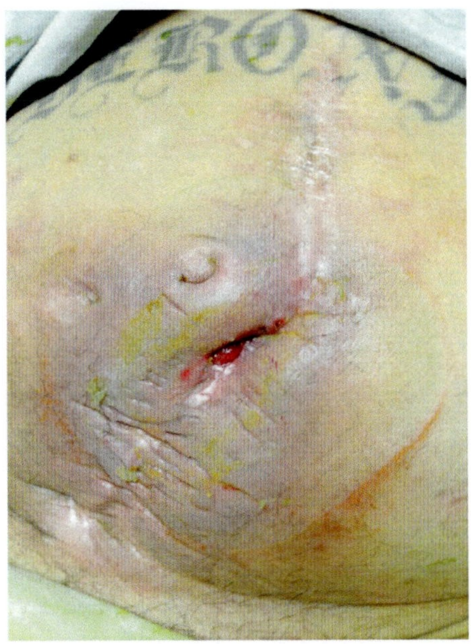

Fig. 25.7 Two months after our initial closure, Malecot tube had been dislodged (*black arrow head*) but the fistula was now draining through the lower incision (*black arrow*) that was well managed with a colostomy appliance

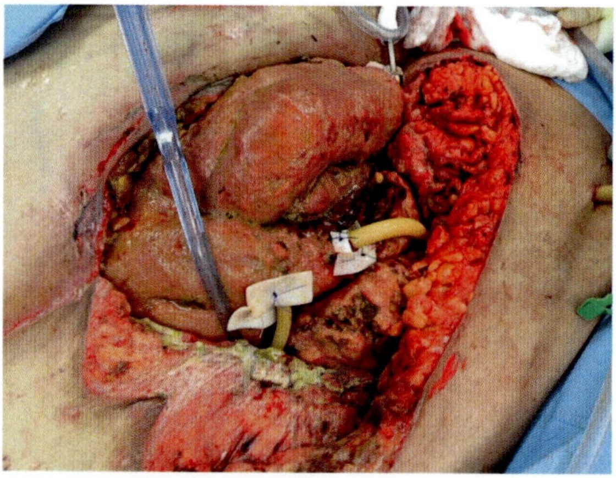

Fig. 25.8 Two EAF developed after anastomotic leak in a super morbidly obese patient with a body mass index of 75. Abdominal wall and skin flaps could not be mobilized due to its thickness and edema. 32-French Malecot tubes (*black arrows*) were used to cannulate the fistula and exteriorized the nearest skin, one was on the left (*black arrow head*), one on the right (not seen in the picture). Due to friable tissue around the fistula, the authors placed purse-string sutures around the Malecot and reinforced with a biological tissue (Strattice, LifeCell, Branchburg, New Jersey)

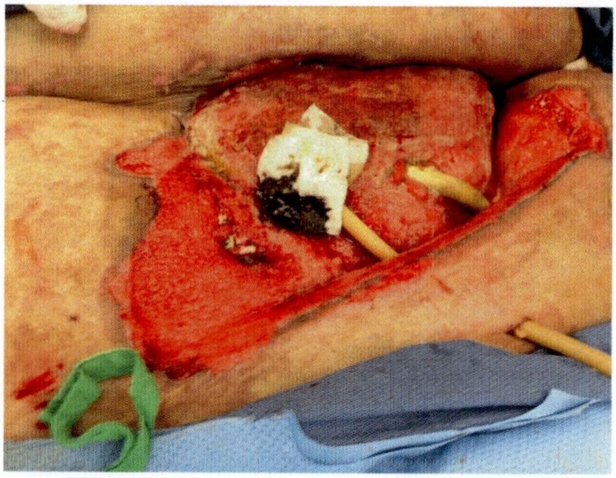

Fig. 25.9 After 1 month, wound was healing with a significant wound contraction

contraction with additional skin graft, the wound healed and fistula can be managed with colostomy appliance (Figs. 25.9, 25.10).

On a similar but a different situation where skin flaps cannot be advanced, the authors rotated a skin flap to cover the fistula and the fistula was cannulated and again exteriorized through the skin (Figs. 25.11, 25.12). Again, the goal of such maneuver was to convert the EAF into ECF, so that fistula effluent control can be achieved.

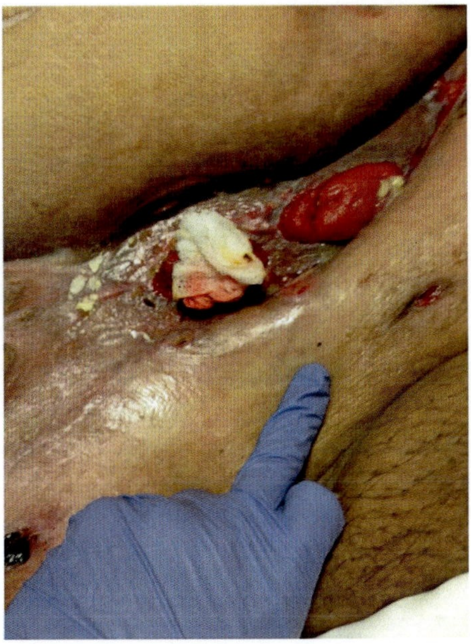

Fig. 25.10 After 3 months and after patient underwent split thickness skin graft, the wound had completely healed and colostomy appliances can now be placed around the fistula to control the effluence

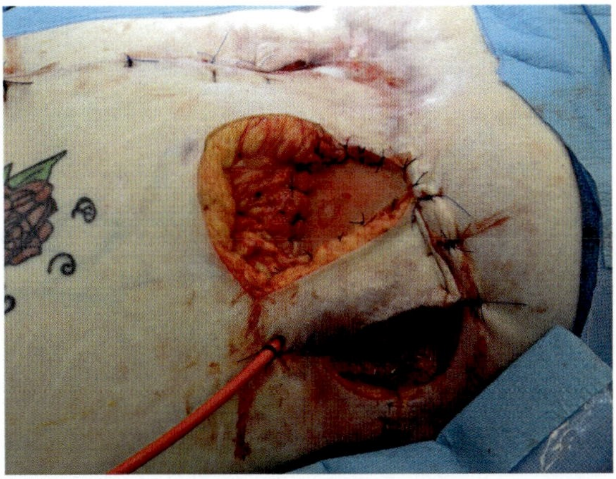

Fig. 25.11 A 46-year-old patient suffered from a self-inflicted gunshot wound with significant abdominal wall domain loss. Post-injury she developed combined gastric and small-bowel fistula. She underwent a successful gastric fistula takedown but her small-bowl fistula recurred postoperatively. No available skin flap could be advanced, so the authors rotated the skin flap to cover the fistula (*black arrow*) and used the red rubber tube to control the fistula effluence

(a) (b)

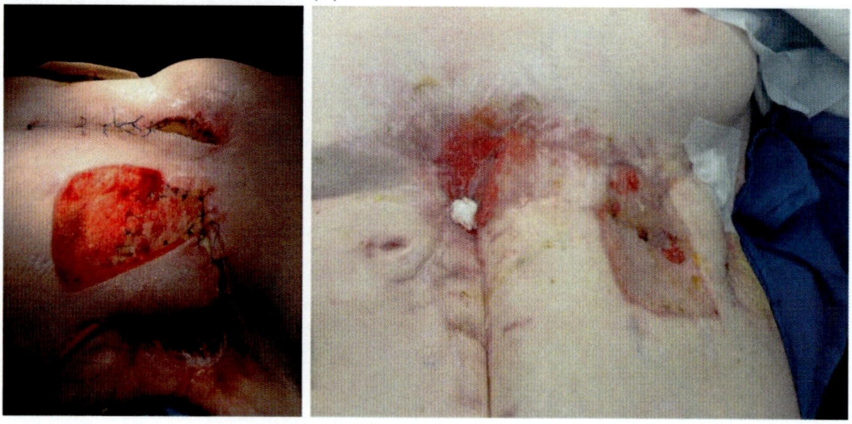

Fig. 25.12 Two months after a combination of wound contraction, skin graft, and low fistula output, EAF spontaneously closed and wound healed

Although our ultimate goal in the management of all EAF is to hope that fistula may close spontaneously, but achieving a goal of non-closure of the fistula that has a good effluent control may still be considered a "success" to a very difficult problem [8]. So if one can achieve good fistula effluent control, then one would wait for the classic teaching of 6–12 months until nutritional status improves and long enough for hostile abdominal environment subsides, or if patient receives skin graft is to wait until skin graft can be pinched between the fingers [7], before patient is taken back for reoperation. Authors would often prefer waiting longer than 12 months because of number of reasons. First, many of these patients have already spent a few months in the hospital from the original complication, and psychologically the longer time away from another hospitalization may prove beneficial. Secondly, nutritional and electrolyte problem is not an issue as this can be supplemented by total parenteral nutrition (TPN). Authors also always allow patient to have intake by mouth for at least self-pleasure and possible minimization of the hepatotoxic effect of the long-term TPN. However in one of our patients and under a somewhat unusual circumstance, the healed skin graft over the abdomen had ruptured and we had to take the patient back to the operating room in less than 6 months. As one can anticipate, this early return to surgery was met with hostile abdomen and significant adhesion. Surgery was, though successful, quite challenging (Figs. 25.13, 25.14).

There has been no prior study predicted in which clinical factors lead to a possible spontaneous EAF closure, but Gunn et al. [8] had suggested that in the presence of any visible intestinal mucosa, EAF closure was unlikely. However in Sarfeh and Jakowatz [4] study, the authors suggested otherwise. In that study, the authors excised the surrounding granulation tissue and the mucosa was primarily

(a) (b)

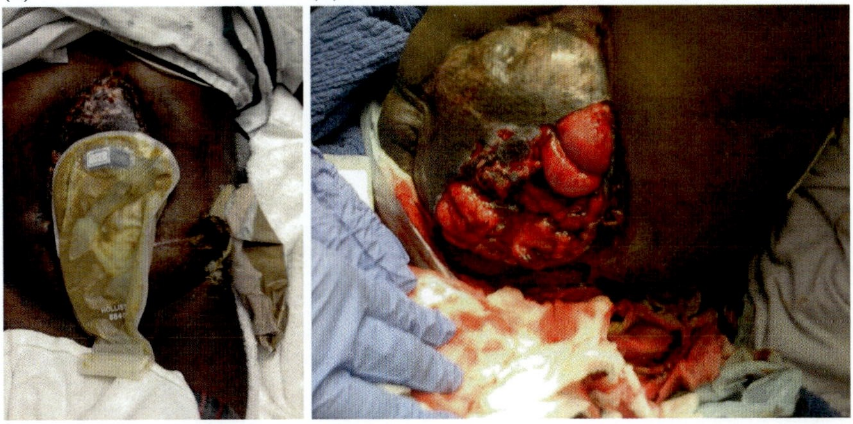

Fig. 25.13 For six months, EAF has been converted to ECF with colostomy appliance and good control of the fistula effluence (**a**). However, skin graft spontaneously ruptured (**b**), forcing the authors having to take the patient back to the operating room in less than 6 months from the original operation

(a) (b) (c)

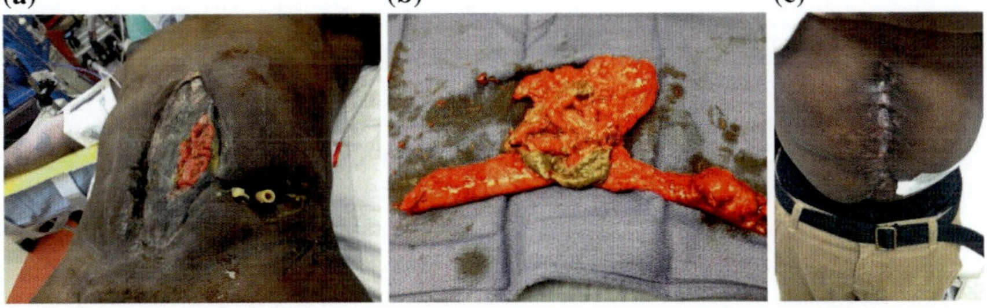

Fig. 25.14 **a** Spontaneous skin graft ruptured resulting in recurrent multiple EAF; **b** specimens of multiple fistula excised en bloc; surgery was 9 h long with difficulty; **c** two weeks postoperative after patient underwent fistula excision, abdominal wall ventral hernia reconstruction with component separation

approximated and then protected with skin graft. Sarfeh and Jakowatz were able to demonstrate fistula closure. We, ourselves, have never had success with attempt fistula closure in the presence of intestinal mucosa.

Back to Our Clinical Scenario

Returning to our clinical scenario, what the authors would do is to cannulate the fistula with the Malecot tube (French 32) and exteriorize the tube through the skin, after performing a bilateral, skin and subcutaneous flap mobilization and

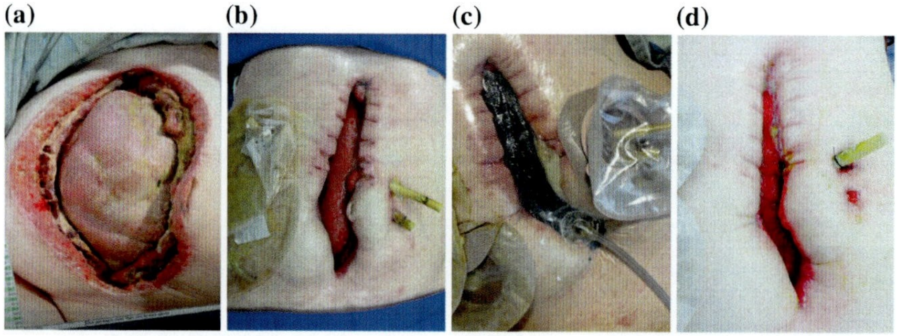

Fig. 25.15 **a** Converting EAF into, **b** ECF using the modified Malecot tube and bilateral, advanced skin and subcutaneous flap, **c** midline was closed with wound vacuum closure and a colostomy appliance was applied over the Malecot tube, **d** 1 month after management, the midline wound continue contraction, most of the effluence was diverted through Malecot tube

advancement toward the midline. In this particular case, the authors could not get the wound to heal at midline leaving the gap which was managed with wound VAC. The colostomy appliance is placed over the Melecot tube to control the fistula effluence. The authors avoid connecting the Malecot tube to Foley gravity bag as this may create traction and may cause Malecot tube to dislodge (Fig. 25.15). Patient was then managed with TPN, oral intake was allowed, and careful weekly monitoring of fluid and electrolyte balance until midline wound had healed with the goal to take the patient back in 12 months or longer for the fistula take down and abdominal wall reconstruction. In essence, the authors have converted EAF in this patient into ECF and continue applying the principle of nutritional support, fluid, and electrolytes balance until wound healing completes.

Conclusion

In conclusion, EAF represents a clinical challenge from the wound management and fistula effluence control. The authors provided a literature review of the existing various novel approaches, including authors' own experience in dealing with this difficult problem. The old idiom "an ounce of prevention is worth a pound of cure" may be true. The goal for all clinicians then should be to avoid the open abdomen if possible, but if one must utilize the open abdomen treatment, the attempt at earlier closure and avoidance of a prolonged intestine exposure and desiccation may help prevent EAF.

Clinical Scenario

Patient, a 45-year-old man, underwent cystoprostatectomy for a focal bladder cancer. His postoperative course was complicated by intra-abdominal sepsis and fascial dehiscence. He required multiple abdominal washout, open abdomen, and later abdominal closure using bridging VICRYL (Polyglactin 910, Ethicon, USA) mesh with negative wound vacuum-assisted closure (VAC). Five days after, there was a copious amount of green fluid drainage from the abdominal wound with an obvious bud of intestinal mucosa identified in the middle of the "bowel ball" below the VICRYL mesh (Fig. 25.1).

Key Questions

1. *How does one decide on the timing to skin graft the open abdominal wound?*
2. *When (and why) consider refeeding of the bilious effluent from a entero-atmospheric fistula?*

References

1. Schecter WP, Hirshberg A, Chang DS, et al. Enteric fistula: principles of management. JACS. 2009;209(4):484–91.
2. Jamshidi R, Schecter WP. Biological dressings for the management of enteric fistula in the open abdomen. Arch Surg. 2007;142(8):793–6.
3. Girard S, Sideman M, Spain DA. A novel approach to the problem of intestinal fistulization arising in patients managed with open peritoneal cavities. Am J Surg. 2002;184:166–7.
4. Sarfeh J, Jakowatz JG. Surgical treatment of enteric 'bud' fistulas in contaminated wound. Arch Surg. 1992;127:1027–31.
5. Al-Khoury G, Kaugman D, Hirshberg A. Improved control of exposed fistula in the open abdomen. JACS. 2008;206:397–8.
6. Subramaniam MH, Liscum KR, Hirshberg A. The floating stoma: a new technique for controlling exposed fistula in abdominal trauma. J Trauma. 2002;53:386–8.
7. Cheesborough JE, Park E, Souza JM, Dumanian GA. Staged management of the open abdomen and enteroatmospheric fistulae using split-thickness skin grafts. Am J Surg. 2014;207:504–11.
8. Gunn LA, Follmar KE, Wong MS, et al. Management of enterocutaneous fistulas using negative-pressure dressings. Ann Plastic Surg. 2006;57:621–5.
9. Layton B, Dubose J, Nichols S, et al. Pacifying the open abdomen with concomitant intestinal fistula: a novel approach. Am J Surg. 2010;199:e48–50.
10. Wang G, Ren J, Liu S, et al. "Fistula patch": making the treatment of enteroatmospheric fistulae in the open abdomen easier. J Trauma ACS. 2013;74:1175–7.

Chapter 26
Unresectable Malignancy and Bowel Obstruction in the Acute Care Surgery Patient

Zara Cooper, Elizabeth Lilley and Gregory J. Jurkovich

Abbreviations

5-HT3	Serotonin type 3 receptor
cm	Centimeter
CT	Computed tomography
D_2	Dopamine type 2 receptor
H_1	Histamine type 1 receptor
L	Liters
MBO	Malignant bowel obstruction
mm	Millimeter
MRI	Magnetic resonance imaging

Background

Malignant bowel obstruction (MBO) is a preterminal condition in patients with advanced, incurable cancer. An international committee on MBO defined it as a bowel obstruction beyond the ligament of Treitz occurring in a patient with either an incurable intra-abdominal primary malignancy or an extra-abdominal primary with clear intraperitoneal spread [1]. Ovarian and colorectal cancers are the most

Z. Cooper (✉)
Harvard Medical School, Boston, MA 02115, USA
e-mail: zcooper@partners.org

E. Lilley
The Center for Surgery and Public Health at Brigham and Women's Hospital, Boston, MA 02120, USA
e-mail: elilley@partners.org

G.J. Jurkovich
Department of Surgery, University of Colorado, 12631 E. 17th Avenue, Aurora, CO 80045, USA
e-mail: gj.jurkovich@comcast.net

J.J. Diaz and D.T. Efron (eds.), *Complications in Acute Care Surgery*,
DOI 10.1007/978-3-319-42376-0_26

common causes of MBO. Other causes include pancreatic, breast, and melanoma. Regardless of the primary cancer, patients with MBO have an underlying non-curable malignancy and present with similar clinical manifestations.

Obstruction may be intra-luminal or extra-luminal. Intra-luminal obstructions are due to direct invasion of tumor into the bowel wall, resulting in intestinal *linitis plastica*. Extra-luminal obstructions are more common and are due to external tethering or compression from metastases or peritoneal carcinomatosis. An inflammatory reaction may occur in the tissue adjacent to the tumor, leading to edema and further luminal narrowing. In addition, tumor invasion into the bowel wall, mesentery, or nerves may lead to dysmotility. Of note, patients with MBO may have multiple, simultaneous causes of obstruction.

For patients with incurable malignancies, development of MBO portends poor prognosis. Estimated survival after initial MBO diagnosis presentation ranges from 1 to 9 months [2]. The high symptom burden and frequent need for inpatient hospitalization during treatment for MBO contribute to high healthcare utilization and impaired quality of life for patients facing terminal illness [3]. Although most patients admitted with MBO are able to be discharged from the hospital, 27–48 % are readmitted with recurrent MBO [4–6]. The majority of patients initially have partial obstructions that gradually worsen. Episodes may be intermittent with spontaneous, symptom-free periods. As the disease process progresses, these intervals become shorter and more frequent, and patients may eventually develop complete obstruction.

Diagnosis

Potential MBO diagnosis should be entertained for patients presenting with signs of obstruction and known intraperitoneal malignancy. MBO presents with symptoms typical of other causes of obstruction, including distension, nausea, emesis, abdominal cramps, dehydration, decreased flatus, and constipation or obstipation. The presence or absence of symptoms may help identify the location of obstruction (see Table 26.1). Prior episodes of obstruction are commonly reported. Over time, patients with long-standing MBO may develop signs of malnourishment related to inadequate nutritional intake, decreased absorption, and the underlying malignancy, so history of recent weight loss may be present in review of systems.

Plain abdominal films will be consistent with bowel obstruction. Although CT is rarely necessary to diagnose bowel obstruction, it may be helpful for identifying malignancy as a potential cause. Moreover, information from CT assists in management decisions and is often helpful for locating the site of obstruction or determining if there is multilevel involvement or a single, discrete segment of bowel that may be amenable to obstruction or bypass. The presence of massive ascites, carcinomatosis, evidence of bowel compromise, or multilevel intestinal involvement will influence surgical decision making if seen on CT. Multidetector CT with thin sections and both oral and intravenous contrast enhancements is the imaging modality

Table 26.1 Clinical signs from history and physical indicating location of obstruction

	Small intestine		Large intestine	
	Proximal	Distal	Competent ileocecal valve	Non-competent ileocecal valve
Anorexia	Present	Variable	Variable	Variable
Vomiting	Present: bilious, large quantity, non-malodorous	Usually present: feculent/particulate, small volume, foul smelling	Absent	May be present
Pain	Peri-umbilical, colicky pain, early symptom	Localized, deep visceral pain with pain-free intervals, late symptom	Localized, deep visceral pain with pain-free intervals, late symptom	Localized, deep visceral pain with pain-free intervals, late symptom
Distension	Usually absent	Present	Present	Present

of choice for detecting carcinomatosis. There are limits to the sensitivity of imaging. For example, peritoneal implants <5 mm and those in certain anatomical locations, including the small intestine serosa, may not be detected on CT, so their absence in imaging does not exclude diagnosis of carcinomatosis [7]. MRI could be considered for some patients. Although MRI has comparable detection sensitivity with multi-detector CT for identifying peritoneal deposits >1 cm, fat-suppressed, delayed gadolinium-enhanced MRI is more sensitive than CT for detecting subcentimeter deposits, including those <5 mm, and deposits on bowel serosa or other anatomically difficult sites [7].

Treatment Decisions and Patient Selection

Surgical decision making for MBO requires the highest degree of clinical judgment and thoughtful communication with patients and families. Perhaps the most fundamental decision is the one regarding the need and benefit of surgical intervention. An algorithm summarizing decision making is presented in Fig. 26.1. Because MBO rarely requires intervention within the first few hours of presentation, there is usually adequate time to counsel the patient and family. Surgical intervention for MBO aims to reduce symptoms and improve the quality of life but does not address the underlying incurable malignancy. However, relieving the obstruction may improve nutritional intake, prevent perforation and ischemia and prolong life. One retrospective, single institution study of a heterogeneous population of patients with MBO compared 324 patients who had surgery with 199 patients who did not. They found that surgical patients had lower rates of reobstruction (18 % vs. 35 %), longer mean time to reobstruction (223 days vs. 36.4 days), and longer duration of

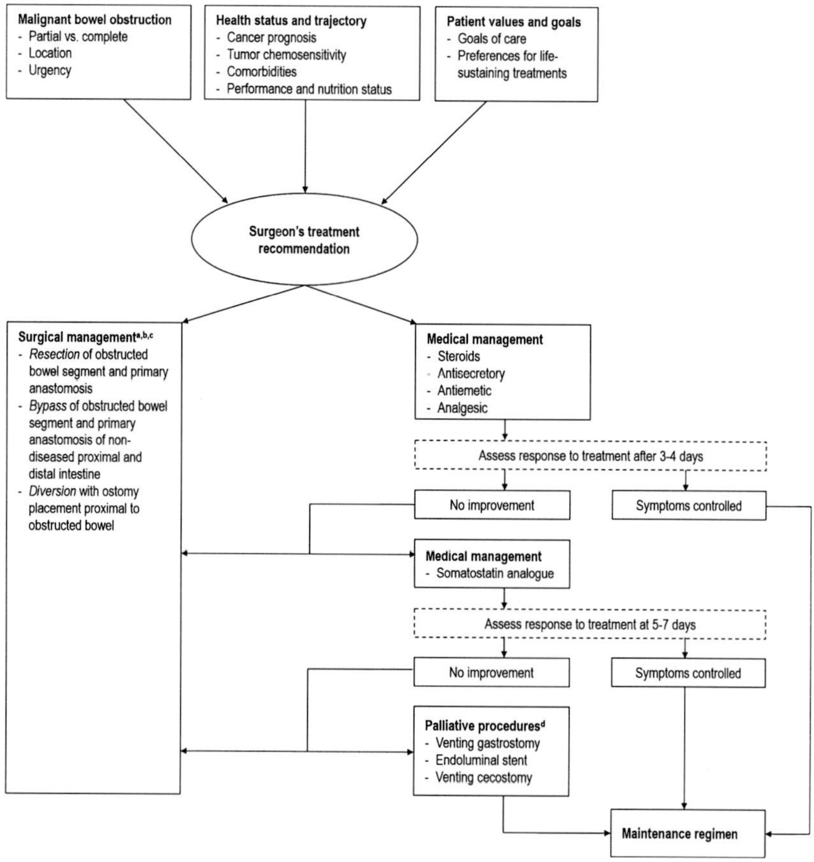

Fig. 26.1 Treatment decision-making algorithm for malignant bowel obstruction

survival (331 days vs. 174 days) [2]. Other studies using population-based data for patients with ovarian and colorectal cancer found increased survival among patients managed surgically, but did not demonstrate a lower rate of reobstruction [5, 6]. Surgery may also act as a bridge to allow further disease-directed treatments, including additional chemotherapy [4]. However, because there are currently are no randomized controlled trials of MBO management, favorable outcomes may be subject to selection bias.

Patient factors associated with worse surgical outcomes include advanced age, poor nutritional status, comorbidities, persistent ascites, poor performance status, prior abdominal radiation therapy, and failed prior surgery for MBO (see Table 26.2). Poor nutritional status and poor performance status are each associated with 3 times higher odds of dying after surgery [8]. Although not absolute contraindications to surgery, these factors greatly increase surgical risk, and potential benefits of surgery must be weighed against increased potential for complications.

Table 26.2 Poor prognostic factors for surgical treatment of bowel obstruction

Patient factors	– Advanced age – Chronic comorbidities – Poor performance status – Poor nutritional status (low albumin, progressive weight loss) – Prior abdominal radiation
Disease factors	– Disease progression despite chemotherapy – Multilevel obstruction – Diffuse peritoneal carcinomatosis – Palpable masses – Persistent ascites – Complete obstruction (vs. partial obstruction)

Patients who have diffuse peritoneal carcinomatosis and those with multilevel obstruction are unlikely to receive benefit from surgical intervention. Peritoneal carcinomatosis is associated with high rates of serious complications (7–44 %), mortality (6–32 %), reobstruction (6–47 %), and readmissions (38–74 %) with limited survival [3]. Therefore, surgery is not recommended for these patients.

Given the overall poor prognosis for patients with incurable cancer and MBO, a thorough discussion should take place before surgery between the surgeon, patient, and family to elicit the patient's goals for treatment and set reasonable expectations for recovery and outcomes. Patients have differing degrees of disease awareness, so it is helpful to initiate the conversation by determining the patient's and family's understanding of their disease and prognosis. This will allow the surgeon to place the acute MBO in the context of underlying disease. The surgeon should then inform the patient and family about the acute problem, explaining the disease course of MBO and its likely impact on the patient's health trajectory. If at all possible, it is advisable to engage other treating clinicians, including the patient's oncologist, in discussions about prognosis, potential outcomes, and treatment decisions [9].

The American College of Surgeons has built an online risk calculator based on NSQIP data to help surgeons and families understand the range of morbidity and mortality associated with certain known comorbidities, urgency of the operation, age, and specifics of the operation. It is worth running the risk calculator to see whether the family's or surgeon's expectations are founded on the data available to this risk calculator, which should evolved over time (http://www.riskcalculator.facs.org/).

The risks, benefits, and burdens associated with each treatment option should be described clearly. Discussing treatment burden is of particular importance because patients may experience prolonged recovery, substantial hospitalization, and discharge to institutional settings which, in the context of limited survival, may be incongruent with their priorities for end-of-life care. Determining the appropriateness of treatment options requires considering the ability of each treatment to achieve the individual patient's goals for care. In addition to speaking about specific treatments for MBO, surgeons should inquire about the patient's general priorities for health care, and goals for comfort, quality, and duration of life. This conversation should identify specific health states or life-sustaining treatments that would be unacceptable to the patient as well as activities and milestones that are most important. Existing advance directives and healthcare proxy designations should be reviewed.

The surgeon should then make a recommendation, synthesizing the patient's goals with clinical data. Patients who consent to surgery must be counseled on the element of uncertainty prior to the operation. Although imaging and history may guide surgical planning, the definitive decision must be made intra-operatively, so their consent or rejection of each potential surgical approach should be determined. The care plan for patients managed non-surgically should include a plan to evaluate success at specific times and revisit treatment options. This conversation and the treatment plan should be documented in the medical record and shared with other clinicians and the patient's surrogate decision makers.

Surgical Approaches

Surgical intervention in the face of MBO should be directed at achieving the lowest risk of complications with the highest chance of meeting patients' goals for care (see Table 26.3). Decisions about future chemotherapy, including intraperitoneal regimens after cytoreductive operations, will be guided by the patient's performance status, prior experience with chemotherapy, and tumor type. Thus, surgical decisions predicated on future chemotherapy should be made in consultation with the patient's oncologist. For patients with MBO from a colorectal primary and unresectable metastatic disease, resection of the primary tumor is associated with longer survival compared with endoluminal stenting. Therefore, tumor resection with negative margins is the procedure of choice for patients with MBO due to a single lesion. If this is not possible, there is little benefit conferred from tumor debulking in regard to overall prognosis for patients with incurable disease.

In patients with an unresectable cancer causing a single point of obstruction that cannot be safely resected, the segment of bowel should be bypassed using a side-to-side anastomosis. The unresected tumor will remain intact, but intestinal contents will be permitted to flow around it. This procedure should be considered for patients who have normal-appearing, disease-free proximal and distal bowel. In addition, the surgeon should consider the patients' nutritional status, any history of vasculopathy, or prior abdominal radiation that would impair healing at the anastomosis. Neither resection nor bypass would be appropriate for patients with signs of bowel compromise, distal points of obstruction, inadequate intestinal perfusion, or multiple risk factors for poor healing capacity.

Another surgical option is proximal diversion by creation of a stoma. This procedure is most suitable for patients who have multiple points of obstruction in the distal small intestine or colon and normal, healthy bowel proximal to the transition point. Proximal diversion is also favored for patients with high risk of

Table 26.3 Surgical approaches to malignant bowel obstruction

Technique	Considerations
Cytoreductive surgery	– Should be performed if complete resection with negative margins is possible (as in obstructing colon cancers) – May be performed for patients with ovarian cancer if residual disease is <1 cm and the patient plans to receive intraperitoneal chemotherapy – Not appropriate in setting of diffuse carcinomatosis (consider bypass, proximal diversion, or venting gastrostomy)
Bypass	– Must have healthy, normal bowel proximal and distal to the site of obstruction – Must have adequate perfusion to heal primary anastomosis – Primary anastomosis may not be appropriate for patients with profound malnourishment or cachexia (consider proximal diversion or venting gastrostomy with or without feeding jejunostomy) – Not appropriate for patients with multiple obstructions throughout the intestine (consider proximal diversion or venting gastrostomy) – Not appropriate in setting of diffuse carcinomatosis (consider venting gastrostomy)
Proximal diversion	– May be helpful in patients with multiple distal obstruction sites not amenable to bypass – Should be considered as an alternative to bypass for patients with high risk of anastomotic leak – Must have ≥100-cm proximal small intestine to maintain nutritional status – Very proximal ostomies may have high output and be difficult to manage and should be avoided (venting gastrostomy with or without feeding jejunostomy) – Not appropriate in setting of diffuse carcinomatosis (consider venting gastrostomy)
Venting gastrostomy	– Can be performed percutaneously with fluoroscopic or endoscopic guidance or as a laparoscopic or open operation – Not appropriate for large bowel obstruction if patient has competent ileocecal valve – Does not address obstruction; patients will not have adequate nutrition (consider feeding jejunostomy in patients with good performance status and reasonable expectation for survival)
Venting cecostomy	– Indicated for patients with large bowel obstruction – Can be performed percutaneously with fluoroscopic or endoscopic guidance or as a laparoscopic or open operation does not address obstruction

anastomotic leak (i.e., prior radiation, poor nutritional status, compromised perfusion) or other factors for whom bypass is deemed inappropriate. The length of proximal healthy bowel should be measured intra-operatively. A minimum of 100 cm of healthy intestine is required for adequate enteral nutrition. Ideally, the proximal ostomy is best if created in the most distal bowel, and proximal jejunostomies are often associated with high output and may lead to significant fluid shifts and metabolic derangements.

Open surgical gastrostomy tube placement can be performed as a palliative procedure for gastric decompression when intra-operative findings preclude other surgical interventions. Similarly, cecostomy tube placement can be performed for palliation of large bowel obstruction for patients if the distal colon cannot be adequately mobilized to create a tension-free colostomy. These procedures and their minimally invasive correlates are discussed in further detail in the section on other palliative procedures.

In cases of acute large bowel obstruction where the patient is a poor candidate for emergent surgery (i.e., would benefit from optimizing medical comorbidities beforehand), a bare metal stent (see below section on palliative procedures) may be used as a temporary bridge to an elective procedure. In some cases, a stoma can be avoided once the patient is more physiologically fit for surgery.

Non-surgical Management

Non-surgical treatment options are available for patients with carcinomatosis or as an alternative option for those who do not want surgery. Medications may reduce symptoms and relieve early obstructions. If these are not successful at controlling symptoms, other palliative procedures may be appropriate.

Medications

Medication regimens for patients with non-operable MBO should include antiemetics, antisecretory agents, steroids, and analgesics (see Table 26.4). Medications alone can control symptoms in 60–80 % of patients with MBO due to peritoneal carcinomatosis [10].

Antiemetics help to reduce nausea and vomiting. Dopamine type 2 (D_2) receptor antagonists, including haloperidol and chlorpromazine, are effective centrally acting antiemetics that reduce nausea and vomiting and should be initiated as first-line therapy. Histamine type 1 (H_1) receptor antagonists such as dexamethasone, diphenhydramine, and promethazine can also reduce stimulation of peripheral pathways and may be used in concert with D_2 blockers. If these are not effective, 5-HT3 receptor antagonists, such as ondansetron, can be used in combination or as a single agent. Metoclopramide should not be administered to patients with complete obstructions, as its prokinetic effects may worsen pain.

Corticosteroids may decrease inflammation and reduce or relieve early or incomplete obstructions. Despite the lack of high-quality evidence, expert consensus recommendations favor a short course of methylprednisolone or dexamethasone, administered intravenously or subcutaneously, starting on the first day of treatment [10]. Patients with partial obstructions should receive a peristaltic agent (i.e., metoclopramide, amidotrizoate) along with corticosteroids.

Table 26.4 Medications commonly used in management of malignant bowel obstruction

Category	Medications
Antiemetics	*Neuroleptic* – Metoclopramide: 10–15 mg IV, SC, or IM q 6–8 h (contraindicated for patients with complete obstruction) – Haloperidol: 1–5 mg SC or IM q 8 h – Chlorpromazine: 25–50 mg IV or IM q 4–6 h *5-HT3 receptor antagonists* – Ondansetron: 4–8 mg IV q 12 h – Granisetron: 3 mg IV q 24 h
Steroids	– Methylprednisolone: 1–4 mg/kg IV q 24 h for 5–10 days – Dexamethasone: 0.25–1 mg/kg IV q 24 h for 5–10 days
Antisecretory	– Hyoscine butylbromide: 20–40 mg SC or IV q 8 h – Scopolamine: 0.25–0.5 mg SC or IV q 8 h – Glycopyrrolate: 0.1–0.2 mg SC or IV q 4–8 h – Pantoprazole: 40–80 mg/d as continuous infusion – Octreotide: 200 μg SC or IV q 8 h or as a continuous infusion – Lanreotide PR: 30 mg IM single injection every 10 days
Analgesics	– Morphine: IV or PCA – Hydromorphone: IV or PCA

Anticholinergic antisecretory medications, including hyoscine butylbromide, or glycopyrrolate, are first-line agents that reduce gastric secretions. Hyoscine butylbromide and glycopyrrolate are peripherally acting muscarinic anticholinergic agents. They do not penetrate the blood–brain barrier; therefore, they are well-tolerated. Scopolamine is also an effective antisecretory, but is associated with side effects due to its central nervous system activity. The utility of gastric antisecretory drugs, including proton pump inhibitors and histamine antagonists, has not been studied for patients with MBO. However, they may be considered as an adjunct to anticholinergic antisecretory agents.

If anticholinergic antisecretory agents do not improve symptoms after 3–4 days of treatment and nasogastric tube output remains high volume (greater than 1 L/24 h), a somatostatin analogue may be initiated as second-line therapy. Octreotide and lanreotide are synthetic somatostatin analogues that decrease gastric, pancreatic, and enteric secretions and increase water and electrolyte resorption. Both are available in long-acting forms. They are more effective at reducing secretions and controlling nausea and vomiting than anticholinergic agents, but are expensive, and should be reserved for patients who fail first-line treatment or develop an early recurrence.

At this stage, surgery may still be a reasonable option if medical management fails, and if surgery is still aligned with the patient's goals of care and technically feasible. However, it is our experience that a prolonged trial of failing medical management leads to a malnourished, weakened patient who is less able to withstand the demands of surgery and more likely to experience complications. Therefore, surgery, if it is to be offered, should be offered early in the patient's episode.

Other Palliative Procedures

If medications fail to control symptoms, or the patient is not a candidate for surgery, other palliative procedures such as self-expanding metal stent placement, venting gastrostomy, and cecostomy should be considered. Self-expanding metal stents can be placed endoscopically and are useful for colonic obstructions as either a bridge to surgery, or as an alternative to colostomy in patients with less than 6 months of life expectancy [11]. Stents are fairly well-tolerated; however, patients may experience bleeding, pain, fecal impaction or incontinence, which can all be treated supportively. Complications from stents include stent failure because the stent is too short, perforation, migration, and reocclusion from tumor ingrowth.

Venting gastrostomy placement for small bowel obstruction is associated with low rate of complications and leads to symptom resolution in over 80 % of patients. Patients may be able to resume oral intake (for comfort) and those with intermittent symptoms can be managed at home and avoid hospitalization. Percutaneous approaches to venting gastrostomy placement are contraindicated in patients with copious ascites or unfavorable anatomy due to the increased risk of bowel injury. Adhesions from prior surgery, and carcinomatosis, may prevent mobilization of the stomach to the anterior abdominal wall. An abdominal CT scan can assist in determining feasibility of the procedure. Complications from venting gastrostomy include leak, peritonitis, gastrointestinal bleeding, injury to adjacent intestine, and aspiration.

For patients with a large bowel obstruction causing cecal dilatation, a venting cecostomy tube can be placed percutaneously, laparoscopically, or during laparotomy. Tube placement creates a controlled fistula allowing decompression of the colon. Complications include soft tissue infection, peritonitis, gastrointestinal bleeding, abdominal wall bleeding, and tube occlusion by solid feces.

Conclusion

Regardless of the desired outcome and treatment approach, it is important to remember that MBO is a by-product of the underlying, incurable disease process. As such, all management of MBO is palliative. Treatment should focus on providing comfort and quality of life for the patient. As such, any procedure should be performed with the intention of achieving the individual patient's priorities for the time they have left. When available, focused pain and palliative care providers are often useful in helping the patient and family understand their goals and achieving reasonable expectations the entire healthcare team and family can accept. Regardless of treatment, referral to hospice may be appropriate for patients with less than 6 months of life expectancy.

Clinical Scenario

A 62-year-old woman presents with 5 days of progressive obstipation and mild abdominal distension, and worsening pain. She has experienced occasional left-lower quadrant "crampy" pain, anorexia, and 20-lb weight loss over the last several months. She has a history of ovarian carcinoma diagnosed 3 years prior and underwent hysterectomy with bilateral salpingo-oophorectomy at that time. Her cancer recurred with intraperitoneal metastases 18 months ago, for which she underwent cytoreductive surgery, involving a pelvic lymphadenectomy, partial cystectomy, and recto-sigmoidectomy with primary end-to-end coloanal anastomosis. This was followed by placement of an intraperitoneal chemotherapy port and six cycles of intravenous and intraperitoneal chemotherapy per the latest protocols available. Her port was removed 7 months ago and she has since been maintained on a single-agent regimen. Surveillance abdominal CT scan, completed one month ago, showed disease progression with metastatic disease in the pleura and multiple nodules in her abdomen suggesting extensive peritoneal carcinomatosis.

CT scan today demonstrates normal-appearing small intestine, dilated ascending and transverse colon, mild ascites, more extensive carcinomatosis compared to her prior CT and a transition point at the splenic flexure. The cecum is dilated, measuring 14 cm.

Key Questions

1. *What governs the decision to perform a diverting loop ileostomy versus a diverting end ostomy with a mucous fistula?*
2. *Is there a role for the tube cecostomy?*

References

1. Anthony T, Baron T, Mercadante S, Green S, Chi D, Cunningham J, et al. Report of the clinical protocol committee: development of randomized trials for malignant bowel obstruction. J Pain Symptom Manage. 2007;34(1 Suppl):S49–59.
2. Henry JC, Pouly S, Sullivan R, Sharif S, Klemanski D, Abdel-Misih S, et al. A scoring system for the prognosis and treatment of malignant bowel obstruction. Surgery. 2012;152(4):747–56; discussion 56–7.
3. Paul Olson TJ, Pinkerton C, Brasel KJ, Schwarze ML. Palliative surgery for malignant bowel obstruction from carcinomatosis: a systematic review. JAMA Surg. 2014;149(4):383–92.
4. Chakraborty A, Selby D, Gardiner K, Myers J, Moravan V, Wright F. Malignant bowel obstruction: natural history of a heterogeneous patient population followed prospectively over two years. J Pain Symptom Manage. 2011;41(2):412–20.
5. Mooney SJ, Winner M, Hershman DL, Wright JD, Feingold DL, Allendorf JD, et al. Bowel obstruction in elderly ovarian cancer patients: a population-based study. Gynecol Oncol. 2013;129(1):107–12.

6. Winner M, Mooney SJ, Hershman DL, Feingold DL, Allendorf JD, Wright JD, et al. Management and outcomes of bowel obstruction in patients with stage IV colon cancer: a population-based cohort study. Dis Colon Rectum. 2013;56(7):834–43.
7. Patel CM, Sahdev A, Reznek RH. CT, MRI and PET imaging in peritoneal malignancy. Cancer imaging: Official Publ Int Cancer Imaging Soc. 2011;11:123–39.
8. Helyer L, Easson AM. Surgical approaches to malignant bowel obstruction. J Support Oncol. 2008;6(3):105–13.
9. Cooper Z, Koritsansky LA, Cauley CE, Frydman JL, Bernacki RE, Mosenthal AC, et al. Recommendations for best communication practices to facilitate goal-concordant care for seriously ill older patients with emergency surgical conditions. Ann Surg. Accepted July 2015, Forthcoming.
10. Laval G, Marcelin-Benazech B, Guirimand F, Chauvenet L, Copel L, Durand A, et al. Recommendations for bowel obstruction with peritoneal carcinomatosis. J Pain Symptom Manage. 2014;48(1):75–91.
11. Simmons DT, Baron TH. Technology insight: enteral stenting and new technology. Nat Clin Prac Gastroenterol Hepatol. 2005;2(8):365–74; quiz 1 p following 74.

Chapter 27
Jehovah's Witness and the Bleeding Surgical Patient

L.D. Britt

The religion named Jehovah's Witness was founded by Charles Russell in Allegheny, Pennsylvania, in 1869. Members of this religion do not accept blood transfusions based on passages from the Bible, such as Genesis 9:3-4, Leviticus 17:10-11, and Acts 15:28-29. "As for any man who eats any sort of blood, I shall certainly set my face against the soul that is eating the blood, and I shall in deed cut him off from among 'his people.'" Interpreting blood transfusions as "eating the blood," Jehovah's Witnesses believe that hope for an eternal life would be denied if blood transfusion is allowed.

Worldwide, there are approximately 6 million Jehovah's Witnesses, with approximately 1 million residing in the USA [1]. Many of whom do not accept homologous or autologous whole blood, packed red blood cells, white blood cells, or platelets [2]. Some will agree to the use of dialysis, heart-lung, or similar technology if the extracorporeal circulation is uninterrupted. Reportedly, the religion's belief of Jehovah's Witnesses does not absolutely prohibit the use of all component therapies, such as hemophiliac preparations, albumin, and immune globulins.

Unfortunately, a substantial percentage of bleeding surgical patients present in hemorrhagic shock and are in need of multiple transfusions [3]. This becomes a major impediment if the patient is a Jehovah's Witness, who abstains from receiving blood transfusions and blood product infusions based on his/her religious beliefs. The literature has been sparse regarding the determination of the risks of death after severe injury. Varela, Gomez-Marin, Fleming, and Cohn studied a cohort of 556 trauma patients, with 82 (14.7 %) being Jehovah Witnesses [4]. The authors concluded that after controlling for age, race, systolic blood pressure, Glasgow coma score, and type of trauma, Jehovah's Witnesses had a "nonsignificant increase risk of death after major trauma compared with other religious

L.D. Britt (✉)
Department of Surgery, Eastern Virginia Medical School,
825 Fairfax Ave. Suite 610, Norfolk, VA 23507, USA
e-mail: brittld@evms.edu

J.J. Diaz and D.T. Efron (eds.), *Complications in Acute Care Surgery*,
DOI 10.1007/978-3-319-42376-0_27

Table 27.1 Injury and mortality data[a]

Religion	Mean ISS	Type of injury	Case of injury (%)	Mortality (%)
Jehovah's Witnesses	10.3 ± 9 (NS)	Blunt (82)	MC (39)	11.0 (NS)
Catholic	10.3 ± 11	Blunt (68)	MVC (39)	6.9
Baptist	8.9 ± 10	Penetrating (56)	GSW (31)	5.8

Mean ISS for other religious groups was 11.3 ± 14. No statistically significant associations between religion and injury severity scores were identified by x^2 analysis

ISS injury severity score; *MVC* motor vehicle crash; *GSW* gunshot wound; *NS* not significantly different when compared to Catholics or Baptists by one-way analysis of variance

[a]Mean injury severity score for 433 injured patients, type, and cause of injuries, and mortality by religion

groups" (Table 27.1). While Catholics and Baptists were the other major religious groups, the full spectrum of religions was represented; however, the groups did not have a sufficient number of individuals for statistical analysis. Ott and Cooley [5] reported a similar finding when they documented that the Jehovah's Witness patients did not have a substantially higher death rate than other religious groups when elective surgery was being performed. The literature is replete with reports from other authors that compared to non-Jehovah's Witness groups, Jehovah's Witnesses do not have a statistically increased risk of death after major trauma when demographics, severity, and type of injury are taken into account [6–8]. However, there are some important baselines that must be considered when refraining from using blood transfusions and blood product infusion. Carson et al. reported in Lancet, on the operative mortality rate in surgical patients who refused blood transfusion, that there was a 61.5 % mortality rate for those with levels less than 6 mg/dL and the overwhelming majority of patients with hemoglobin levels less than 5 md/dL did not survive [9].

Under the autonomy principle, a competent patient can refuse any interventions, including one that is considered lifesaving. Refusal of treatment that ultimately results in the death of the patient who exercised his/her right to make such decisions is broadly supported by the courts—based on the patient's autonomy principle. The prototypical situation occurs when the proposed treatment/therapy violates someone's cultural or religious beliefs (e.g., the Jehovah's Witness patient). However, when there are situations when parents or guardians are the ones who refuse treatment of a minor, the courts have routinely intervened to balance the interests of the child with wishes of the parents/guardians—allowing blood/blood product transfusions to be given to the minor.

It has been reported in the past that the majority (two-thirds) of the European physicians working in intensive care units would give transfusions to an unconscious Jehovah's Witness who is losing blood, with 41 % indicating that they would not inform the patient later [10].

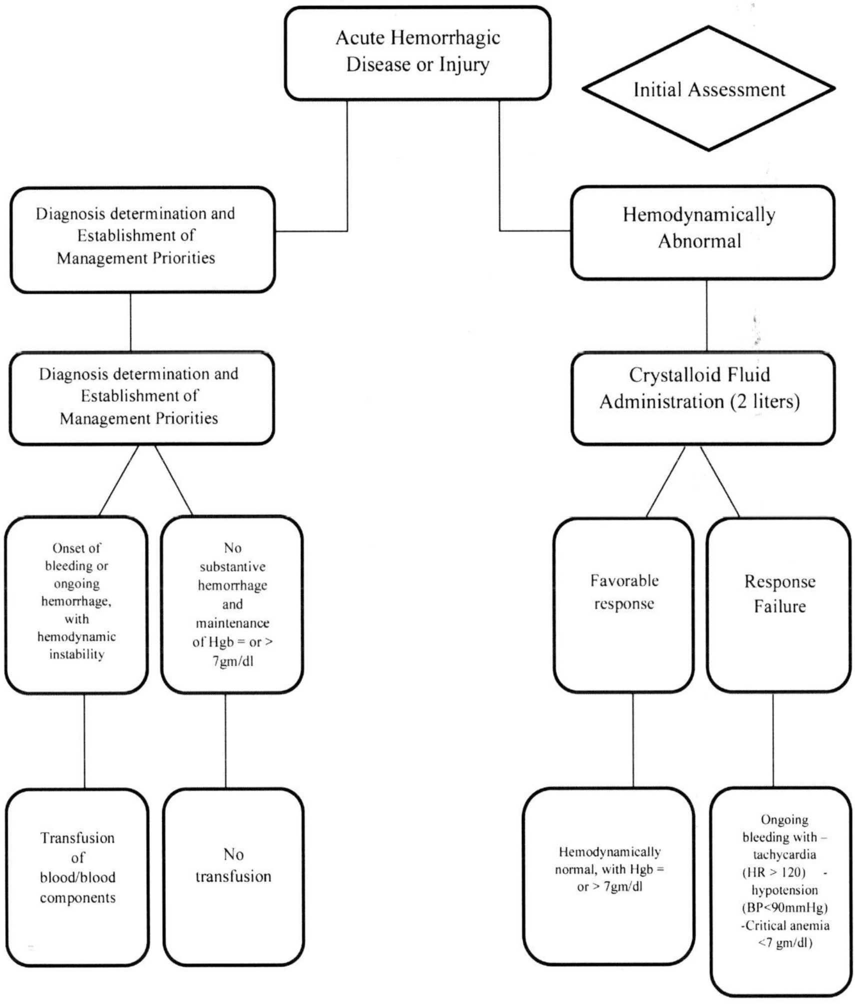

Fig. 27.1 Intravascular volume restoration after acute hemorrhage disease or injury

It is imperative that acute care surgeons not be dismissive of the legal liability if they choose to ignore a Jehovah's Witness' advance directive not to receive blood.

The practice guideline or algorithm for restoring intravascular volume after bleeding secondary to injury or hemorrhagic diseases is well chronicled (Fig. 27.1). The decision branches leading to the transfusion of blood/blood products are <u>not</u> an option for the competent patient who is a Jehovah's Witness and refuses blood/blood product transfusion. However, there is a spectrum of management strategies for the Jehovah's Witnesses with severe blood loss (Table 27.2).

Table 27.2 Armamentarium of management strategies

For Jehovah's Witnesses with acute severe blood loss
• Maximizing oxygen delivery (maintain O_2 saturation >98 %)
• Minimize metabolic demand (oxygen demand)
• Blood conservation and minimizing diagnostic phlebotomies
• Establishing optimal oxygen delivery
• Preventing iatrogenic injury and associated blood loss
• Stimulation of hematopoiesis
• Increasing the production of red blood cells (enhancement of erythropoiesis)
• Intravenous iron infusion
• Recombinant human erythropoietin (rHuEPO)
• Red cell substitutes[a] (or alternative oxygen-carrying agents)
• Meticulous and limited surgical dissection

[a]Artificial substitutes for human hemoglobin are still being studied. However, known limitations of these products include short half-life, poor oxygen-carrying capacity, and suboptimal release of oxygen to the tissue

Management Controversy

Recombinant Human Erythropoietin

After illness or injury-induced severe blood loss, the erythropoietin response is less than optimal secondary to release of inflammatory cytokines that down-regulate the erythropoietin gene, along with inhibition of bone marrow and modification of iron metabolism [11, 12]. The controversy has always revolved around some documentation that erythropoietin levels are actually preserved and that there is failure of the bone marrow to respond to erythropoietin—calling into question the utility of exogenous erythropoietin. Proponents for erythropoietin administration realize that beneficial effects take ten days to three weeks [13, 14]. Also, because some Jehovah's Witness patients will not accept any blood product, erythropoietin might not be considered a viable option due to the fact that it does contain small amounts of human albumin, which is a blood product [15].

Special Consideration and Circumstances

Although not included, one of the key underlying trends affecting optimal health care as outlined in Table 27.3, tailoring medical management based on religious beliefs, can also affect optimal health care.

Table 27.3 Key underlying trends affecting optimal healthcare

• Healthcare disparities of the population
• Aging of the population
• Increasing rates of utilization
• Economic growth of the nation
• End-of-life issues
• Advances in genetics screening
• Changes in health services delivery system
• Efforts to weed out unnecessary or marginally beneficial services
• Cost containment efforts

Table 27.4 Institute of Medicine

Six aims of care
• Safe
• Effective
• Patient-centered
• Timely
• Efficient
• Equitable

In its report on health literacy, the Institute of Medicine (IOM) highlighted that 90 million adults have trouble understanding and acting on health information. A patient who is fully informed regarding the full spectrum of management options, electing not to accept a potentially lifesaving intervention due to his/her religious belief, is the antithesis of someone whose "health literacy" is challenged. On the contrary, such a patient is fully informed and an active participant in his/her care. The Jehovah's Witness represents such a cohort of patients. Even the highly touted six aims of care by the IOM (Table 27.4) the patient can completely affect whether the care is, indeed, "equitable" by refusal of the prescribed or recommended care.

While others have reported on the role of nonoperative management of a splenic injury in a Jehovah's Witness patient with a bleeding disorder (hemophilia), an admonition should be made that the overall approach to nonoperative and selective management of solid organ injuries is predicated on the possible utilization of blood transfusion and/or blood product infusion [16, 17]. More prudent strategy would be to expeditiously address the solid organ (liver or spleen) injuries with more aggressive intervention by either angiography/embolization of surgical extirpation (e.g., splenectomy).

The increasing healthcare expenditures have been on a consistent trajectory, with a projected four trillion dollar price tag by 2018. In addition to providing quality patient care, each healthcare provider has a fiduciary responsibility to be good stewards of the finances of medicine. Some of the strategic options for the Jehovah's Witness patients are, indeed, expensive. A difficult question can be posed, asking the following: Who should be financially responsible for such excess expenses, incurred by those choosing not to accept blood transfusions and blood product infusions? Of course, one could entertain the same argument for alcohol and smoke-related illnesses.

In a recent article by Peitzman et al. [18], it was reported that a potential expanded role for acute care surgery is "surgical rescue". The authors stated that "it has become apparent to us that a crucial service we provide to both our hospital and regions is that of surgical rescue." Ninety percent of operative deaths occur in the highest risk quintile, with 20 % of patients with the greatest risk for developing postoperative complications accounting for approximately 90 % of failure to rescue. In a landmark article by Ghaferi et al. [19] in Med Care, the authors underscore the advantages of establishing strategies that focus on the timely recognition and management of complications once they occur. With the postoperative complication of medical or surgical care being one of the most frequent hospital-based diagnoses (exceeding even cholocystitis, intestinal obstruction, and appendicitis), acute care surgery, undoubtedly, offers the specialty expertise needed to provide the hospital surgical rescues to optimally address these complications. Such management often necessitates volume resuscitation and the administration of blood products. Consequently, this expanded role of the specialty, acute care surgery, would likely not be applicable for a patient who is a Jehovah's Witness.

Irrespective of such an intervention, if any rescue strategy involves blood transfusion, it would not be an advantage for the Jehovah's Witness patient. The legal precedent is set in upholding the right of a competent patient to refuse blood transfusion, and the standard-of-care practice is established that there should be an informal consent for blood and blood component transfusion [20]. Healthcare providers should be knowledgeable of the fact that many Jehovah's Witnesses have an advance medical directive/release form (Fig. 27.2). In addition, there is a current classification of what is unacceptable and specific blood products that are available for the "Christian to Decide"—on an individual basis (Fig. 27.3).

The four major ethical principles that any healthcare provider should incorporate in his/her clinical practice include the following:

- autonomy—respecting the values of the patient
- beneficence—acting to benefit patients by sustaining life and treating illnesses
- non-maleficence—meaning to refrain from harm, a correlative principle to beneficence
- justice—the balance between the personal needs of the patient and societal resources

Justice underscores the fact that there must be recognition that resources are finite. Necessary stewardship must focus on the methods of cost containment, including attempts to limit care when it is deemed futile—either based on the status of the patient or on the restrictions imposed by the patient. While "futile care" can be rejected based upon the principles of non-maleficence and beneficence, such care can also be opposed due to the principle of distributive justice. Futile care is usually defined as a treatment that merely preserves permanent unconsciousness and/or

ADVANCE MEDICAL DIRECTIVE/RELEASE

I, ____________, make this advance directive as a formal statement of my wishes. These instruction reflect my resolute decision.

I direct that *no blood transfusions* (whole blood, red cells, white cells, platelets, or blood plasma) be given to me under any circumstances, even if physicians deem such necessary to preserve my life or health. I will accept nonblood volume expanders (such as dextran, saline or Ringer's solution, or hetastarch) and other nonblood management.

This legal directive is an exercise of my right to accept or to refuse medical treatment in accord with my deeply held value and convictions. I am one of Jehovah's Witnesses, and I make this directive out of obedience to commands in the Bible, such as "Keep abstaining…from blood." (Acts 15:28, 29). This is, and has been, my unwavering religious stand for ______ years. I am ______ years old.

I also know that there are various dangers associated with blood transfusions. So I have decided to avoid such dangers and, instead, to accept whatever risks may seem to be involved in my choicer of alternative nonblood management.

I release physicians, anesthesiologists, and hospitals and their personnel from liability for any damages that might be caused by my refusal of blood, despite their otherwise competent care.

I authorize the person(s) named on the reverse to see that my instructions set forth in this directive are upheld and to answer any questions about my absolute refusal of blood.

____
Signature

____
Address Date

____
Telephone

____
Witness

____
Witness

Fig. 27.2 Advance medical directive/release

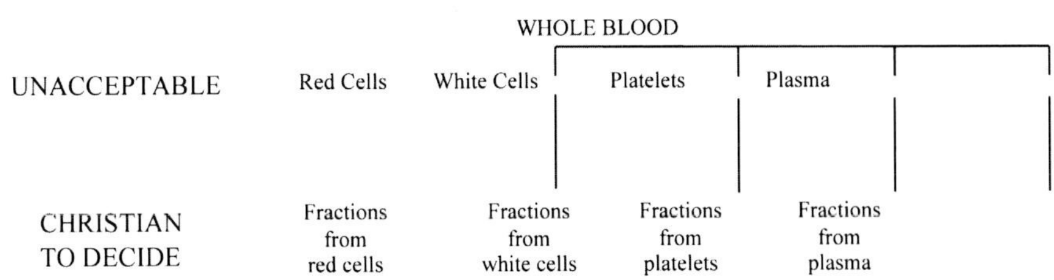

Fig. 27.3 The Watchtower Bible and Tract Society's current classification of blood products' acceptability

cannot end dependence on critical care. Table 27.5 depicts the proportional contribution to premature death. If a patient succumbs to an illness injury as a result of refusal of a potential lifesaving resource or intervention, the resulting premature death is the result of "social circumstances," as opposed to health care.

Although the surgeon of the future will lead safe high-performance teams and will implement evidenced-based effective practices with outcomes that are publicly reported (Table 27.6), the decision by the fully aware patient who exercises his or her will to reject specific elements of care.

Table 27.5 Proportional contribution to premature death

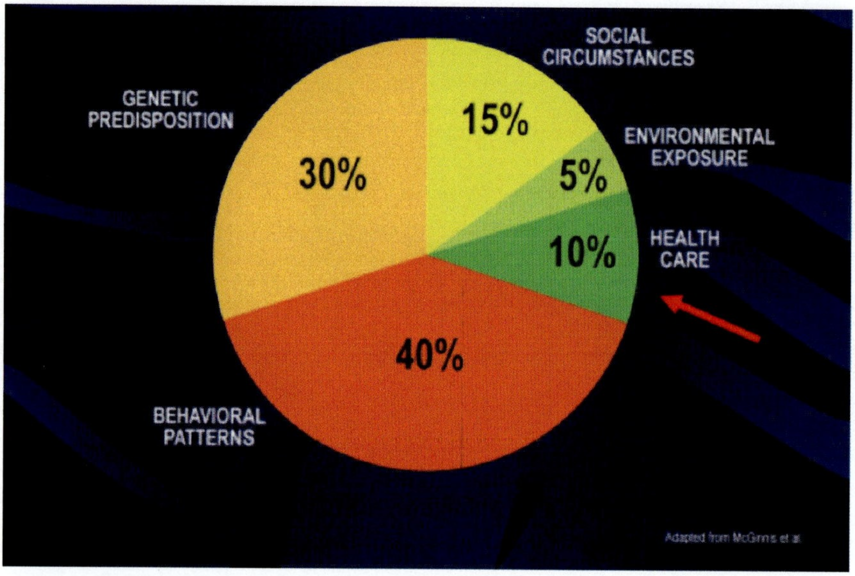

Table 27.6 The surgeon of the future

• Lead safe high-performance teams
– Integration of surgical/nonsurgical skills
– Part of systems of care
– Communication, respect for others
• *Evidence-based effective practice*
• Outcomes data—publicly reported
• Continuous, professional development
– Recertification based on practice
• Payment—performance-based

Clinical Scenario

69-year old man with a history of HTN and CAD has 6 weeks s/p large left hemispheric stroke. He underwent carotid artery stenting and was placed on Plavix and ASA. He recovers reasonably with mild residual deficit (right upper and lower extremity weakness). In rehab, he is noted to be short of breath and occasionally lightheaded. He is noted to have dark stools, and HGB check demonstrates a new level of 6.1 (previously 12). Colonoscopy demonstrates a friable cecal mass.

Response:

Confirmation that this 69-year-old man is a devout Jehovah Witness (who will refuse transfusion of any blood or blood products) should dictate addressing this patient's precipitous decline of his hemoglobin, with the associated symptomatology (shortness of breath and weakness). Even with the patient's comorbidities, the likely source of bleeding must be addressed. Consequently, this patient should be expeditiously prepared for extirpation of the documented "friable cecal mass." In addition to being the source of bleeding, the colon mass is likely a harbinger for a malignant neoplasm. Although clopidogrel should be stopped 5 days before surgery, this patient should remain on ASA throughout the perioperative period. The clopidogrel can be restarted on postoperative day 2—using a loading dose.

Key Questions

1. *In acute care surgery setting does having a Jehovah's Witnesses necessarily make them a high-risk patient?*
2. *As opposed to an elective procedure, can an acute care surgeon refuse to be involved in the emergency care of a patient who's refusal of transfusion makes intervention almost assuredly prohibitive?*

References

1. Ridley DT. Jehovah's Witnesses refusal of blood: obedience to scripture and religious conscience. J Med Ethics. 1999;25:469–72.
2. Singelenberg R. The blood transfusion taboo and Jehovah's Witnesses: origin, development and function of a controversial doctrine. Soc Sci Med. 1990;31:515–23.
3. Pedowitz RA, Shakford SR. Non-cavitary hemorrhage producing shock in trauma patients: incidents and severity. J Trauma. 1989;29:219–23.
4. Varela JE, Gomez-Marin O, Fleming LE, Cohn SM. The risk of death for Jehovah's Witnesses after major trauma. J Trauma. 2002;54:967–72.
5. Ott DA, Cooley DA. Cardiovascular surgery in Jehovah's Witnesses. JAMA. 1979;238:1251–8.
6. Collins SL, Timberlake GA. Severe anemia in the Jehovah's Witness: case report and discussion. Am J Crit Care. 1993;2:256–9.
7. Hershman H. Treating the Jehovah's Witness. Emerg Med. 1980;12:73–6.

8. Victorina G, Wisner DH. Jehovah's Witnesses: unique problems in a unique trauma population. J Am Coll Surg. 1997;184:458–68.
9. Carson JL, Poses RM, Spark RK, et al. Severity of anemia and operative mortality and morbidity. Lancet. 1988;331:727–9.
10. Vincent JL. Transfusion in the exsanguinating Jehovah Witness patient—attitude of intensive care doctor. Eur J Anaesthesiol. 1991;8:297–300.
11. Hobisch-Hagen P, Wiedorman F, Mayr A, et al. Blunted erythropoietic response to anemia in multiple traumatized patients. Crit Care Med. 2001;29:743–7.
12. Livingston DH, Anjaria D, Wu J, et al. Bone marrow failure following sever injury in humans. Ann Surg. 2003;238:748–53.
13. Gabriel A, Kozek S, Chiari A, et al. High-dose recombinant human erythropoietin stimulates reticulocyte production in patients with multiple organ dysfunction syndrome. J Trauma. 1998;44:361–7.
14. Van Iperon CE, Gaillard CA, Kraaljehagan RJ, Braam BG, Marx JJ, van de Wiel A. Response of erythropoiesis and iron metabolism to recombinant human erythropoietic in intensive care unit patients. Crit Care Med. 2000;28:2773–8.
15. McGraw JP. Use of recombinant human erythropoietin in a Jehovah's Witness. J Trauma. 1991;31:1017–8.
16. Zeig PM, Cohn SM, Bearlsley DS. Nonoperative management of a splenic tear in a Jehovah's Witness with hemophilia. J Trauma. 1996;40(2):299–301.
17. Mackenzie CF, Morrison C, Genuit T, Katamuluma S. Management of hemorrhagic shock when blood is not an option. J Clinic Anesth. 2008;20:530–41.
18. Peitzman AB, Sperry JL, Kutcher ME, et al. Redefining acute care surgery: surgical rescue. J Trauma. 2015;79:327.
19. Ghaferi AA, Birkmeyer JD, Dimick JB. Hospital volume and failure to rescue with high-risk surgery. Med Care. 2011;49:1076–81.
20. Goldman EB, Oberman HA. Legal aspects of transfusion of Jehovah's Witnesses. Transfuse Med Rev. 1991;5:263.

Index

Note: Page numbers followed by *f* and *t* refer to figures and tables, respectively

J.J. Diaz and D.T. Efron (eds.), *Complications in Acute Care Surgery*,
DOI 10.1007/978-3-319-42376-0

O

P